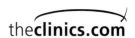

CARDIOLOGY CLINICS

Chest Pain Units

GUEST EDITORS
Ezra A. Amsterdam, MD, FACC
J. Douglas Kirk, MD, FACEP

CONSULTING EDITOR
Michael H. Crawford, MD

November 2005 • Volume 23 • Number 4

SAUNDERS

An Imprint of Elsevier, Inc.
PHILADELPHIA   LONDON   TORONTO   MONTREAL   SYDNEY   TOKYO

W.B. SAUNDERS COMPANY
A Division of Elsevier Inc.

Elsevier Inc. • 1600 John F. Kennedy Blvd., Suite 1800 • Philadelphia, Pennsylvania 19103-2899

http://www.theclinics.com

CARDIOLOGY CLINICS	**Volume 23, Number 4**
November 2005	**ISSN 0733-8651**
Editor: Karen Sorensen	**ISBN 1-4160-2701-7**

Reprints. For copies of 100 or more, of articles in this publication, please contact the Commercial Reprints Department, Elsevier Inc., 360 Park Avenue South, New York, New York 10010-1710. Tel. (212) 633-3813 Fax: (212) 462-1935 email: reprints@elsevier.com.

The ideas and opinions expressed in *Cardiology Clinics* do not necessarily reflect those of the Publisher. The Publisher does not assume any responsibility for any injury and/or damage to persons or property arising out of or related to any use of the material contained in this periodical. The reader is advised to check the appropriate medical literature and the product information currently provided by the manufacturer of each drug to be administered to verify the dosage, the method and duration of administration, or contraindications. It is the responsibility of the treating physician or other health care professional, relying on independent experience and knowledge of the patient, to determine drug dosages and the best treatment for the patient. Mention of any product in this issue should not be construed as endorsement by the contributors, editors, or the Publisher of the product or manufacturers' claims.

Cardiology Clinics (ISSN 0733-8651) is published quarterly by W.B. Saunders Company; Corporate and editorial Offices: Elsevier Inc., 1600 John F. Kennedy Blvd., Suite 1800, Philadelphia, PA 19103-2899. Accounting and circulation offices: 6277 Sea Harbor Drive, Orlando, FL 32887-4800. Periodicals postage paid at Orlando, FL 32862, and additional mailing offices. Subscription prices are $180.00 per year for US individuals, $280.00 per year for US institutions, $90.00 per year for US students and residents, $220.00 per year for Canadian individuals, $340.00 per year for Canadian institutions, $240.00 per year for international individuals, $340.00 per year for international institutions and $120.00 per year for Canadian and foreign students/residents. To receive student/resident rate, orders must be accompanied by name of affiliated institution, data of term, and the *signature* of program/residency coordinator on institution letterhead. Orders will be billed at individual rate until proof of status is received. Foreign air speed delivery is included in all *Clinics* subscription prices. All prices are subject to change without notice. POSTMASTER: Send address changes to *Cardiology Clinics*, W.B. Saunders Company, Periodicals Fulfillment, Orlando, FL 32887-4800. **Customer Service: 1-800-654-2452 (US). From outside of the US, call 1-407-345-1000.**

Cardiology Clinics is also published in Spanish by McGraw-Hill Interamericana Editores S. A., P.O. Box 5-237, 06500, Mexico D. F., Mexico; in Portuguese by Reichmann and Alfonso Editores Rio de Janeiro, Brazil; and in Greek by Dimitrios P. Lagos, 8 Pondon Street, GR115-28 Ilissia, Greece.

Cardiology Clinics is covered in *Index Medicus, Excerpta Medica, The Cumulative Index to Nursing and Allied Health Literature* (INAHL).

Printed in the United States of America.

CONSULTING EDITOR

MICHAEL H. CRAWFORD, MD, Professor of Medicine, Lucie Stern Chair in Cardiology, University of California, San Francisco; Chief of Clinical Cardiology, University of California, San Francisco Medical Center, San Francisco, California

GUEST EDITORS

EZRA A. AMSTERDAM, MD, FACC, Professor, Department of Internal Medicine; Associate Chief (Academic Affairs), Division of Cardiovascular Medicine, University of California School of Medicine (Davis) Medical Center, Sacramento, California

J. DOUGLAS KIRK, MD, FACEP, Associate Professor and Vice Chair, Department of Emergency Medicine; Medical Director, Chest Pain Service, University of California School of Medicine (Davis) Medical Center, Sacramento, California

CONTRIBUTORS

WAEL A. ALJAROUDI, MD, MS, Resident in Medicine, Department of Medicine, Duke University Medical Center, Durham, North Carolina

EZRA A. AMSTERDAM, MD, FACC, Professor, Department of Internal Medicine; Associate Chief (Academic Affairs), Division of Cardiovascular Medicine, University of California School of Medicine (Davis) Medical Center, Sacramento, California

ANDRA L. BLOMKALNS, MD, Assistant Professor, Department of Emergency Medicine, University of Cincinnati College of Medicine, Cincinnati, Ohio

CHRISTOPHER P. CANNON, MD, Senior Investigator, TIMI Study Group, Cardiovascular Division, Department of Medicine, Brigham and Women's Hospital and Harvard Medical School, Boston, Massachusetts

DENISE H. DAUDELIN, RN, MPH, Instructor of Medicine, Tufts University School of Medicine; Project Director, Medical Error Prevention, Institute for Clinical Research and Health Policy Studies, Tufts-New England Medical Center, Boston, Massachusetts

DEBORAH B. DIERCKS, MD, Associate Professor, Department of Emergency Medicine, University of California School of Medicine (Davis) and Medical Center, Sacramento, California

W. BRIAN GIBLER, MD, Professor and Chairman, Department of Emergency Medicine, University of Cincinnati College of Medicine, Cincinnati, Ohio

ALLAN S. JAFFE, MD, Consultant in Cardiology and Laboratory Medicine, Mayo Clinic and Mayo Medical School, Rochester, Minnesota

J. DOUGLAS KIRK, MD, FACEP, Associate Professor and Vice Chair, Department of Emergency Medicine; Medical Director, Chest Pain Service, University of California School of Medicine (Davis) Medical Center, Sacramento, California

MICHAEL C. KONTOS, MD, Associate Director, Acute Cardiac Care; Assistant Professor, Departments of Internal Medicine, Radiology, and Emergency Medicine, Virginia Commonwealth University, Richmond, Virginia

GERALD J. KOST, MD, PhD, MS, FACB, Director, Point-of-Care Testing Center for Teaching and Research; Professor, Pathology and Laboratory Medicine, School of Medicine; Faculty, Biomedical Engineering; Director, Clinical Chemistry, UCD Health System; University of California, Davis, California; and Affiliate Faculty, Chulalongkorn University, Bangkok, Thailand

AMIR LERMAN, MD, Professor of Medicine, Center of Coronary Physiology, Division of Cardiovascular Diseases, Mayo College of Medicine, Rochester, Minnesota

WILLIAM R. LEWIS, MD, Associate Professor, Department of Internal Medicine, Division of Cardiovascular Medicine, University of California School of Medicine (Davis) and Medical Center, Sacramento, California

JAMES MCCORD, MD, Henry Ford Health System, Heart & Vascular Institute, Detroit, Michigan

L. KRISTIN NEWBY, MD, MHS, Associate Professor of Medicine/Cardiology, Duke Clinical Research Institute, Durham, North Carolina

W. FRANK PEACOCK, MD, FACEP, Vice Chief of Research, Department of Emergency Medicine; Medical Director, Event Medicine, The Cleveland Clinic, Cleveland, Ohio

J. HECTOR POPE, MD, Assistant Professor of Emergency Medicine, Tufts University School of Medicine, Boston, Massachusetts

HARRY P. SELKER, MD, MSPH, Professor of Medicine, Tufts University School of Medicine; Executive Director, Institute for Clinical Research and Health Policy Studies, Tufts-New England Medical Center, Boston, Massachusetts

SANDRA SIECK, RN, MBA, Health Care Reform Field Specialist, Sieck HealthCare Consulting, Mobile, Alabama

JAMES L. TATUM, MD, Director, Molecular Imaging Center; Professor, Departments of Radiology and Internal Medicine, Virginia Commonwealth University, Richmond, Virginia

NAM K. TRAN, BS, Research Specialist, Point-of-Care Testing Center for Teaching and Research, University of California School of Medicine (Davis), Sacramento, California

SAMUEL D. TURNIPSEED, MD, Associate Professor, Department of Emergency Medicine, University of California School of Medicine (Davis) and Medical Center, Sacramento, California

TRACY Y. WANG, MD, MS, Fellow in Cardiology, Division of Cardiology, Duke University Medical Center, Durham, North Carolina

ERIC H. YANG, MD, Fellow in Interventional Cardiology, Center of Coronary Physiology, Division of Cardiovascular Diseases, Mayo College of Medicine, Rochester, Minnesota

CONTENTS

Foreword   xi
Michael H. Crawford

Preface   xiii
Ezra A. Amsterdam and J. Douglas Kirk

Acute Coronary Syndromes: Risk Stratification and Initial Management   401
Christopher P. Cannon

> For patients who have acute coronary syndromes (ACS), risk stratification is key to ini-
> tiating appropriate treatment. For ST-segment elevation MI, immediate reperfusion
> therapy is needed, and thus rapid identification of ST elevation on the ECG is critical.
> Then, having a standardized protocol for rapid treatment—with either primary percuta-
> neous coronary intervention or thrombolysis—is critical. For unstable angina/non–ST
> elevation ACS, after first identifying the patients who have a higher likelihood of actu-
> ally having an ACS (as opposed to noncardiac chest pain) stratification to high versus
> lower risk is needed to choose appropriate therapies. Thus, it is important for risk stra-
> tification to be a central part of all management of patients who have ACS.

Chest Pain Unit Concept: Rationale and Diagnostic Strategies   411
Andra L. Blomkalns and W. Brian Gibler

> Each year in the United States, over 8 million patients present to the emergency depart-
> ment (ED) with complaints of chest discomfort or other symptoms consistent with pos-
> sible acute coronary syndrome (ACS). While over half of these patients are typically
> admitted for further diagnostic evaluation, fewer than 20% are diagnosed with ACS.
> With hospital beds and inpatient resources scarce, these admissions can be avoided by
> evaluating low- to moderate-risk patients in chest pain units. This large, undifferentiated
> patient population represents a potential high-risk group for emergency physicians re-
> quiring a systematic approach and specific ED resources. This evaluation is required
> to appropriately determine if a patient is safe to be discharged home with outpatient
> follow-up versus requiring admission to the hospital for monitoring and further testing.

**Acute Coronary Syndromes in the Emergency Department: Diagnostic
Characteristics, Tests, and Challenges**   423
J. Hector Pope and Harry P. Selker

> Failure to diagnose patients who have acute coronary syndromes (ACSs)—either acute
> myocardial infarction (AMI) or unstable angina pectoris (UAP)—who present to the

emergency department (ED) remains a serious public health issue. Better understanding of the pathophysiology of coronary artery disease has allowed the adoption of a unifying hypothesis for the cause of ACSs: the conversion of a stable atherosclerotic lesion to a plaque rupture with thrombosis. Thus, physicians have come to appreciate UAP and AMI as parts of a continuum of ACSs. This article reviews the state of the art regarding the diagnosis of ACSs in the emergency setting and suggests reasons why missed diagnosis continues to occur, albeit infrequently.

Use of Biomarkers in the Emergency Department and Chest Pain Unit

453

Allan S. Jaffe

The use of biomarkers of cardiac injury in the emergency department (ED) and observation unit settings has several nuances that are different and, therefore, worthy of its own set of use guidelines. The markers that are used, however, are the same. The primary marker of choice continues to be cardiac troponin (Tn). Other markers that have been used because of the need in the ED for rapid triage have been myoglobin and fatty acid binding protein. In addition, some centers still prefer less sensitive and less specific markers such as creatine kinase myocardial band (CK-MB). More recently, a push has occurred to develop markers of ischemia, such as ischemia modified albumin (IMA), to determine which patients have ischemia, even in the absence of cardiac injury. As troponin assays become more sensitive and method for use becomes better understood, the use of these other markers are being relegated to lesser and lesser roles. Markers of ischemia are useful, but at present, despite some enthusiasm, are not ready for routine use. Before describing the recommendations for clinical use of biomarkers in the ED, a basic understanding of some of the science and measurement issues related to these analytes is helpful.

Point-of-Care Testing and Cardiac Biomarkers: The Standard of Care and Vision for Chest Pain Centers

467

Gerald J. Kost and Nam K. Tran

Point-of-care testing (POCT) is defined as testing at or near the site of patient care. POCT decreases therapeutic turnaround time (TTAT), increases clinical efficiency, and improves medical and economic outcomes. TTAT represents the time from test ordering to patient treatment. POC technologies have become ubiquitous in the United States, and, therefore, so has the potential for speed, convenience, and satisfaction, strong advantages for physicians, nurses, and patients in chest pain centers. POCT is applied most beneficially through the collaborative teamwork of clinicians and laboratorians who use integrative strategies, performance maps, clinical algorithms, and care paths (critical pathways). For example, clinical investigators have shown that on-site integration of testing for cardiac injury markers (myoglobin, creatinine kinase myocardial band [CK-MB], and cardiac troponin I [cTnI]) in accelerated diagnostic algorithms produces effective screening, less hospitalization, and substantial savings. Chest pain centers, which now total over 150 accredited in the United States, incorporate similar types of protocol-driven performance enhancements. This optimization allows chest pain centers to improve patient evaluation, treatment, survival, and discharge. This article focuses on cardiac biomarker POCT for chest pain centers and emergency medicine.

Markers of Cardiac Ischemia and Inflammation

491

Tracy Y. Wang, Wael A. AlJaroudi, and L. Kristin Newby

Because biomarkers of myocardial necrosis only become positive in the setting of myocardial necrosis and disruption of cellular integrity, the diagnosis of myocardial infarction can only be made in retrospect. Ideally, one would like to identify patients at risk for complications before myocardial necrosis occurs. Insights into the pathophysiology of atherothrombosis have allowed development of novel markers to detect not only early ischemia without myocyte death but also early indicators of coronary inflammation in patients who have preclinical atherosclerosis.

Exercise Testing in Chest Pain Units: Rationale, Implementation, and Results   503

Ezra A. Amsterdam, J. Douglas Kirk, Deborah B. Diercks, William R. Lewis, and Samuel D. Turnipseed

Chest pain units are now established centers for assessment of low-risk patients presenting to the emergency department with symptoms suggestive of acute coronary syndrome. Accelerated diagnostic protocols, of which treadmill testing is a key component, have been developed within these units for efficient evaluation of these patients. Studies of the last decade have established the utility of early exercise testing, which has been safe, accurate, and cost-effective in this setting. Specific diagnostic protocols vary, but most require 6 to12 hours of observation by serial electrocardiography and cardiac injury markers to exclude infarction and high-risk unstable angina before proceeding to exercise testing. However, in the chest pain unit at UC Davis Medical Center, the approach includes "immediate" treadmill testing without a traditional process to rule out myocardial infarction. Extensive experience has validated this approach in a large, heterogeneous population. The optimal strategy for evaluating low-risk patients presenting to the emergency department with chest pain will continue to evolve based on current research and the development of new methods.

Imaging in the Evaluation of the Patient with Suspected Acute Coronary Syndrome   517

Michael C. Kontos and James L. Tatum

Over the last decade, major advances have been made in the treatment of acute coronary syndromes (ACSs). However, effective implementation of these treatments requires timely and accurate identification of the high-risk patient among all those presenting to the emergency department (ED) with symptoms suggestive of ACS. The opportunity for improving outcomes is time-dependent, so that early identification of the patient who has true ACS is essential. This necessity further increases the need for rapid triage tools, especially in the current setting of ED and hospital overcrowding that has become the norm in large urban centers.

Echocardiography in the Evaluation of Patients in Chest Pain Units   531

William R. Lewis

Using percutaneous angioplasty to induce the ischemic cascade in the cardiac catheterization laboratory, echocardiographic wall motion abnormalities have been documented to precede electrocardiographic abnormalities and angina. Therefore, detection of cardiac wall motion abnormalities is potentially more sensitive than the history, physical examination, and ECG for identification of myocardial ischemia. Echocardiography is highly reliable for assessing cardiac wall motion and, thus, it has been used for diagnosis and risk assessment in patients presenting to the emergency department (ED) with symptoms suggestive of myocardial ischemia. In patients who have acute ST-elevation myocardial infarction (MI), echocardiography is comparable to invasive left ventriculography for detecting wall motion abnormalities. However, the usefulness of echocardiography in the low-risk population that has chest pain of uncertain origin and a nondiagnostic initial presentation is less well established.

Newer Imaging Methods for Triaging Patients Presenting to the Emergency Department with Chest Pain   541

James McCord and Ezra A. Amsterdam

The usefulness of electron beam CT (EBCT) for the risk stratification of patients in the emergency department (ED) who have possible acute coronary syndrome has been evaluated in three small studies. The results of these studies are promising, as patients who have no coronary calcium detected by EBCT essentially had no adverse cardiac events.

Although the negative predictive value of EBCT was excellent, the limited positive predictive value that would lead to further diagnostic testing makes this strategy less attractive if applied to a broad population. Further larger studies may help define which patients in the ED who have chest pain and nondiagnostic ECGs can be effectively evaluated by EBCT. Recent advances in noninvasive coronary angiography by multislice computed tomography are of considerable interest in the ED evaluation of patients with undefined chest pain, but the utility of this method in this setting awaits clinical studies.

Chest Pain Units: Management of Special Populations

549

Deborah B. Diercks, J. Douglas Kirk, and Ezra A. Amsterdam

Chest pain units provide an important alternative to traditional hospital admission for patients who present to the emergency department with symptoms compatible with acute coronary syndrome and a normal or inconclusive initial evaluation. Although patient subgroups such as women, diabetics, those with established coronary artery disease, and those with symptoms related to stimulant use present unique challenges, management in a chest pain unit appears to be appropriate in these populations. Judicious application of accelerated diagnostic protocols and current testing methods can promote safe, accurate, and cost-effective risk stratification of special populations to identify patients who can be safely discharged and patients who require hospital admission for further evaluation.

Management of the Patient with Chest Pain and a Normal Coronary Angiogram

559

Eric H. Yang and Amir Lerman

Angina in the setting of a normal coronary angiogram (NOCAD) occurs in 20% to 30% of patients undergoing coronary angiography. The management of these patients can be challenging and requires a correct diagnosis of the etiology. The differential diagnosis of NOCAD can be classified anatomically into three categories: (1) epicardial disease, (2) coronary microvascular dysfunction, and (3) noncoronary disease. The pathophysiology of NOCAD and a systematic diagnostic approach to these patients is reviewed. Potential therapeutic options and prognosis are also discussed.

Using the Emergency Department Clinical Decision Unit for Acute Decompensated Heart Failure

569

W. Frank Peacock

Acute decompensated heart failure (ADHF) is a complex disease of epidemic proportions. In the United States, it accounts for more than 1 million hospitalizations annually, and heart failure represents the single greatest cost to the Centers for Medicaid and Medicare Studies. Half of the annual costs are estimated to be the result of hospitalization. Compared with other pathology, heart failure has a very high hospitalization rate, with 80% of emergency department ADHF patients being admitted. This high rate has resulted from the lack of successful management predictors available to the emergency physician and the lack of any disposition option other than hospitalization for the ADHF patient. The emergency department observation unit offers an alternative to hospitalization for patients with ADHF. Validated protocols have demonstrated that in ADHF, intensive short-term therapeutic, diagnostic, and educational protocols result in a marked improvement in hospitalization rates, while at the same time decreasing costs. New risk stratification data can aid in the identification of the appropriate candidate. The observation unit now represents a nonhospitalization disposition option for patients presenting to the emergency department with ADHF.

Cost Effectiveness of Chest Pain Units   589

Sandra Sieck

Health care facilities face many challenges in their attempts to provide cost-effective care without sacrificing quality. One key factor in producing quality outcomes while maintaining economic profitability is the establishment of a cost-effective outpatient care environment. Chest Pain Units (CPUs) have evolved to provide a streamlined approach to acute cardiac care that emphasizes optimal efficiency initiated at the point of entry. The Centers for Medicare and Medicaid Services have structured new reimbursement approaches designed to shift care from the inpatient setting and "reward" efficient and appropriate care delivered in the outpatient arena. These new reimbursement strategies have transformed the CPU into an economically viable entity for the acute care facility and also have afforded opportunities to enhance the quality of care delivered to the acute cardiac patient.

Medical Error Prevention in ED Triage for ACS: Use of Cardiac Care Decision Support and Quality Improvement Feedback   601

Denise H. Daudelin and Harry P. Selker

Medical errors in the care of patients who present with acute coronary syndrome (ACS) include errors in emergency department (ED) triage, such as the decision to send home a patient who presents with ACS or to hospitalize a patient who does not have ACS to the cardiac care unit (CCU), and errors in treatment, such as the failure to promptly use reperfusion therapy for patients who present with ST-elevation acute myocardial infarction (AMI). ECG-based acute cardiac ischemia time-insensitive predictive instrument (ACI-TIPI) and thrombolytic predictive instruments (TPIs), with a linked TIPI information system (TIPI-IS), provide real-time, concurrent, and retrospective decision support tools and feedback for the prevention of medical errors in the care of patients who present with ACS. In real-time, ACI-TIPI probabilities printed on the ECG header for the ED physician, provide an additional piece of information for triage decision making, and the ACI-TIPI Risk Management form reduces liability risk by prompting consideration and documentation of key clinical factors in the diagnosis of ACI. Also in real-time, the TPI increases overall coronary reperfusion therapy use. Concurrent flagging by TIPI-IS uses electronically acquired ECG and hospital data to provide concurrent alerts about potential misdiagnosis or mis-triage of patients with ACS. Retrospectively TIPI-IS-based feedback reports allow performance improvement. These examples of information technology tools integrated into ECG equipment already used in hospitals to deliver patient care demonstrate the potential to adapt other existing equipment or other patient care activities to enhance patient safety and error reduction.

Cumulative Index 2005   615

FORTHCOMING ISSUES

February 2006

Emergency Cardiac Care: From ED to CCU
Amal Mattu, MD, and Mark Kelemen, MD, MSc
Guest Editors

May 2006

Interventional Cardiology
Samin K. Sharma, MD, *Guest Editor*

August 2006

Advanced 12-Lead Electrocardiography
S. Serge Barold, MD, *Guest Editor*

RECENT ISSUES

August 2005

Cardio-Renal Disease

Ragavendra R. Baliga, MD, MBA, FACC, FRCP(Edin),
Sanjay Rajagopalan, MD, and
Rajiv Saran, MD, MS, MRCP, *Guest Editors*

May 2005

**Therapeutic Strategies in Diabetes
and Cardiovascular Disease**

Prakash C. Deedwania, MD, FACC, FACP, FCCP, FAHA
Guest Editor

February 2005

Patent Foramen Ovale

Edward A. Gill, Jr, MD, and John D. Carroll, MD
Guest Editors

Cardiol Clin 23 (2005) xi

Foreword

Chest Pain Units

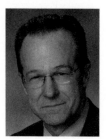

Michael H. Crawford, MD
Consulting Editor

Chest pain units have been enthusiastically embraced by some medical centers and disdained as marketing ploys by critics. Whether you have one or not, this issue should be of interest. If you already have one, you may get some ideas for improvement or widening the scope of your operation. If you don't have one, this issue will help with the decision of whether to pursue establishing one. One clear benefit of chest pain centers is that they decrease unnecessary hospital admissions by allowing patients to be evaluated further without bogging down the emergency department or being admitted. As pointed out in one of the articles, this concept is not unique to chest pain but can also be applied to heart failure exacerbation patients.

Drs. Amsterdam and Kirk from cardiology and emergency medicine, respectively, at the University of California at Davis School of Medicine are leaders in this area and both are very active in the growing Society of Chest Pain Centers. They have assembled a panel of experts to cover every aspect of chest pain centers,

including articles on cost effectiveness, medical errors, and the employment of various types of diagnostic imaging. New noninvasive methods for imaging the coronary arteries are adding a new dimension to the evaluation of chest pain patients. Newer biomarkers are also changing the triage of patients with chest pain. They are discussed in three articles. After more than 102 years of use, is the ECG ready for the medical museum? Will biomarkers and imaging replace the ECG in triaging chest pain patients? Read on.

Michael H. Crawford, MD
Division of Cardiology
Department of Medicine
University of California
San Francisco Medical Center
505 Parnassus Avenue, Box 0124
San Francisco, CA 94143-0124, USA

E-mail address: michael.crawford@
ucsfmedctr.org

Preface

Chest Pain Units

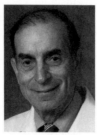 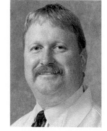

Ezra A. Amsterdam, MD, FACC   J. Douglas Kirk, MD, FACEP
Guest Editors

Although time-dependent therapy is an over-arching principle of the management of acute coronary syndromes (ACS), fulfillment of this concept remains incomplete [1]. Delays in recognition of ACS and initiation of therapy entail patient, physician, and systemic factors [2]. This problem is particularly pertinent to the treatment of non-ST elevation (non-STE) ACS in which the history and ECG may be ambiguous. Although the high-risk patient is the primary clinical focus, most patients who present with chest pain have a noncardiac etiology that is frequently benign. The clinical dilemma posed by this situation has often been resolved by unnecessary admissions to avert missed diagnoses of ACS, resulting in suboptimal patient care and resource use [3]. The development and growth of chest pain units (CPUs) is a response to this problem by application of a systematic approach to optimize management of patients presenting with symptoms compatible with ACS by affording: (1) prompt identification and treatment of those with an ischemic syndrome and (2) early and accurate discharge of individuals without evidence of myocardial ischemia.

Through its recently implemented process, the Society of Chest Pain Centers has accredited almost 150 CPUs in this country [4] and, based on the current growth rate, it is anticipated that this number will reach 200 or more by the end of this year. Although these units differ in certain respects, their common basis is a protocol-driven patient evaluation by an accelerated diagnostic strategy, including clinical observation, sequential ECGs, and serial cardiac injury markers. These basic methods are being extended by rapidly emerging technologies with the promise of earlier and more accurate diagnostic capability, thereby further enhancing the use of CPUs. This volume of *Cardiology Clinics* encompasses these advances in presenting the contemporary status of CPUs and associated methodology from the perspectives of an outstanding group of clinician scientists who have made major contributions to this field.

In his introductory chapter, Cannon synthesizes current understanding of ACS in terms pathophysiology, clinical presentation, and risk stratification. To achieve the latter goal, he considers the roles of basic clinical tools, guidelines, and critical pathways while maintaining focus on the individual patient for optimal management. Blomkalns and Gibler elucidate the rationale of the CPU concept and the practical aspects of its implementation. They relate how these strategies can differ based on institutional variation in methods of staffing, structure, and administration to meet the CPU goals. In the next two articles, Pope and Selker (1) delve further into the diagnostic challenges and current systems for evaluating patients presenting with chest pain and (2)

0733-8651/05/$ - see front matter © 2005 Elsevier Inc. All rights reserved.
doi:10.1016/j.ccl.2005.08.017

explore the crucial problem of missed ACS and inadvertent discharge from the emergency department. In the latter context, they identify the principal factors associated with these clinical errors and methods to prevent them. The pivotal role of cardiac injury markers is developed by Jaffe who describes the most recent advances in this area and charts a rational application based on an understanding of the value and limitations of these essential clinical tools. These concepts are extended by Kost and Tran who analyze the rapidly advancing area of point-of-care testing for cardiac injury markers and the remarkably rapid results while maintaining diagnostic accuracy. Wang, Aroudi, and Newby then explore the increased understanding of inflammation in ACS and the growing body of markers that reflect this process, some of which are already being applied clinically.

The next series of articles is devoted to the varieties of cardiac stress testing and imaging as applied in the CPU setting. Our group reviews the extensive clinical experience in multiple centers confirming the utility of treadmill testing as the final element of accelerated diagnostic protocols and we note our results with the immediate exercise test in low-risk patients. The central role of myocardial scintigraphy in many CPUs is addressed by Kontos and Tatum who demonstrate the efficacy of this method in their innovative approach to risk stratification. Rest and stress echocardiography has had substantial application in the assessment of patients who present with chest pain and the indications and accuracy of this technique are evaluated by Lewis. New imaging methods, such as coronary artery calcium scoring and the emergence of noninvasive coronary angiography by computed tomography, are receiving major attention and McCord and Amsterdam provide a perspective on the potential of these techniques.

Because of their unique clinical characteristics, populations such as women, the elderly, and those with documented coronary heart disease, have required specific investigation to determine if the CPU concept applies to their presentations. Diercks and colleagues demonstrate that the CPU strategy is appropriate in these other groups with special clinical features. A large proportion of patients who present to the emergency department with chest pain do not have obstructive coronary artery disease. Yang and Lerman delineate these distinctive syndromes and impart a systematic approach to their etiology, prognosis, and management. A new dimension that has recently been added to the CPU is the management of patients with acute decompensated heart failure, which is detailed by Peacock in his presentation of the rationale, indications, and results of this innovation.

Reduction of medical errors is an imperative of the CPU and Daudelin and Selker clarify current research in this area. Although their clinical utility has been demonstrated, the complex question of whether CPUs are cost-effective has received limited attention. Sieck reviews this issue in terms of its medical and administrative aspects and their relation to the larger framework of the health care system.

This volume provides a current understanding of the implementation and efficacy of CPUs and the integration of new technology into this approach. These results have provided the basis for continuing advances toward the optimal strategy for the management of patients presenting to the emergency department with chest pain.

Ezra A. Amsterdam, MD, FACC
Professor, Department of Internal Medicine
Associate Chief (Academic Affairs)
Division of Cardiovascular Medicine
University of California School of Medicine
(Davis) Medical Center, Sacramento, CA, USA
E-mail address: eaamsterdam@ucdavis.edu

J. Douglas Kirk, MD, FACEP
Associate Professor and Vice Chair
Department of Emergency Medicine
Medical Director, Chest Pain Service
University of California School of Medicine
(Davis) Medical Center, Sacramento, CA, USA
E-mail address: jdkirk@ucdavis.edu

References

[1] Braunwald E, Antman EM, Beasley JW, et al. ACC/AHA 2002 guideline update for the management of patients with unstable angina and non-ST-segment elevation myocardial infarction. Available at: http://www.acc.org/clinical/guidelines/unstable/unstable.pdf.

[2] Gibler WB, Cannon CP, Blomkalns AL, et al. Practical implementation of the guidelines for unstable angina/non-ST-segment elevation myocardial infarction in the emergency department. Ann Emerg Med 2005;46:185–97.

[3] Amsterdam EA, Lewis WR, Kirk JD, et al. Acute ischemic syndromes. Chest pain center concept. Cardiol Clin 2002;20:117–36.

[4] Society of Chest Pain Centers. Available at: http://www.scpcp.org/accreditation/accreditedlist.html

ELSEVIER
SAUNDERS

Cardiol Clin 23 (2005) 401–409

CARDIOLOGY
CLINICS

Acute Coronary Syndromes: Risk Stratification and Initial Management

Christopher P. Cannon, MD

Cardiovascular Division, Brigham and Women's Hospital, 75 Francis Street, Boston, MA 02115, USA

In the United States, there are approximately 1.68 million patients admitted every year to hospitals with acute coronary syndromes (ACSs) [1]. Of these, one quarter present with acute myocardial infarction (MI) associated with ECG ST-segment elevation (STEMI), whereas three quarters, or approximately 1.3 million patients, have unstable angina/non–ST elevation MI (UA/NSTEMI) [1]. The former is most commonly caused by acute total occlusion of a coronary artery and therefore urgent reperfusion is the mainstay of therapy, whereas UA/NSTEMI is usually associated with a nonocclusive thrombus [2]. Among patients who have UA/NSTEMI, between 40% and 60% will have evidence of myocardial necrosis with elevated troponin, and are thus diagnosed with a NSTEMI [3,4].

In the past several years, there have been many advances in the diagnosis and management of this patient population, as summarized in part in the 2002 update of the American College of Cardiology (ACC) and the American Heart Association (AHA) UA/NSTEMI guidelines, and the 2004 ACC/AHA STEMI guidelines.

The approach to the patient, especially at the first presentation in the emergency department (ED) or chest pain unit, involves careful risk stratification. This assessment actually involves two steps: assessment of the likelihood that the patient's symptoms represent ACS (as opposed to noncardiac chest pain), and risk stratification of the patients who have ACS to identify high- versus lower-risk patients. The guidelines recommend that specific therapies and treatment can be targeted to only high-risk patients, with other treatments recommended for all patients. The treatments recommended include anti-ischemic, antithrombotic therapy and what strategy should be followed (ie, whether to pursue an invasive versus conservative approach), and reperfusion therapy for STEMI.

Assessment of likelihood of coronary artery disease

Approximately 6 to 7 million persons per year in the United States present to EDs or chest pain units with a complaint of chest pain or other symptoms suggestive of possible ACS. Of these, approximately 20% to 25% have a final diagnosis of unstable angina or MI [5,6]. Thus, the first step in evaluating patients who have possible UA/NSTEMI is to determine the likelihood that coronary artery disease (CAD) is the cause of the presenting symptoms. The 2002 ACC/AHA guidelines list factors associated with increased likelihood that the patient actually has unstable angina (Table 1).

Numerous prediction rules using clinical and ECG variables have also been developed to assess the likelihood of CAD in patients presenting to the ED with chest pain [7–14]. One algorithm, the acute cardiac ischemia time-insensitive prediction instrument (ACI-TIPI) has been integrated into ECG devices. It provides a quantitative likelihood of the patient having ACSs (ie, STEMI and UA/NSTEMI) [12,13]. One randomized trial has shown that ACI-TIPI reduced unnecessary hospital and coronary care unit admissions [13]. Other studies have suggested that good clinical judgment is as good as the computer algorithms [9,10], emphasizing the importance of obtaining a good

E-mail address: cpcannon@partners.org

Table 1
Estimating the likelihood that the suspected acute coronary syndrome event is secondary to coronary artery disease

	High likelihood	Intermediate likelihood	Low likelihood
Feature	Any below:	No high-likelihood features but any below:	No high- or intermediate-likelihood features but may have:
History	Typical angina; known history of coronary artery disease including myocardial infarction	Probable angina; age >70 years; male diabetes mellitus	Atypical symptoms
Examination	Congestive heart failure	Peripheral vascular disease, cerebrovascular accident	Pain on plapation
ECG	New ECG changes	Old ECG abnormalities	Normal ECG
Cardiac markers	Positive	Normal	Normal

From Braunwald E, Mark DB, Jones RH, et al. Unstable angina: diagnosis and management. Rockville MD: Agency for Health Care Policy and Research and the National Heart, Lung, and Blood Institute, US Public Health Service, US Department of Health and Human Services; 1994; AHCPR Publication No. 94-0602.

clinical history when assessing patients who have chest pain.

Risk stratification

Based on data from a global registry, the outcomes of patients who have ACS fall on a spectrum of risk, ranging from 30-day mortality of 1.7% for patients who have unstable angina to 7.4% for those who have NSTEMI and 11.1% for those who have STEMI [15]. Within clinical trials in which inclusion criteria select higher-risk patients, rates of death by 30 days ranged from 3.5% to 4.5% and of new MI from 6% to 12% [16–18]. However, patents who have UA/NSTEMI constitute a wide spectrum of patients and risk [19–21]; thus, the ACC/AHA guidelines strongly recommend risk stratification as important to characterize the patient's prognosis and to select appropriate therapy. Boxes 1 through 3 list the three recommended stratifications for risk of death/MI in UA/NSTEMI.

The rationale for risk stratification is to target some of the more aggressive therapies to the higher-risk patients. This approach has been seen in multiple studies with several of the agents for management of UA/NSTEMI. In STEMI, most of the treatments are similar based on the patient's risk, beginning with reperfusion therapy and including antithrombotic and anti-ischemic therapies, which are similar to that of UA/NSTEMI.

Thus, among patients who have been identified as having a moderate or high likelihood of having an ACS, the ACC/AHA guidelines highlight risk stratification as a key step that can target the intensity of medical and interventional therapies

to higher-risk patients. Factors associated with a high risk for death or nonfatal MI in patients who have UA/NSTEMI are prolonged rest pain, ST-segment changes, elevated cardiac biomarkers (eg, troponin), diabetes, evidence of congestive heart failure, and age over 75 years. Low-risk patients present without rest pain [22], ECG changes, or evidence of heart failure (see Box 3). Other factors are highlighted as markers of long-term risk, such as extent of CAD, left ventricular dysfunction, and elevated markers of inflammation.

In UA/NSTEMI, use of troponin alone has been a powerful tool for risk stratification and targeting of therapies. Studies have found that high-risk patients benefit from the more aggressive treatments. For low molecular weight heparin (LMWH), glycoprotein (GP) IIb/IIIa inhibitors, and an early invasive strategy, there is a greater benefit of these interventions in patients who have a positive troponin, and almost no benefit in patients who have a negative troponin [3,23–26]. For example, with the GP IIb/IIIa inhibitors, there was a 50% to 70% reduction in death or MI in patients who were troponin-positive and were receiving GP IIb/IIIa inhibitors compared with patients not receiving these agents, with no benefit of GP IIb/IIIa inhibitors in those who did not have a positive troponin [24,25]. A different pattern has been seen with the oral antiplatelet agents, in that aspirin and clopidogrel benefit low-, intermediate-, and high-risk patients and those who have positive or negative cardiac markers [27–29]. Thus, aspirin and clopidogrel have been recommended for all patients regardless of risk, whereas GP

Box 1. Short-term high risk for death/ myocardial infarction in unstable angina/NSTEMI

At least one of:
History
  Accelerating tempo of ischemic
    symptoms in preceding 48 hours

Character of pain
  Prolonged ongoing (>20 min)
    rest pain

Clinical findings
  Pulmonary edema, most likely caused
    by ischemia
  New or worsening mitral regurgitation
    murmur
  S_3 or new/worsening rales
  Hypotension, bradycardia, tachycardia
  Age over 75 years

ECG
  Rest angina with transient ST changes
    greater than 0.05 mV
  Bundle branch block
  New sustained ventricular tachycardia

Cardiac markers
  Markedly elevated (eg, Troponin T or
    Troponin I >0.1 ng/mL)

From Braunwald E, Antman EM, Beasley JW, et al. ACC/AHA guidelines for the management of patients with unstable angina and non-ST-segment elevation myocardial infarction: a report of the American College of Cardiology/American Heart Association Task Force on Practice Guidelines (Committee on the Management of Patients With Unstable Angina). J Am Coll Cardiol 2000;36:970–1062; with permission.

Box 2. Short-term intermediate risk for death/myocardial infarction in unstable angina/NSTEMI

No high-risk features, but must have one of:
History
  Prior myocardial infarction, peripheral
    vascular disease, or cerebrovascular
    disease
  Coronary artery bypass grafting
  Prior aspirin use

Character of pain
  Prolonged (>20 min) rest angina,
    now resolved, with moderate or
    high likelihood of coronary artery
    disease
  Rest angina (<20 min) or relieved with
    rest or sublingual nitroglycerin

Clinical findings
  Age over 70 years

ECG
  T-wave inversions greater than 0.2 mV
  Pathologic Q waves

Cardiac markers
  Slightly elevated (eg, Troponin
    T >0.01 ng/mL but <0.1 ng/mL)

From Braunwald E, Antman EM, Beasley JW, et al. ACC/AHA guidelines for the management of patients with unstable angina and non-ST-segment elevation myocardial infarction: a report of the American College of Cardiology/American Heart Association Task Force on Practice Guidelines (Committee on the Management of Patients With Unstable Angina). J Am Coll Cardiol 2000;36:970–1062; with permission.

IIb/IIIa inhibitors are recommended for use only in high-risk patients or those undergoing percutaneous coronary intervention (PCI) (Fig. 1).

Risk scores

Integrating all the risk factors identified in the ACC/AHA guidelines as low-, intermediate-, or high-risk, comprehensive risk scores have been

developed using clinical variables and ECG and initial serum cardiac marker data [30,31]. The Thrombolysis in Myocardial Infarction (TIMI) risk score was developed using multivariate analysis to predict the occurrence of death, MI, or recurrent ischemia leading to urgent revascularization in the TIMI 11B trial. Seven independent risk factors emerged: age over 65 years, more than three risk factors for CAD, documented CAD at

Box 3. Short-term low risk for death/ myocardial infarction in unstable angina

No high or intermediate risk feature, but may have any of:

History
  None indicated

Character of pain
  New-onset Canadian Cardiovascular
    Society class III or IV angina
    in past 2 weeks without prolonged
    (>20 min) rest pain, but with
    moderate or high likelihood of
    coronary artery disease

Clinical findings
  None indicated

ECG
  Normal or unchanged ECG during
    chest discomfort

Cardiac markers
  Normal

From Braunwald E, Antman EM, Beasley JW, et al. ACC/AHA guidelines for the management of patients with unstable angina and non-ST-segment elevation myocardial infarction: a report of the American College of Cardiology/American Heart Association Task Force on Practice Guidelines (Committee on the Management of Patients With Unstable Angina). J Am Coll Cardiol 2000;36:970–1062; with permission.

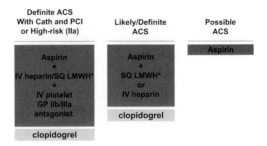

Fig. 1. 2002 American College of Cardiology/American Heart Association guideline recommendations for antithrombotic therapy for unstable angina/non–ST elevation acute coronary syndrome. (*From* Braunwald E, Antman EM, Beasley JW, et al. ACC/AHA guidelines for the management of patients with unstable angina and non-ST-segment elevation myocardial infarction: a report of the American College of Cardiology/American Heart Association Task Force on Practice Guidelines (Committee on the Management of Patients With Unstable Angina). J Am Coll Cardiol 2000;36:970–1062; with permission.)

catheterization, prior ASA, more than two episodes of angina in the last 24 hours, ST deviation more than 0.5 mm, and elevated cardiac markers. This scoring system was able to risk stratify patients across a ten-fold gradient of risk, from 4.7% to 40.9% ($P < .001$) [31]. More importantly, the relative benefit of enoxaparin as compared with unfractionated heparin increased as the risk increased [31]. Similar findings have now been seen using the TIMI risk score to predict the benefit of GP IIb/IIIa inhibitors [32] and an early invasive strategy [3]. Thus, these findings support the ACC/AHA guideline recommendations that risk stratification be the first task in evaluating patients who present with UA/NSTEMI [33].

Antithrombotic and medical therapy

Initial treatment for patients who have UA/NSTEMI should include aspirin, which leads to a 50% to 70% reduction in death or MI as compared with placebo [34]. Current data on aspirin indicate the drug is beneficial for long-term treatment at doses as low as 75 mg/d [27]. New data from the Clopidogrel in Unstable Angina to Prevent Recurrent Events (CURE) trial indicates that lower doses of aspirin (eg, 81 mg) are associated with a 50% lower rate of major bleeding over 1 year of treatment than doses of 200 to 325 mg [35]. Thus, for acute management in-hospital, 160 to 325 mg daily is recommended, but at hospital discharge and during follow-up, the new data suggest a dose of 81 mg may be safer.

The 2002 ACC/AHA guideline included a new Class I recommendation for the use of clopidogrel in addition to aspirin. Clopidogrel blocks the ADP pathway by blocking the P_2Y_{12} component of the ADP receptor, which in turn decreases platelet activation and aggregation. The CURE trial found that clopidogrel plus aspirin led to a 20% relative risk reduction in cardiovascular death, MI, or stroke compared with aspirin alone [28]. This benefit was seen in low- and high-risk patients [29] and was seen as early as 24 hours [36], with the Kaplan-Meier curves for event rate in the two treatment groups diverging after just 2 hours.

This benefit has also been seen in two other trials. In the CREDO trial of patients undergoing PCI, clopidogrel was associated with a significant 27% relative reduction in the combined risk for death, MI, or stroke at 1 year ($P = .02$) [37]. Similarly, in the CAPRIE trial, clopidogrel alone had a significant reduction in these events versus aspirin through 3 years of follow-up in patients who had prior atherothrombotic disease [38]. Thus, there is strong evidence from large double-blind, randomized trials that clopidogrel plus aspirin is the new optimal long-term antithrombotic regimen.

Intravenous GP IIb/IIIa inhibitors have also been shown to be beneficial in treating UA/NSTEMI [39]. For "upstream" management (ie, initiating therapy when the patient first presents to the hospital), the small molecule inhibitors eptifibatide and tirofiban clearly show benefit, whereas abciximab was of no benefit in an unselected UA/NSTEMI patient population [40] and is in fact contraindicated for patients approached with a noninvasive strategy [41].

Unfractionated heparin (UFH) or LMWH is recommended for patients who have UA/NSTEMI [42]. Comparative trials of enoxaparin (a LMWH) versus UFH have demonstrated superiority of enoxaparin in reducing recurrent cardiac events [43,44]. Based on these data, the 2002 Updated ACC/AHA UA/NSTEMI practice guidelines have made a Class IIA recommendation that enoxaparin is the preferred antithrombin over UFH [41].

Anti-ischemic therapy with nitrates is also recommended, with the use of intravenous nitrates for ongoing ischemic pain and beta-blockade early and during long-term follow-up [33].

In STEMI, benefits of early angiotensin-converting enzyme inhibition are considerable. In the GISSI-3 [45] trial, early initiation of lisinopril was associated with a 12% mortality reduction, and in ISIS-4 [46], captopril therapy resulted in a 7% mortality reduction. Benefits were more pronounced in patients who had anterior MI. However, in patients who had NSTEMI, no benefit was observed in the ISIS-4 study.

Invasive versus conservative strategy: non–ST elevation acute coronary syndrome

For patients who have UA/NSTEMI, nine randomized trials have assessed the merits of an invasive strategy involving routine cardiac catheterization with revascularization (if feasible) versus a conservative strategy where angiography and revascularization are reserved for patients who have evidence of recurrent ischemia either at rest or on provocative testing. Of these, six of the last seven have all shown a significant benefit of the invasive strategy (Fig. 2), especially in higher-risk patients [3,35,47]. Accordingly, the 2002 ACC/AHA guideline has added ST-segment changes and positive troponin to the list of high-risk indicators that would lead to a Class I recommendation for an early invasive strategy, as shown in Box 4 [41]. With regard to the timing of an invasive strategy, the results from the Intracoronary Stenting with Antithrombotic Regimen Cooling-Off study found a benefit of an immediate invasive strategy with an average time to catheterization of 2 hours, compared with a delayed invasive strategy with an average time to catheterization of 4 days [48]. Randomized studies have not yet evaluated whether an immediate invasive approach is better than catheterization 24 to 48 hours postadmission.

Summary—acute therapy for non–ST elevation acute coronary syndrome

Summarizing the ACC/AHA guidelines, there are now five baseline therapies for all patients: aspirin; clopidogrel; heparin or LMWH (with enoxaparin the preferred antithrombin); beta-blockers; and nitrates (Fig. 3) [23]. Then there are two treatments that are best targeted by risk

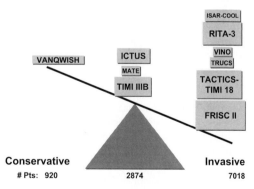

Fig. 2. The "weight of the evidence" showing benefit of an invasive versus conservative strategy in patients who have unstable angina/non–ST elevation acute coronary syndrome. The size of the boxes for each of the nine randomized trials corresponds to the number of patients enrolled. (*Modified from* Cannon CP, Turpie AG. Unstable angina and non-ST-elevation myocardial infarction: initial antithrombotic therapy and early invasive strategy. Circulation 2003;107:2640–5; with permission.)

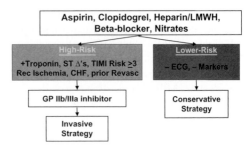

Box 4. ACC/AHA guideline recommendations for an early invasive strategy for unstable angina/non–ST elevation myocardial infarction

Class I
Any of the high-risk indicators (level of evidence: A)

- Recurrent angina at rest/low-level activity despite treatment
- Elevated Troponin T or Troponin I
- New ST-segment depression
- Recurrent angina/ischemia with congestive heart failure symptoms, rales, mitral regurgitation
- Positive stress test
- EF less than 0.40
- Decreased blood pressure
- Sustained tidal volume
- PCI less than 6 months, prior coronary artery bypass grafting

From Braunwald E, Antman EM, Beasley JW, et al. ACC/AHA guidelines for the management of patients with unstable angina and non-ST-segment elevation myocardial infarction: a report of the American College of Cardiology/American Heart Association Task Force on Practice Guidelines (Committee on the Management of Patients With Unstable Angina). J Am Coll Cardiol 2000;36:970–1062; with permission.

Fig. 3. Evidence-based risk stratification to target therapies in unstable angina/non–ST elevation acute coronary syndrome, as recommended in the American College of Cardiology/American Heart Association guidelines. (*From* Cannon CP. Evidence-based risk stratification to target therapies in acute coronary syndromes. Circulation 2002;106:1588–91; with permission.)

stratification: the invasive strategy and the IIb/IIIa inhibitor, where the benefit is in the higher-risk patients.

ECG ST-segment elevation: reperfusion therapy

In STEMI, the coronary artery is in most cases 100% occluded with a fresh thrombus at the site of a ruptured plaque. To restore perfusion to the myocardium, immediate reperfusion of the in-farct-related artery is needed.

There are two approaches: use of fibrinolytic therapy or primary PCI. Time is critical with either therapy, where the sooner reperfusion is achieved, the greater the chance of reducing morbidity and increasing survival.

Primary percutaneous coronary intervention

At present, the preferred method of achieving coronary reperfusion is the use of primary PCI.

Many randomized controlled trials have compared pharmacologic and mechanical reperfusion during STEMI. A meta-analysis of 23 of these trials found that primary PCI was superior to thrombolytic therapy in reducing mortality; nonfatal reinfarction; stroke; and the combined endpoint of death, nonfatal reinfarction, and stroke [49]. The benefits of PCI in reducing mortality and recurrent MI were particularly striking.

At present, however, only 20% to 25% of hospitals have primary PCI capabilities. Therefore, hospitals that do not have PCI capabilities can either treat patients who have STEMI with immediate thrombolysis, or emergently transfer them to a site where PCI can be performed. Recent clinical trials have also found that if door-to-balloon times are within 2 to 3 hours, that primary PCI is superior to fibrinolysis with a 40% to 50% reduction of the combined end point [50–52].

Thrombolysis

Thrombolysis has been shown to reduce mortality in several large placebo-controlled trials using streptokinase (SK) and tissue plasminogen activator (t-PA). These benefits persist through at least 10 years of follow up. The Fibrinolytic Therapy Trialists' overview of all the major placebo-controlled studies showed a 2.6% absolute reduction in mortality for patients who have STEMI treated within the first 12 hours after the onset of symptoms [53]. Patients presenting with new left bundle branch block and a strong clinical history for acute MI also derive a substantial benefit from thrombolysis. Patients who have non–ST elevation ACS, however, do not benefit from thrombolysis.

SK was the initial fibrinolytic drug, with newer agents later developed. The fibrin-specific thrombolytic agents, such as alteplase (t-PA), were seen in the TIMI-1 trial to have twice the rate of infarct-related artery patency as SK [54]. In the GUSTO I trial, accelerated tPA plus heparin led to a highly significant 14% reduction in mortality. Reteplase and tenecteplase are molecular modifications of t-PA designed to have longer plasma half-lives that allow double or single bolus administration, respectively. However, the newer agents did not lead to a further reduction in mortality rates compared with t-PA.

Similarly, use of the combination of half-dose fibrinolysis and GP IIb/IIIa receptor inhibitors did not improve mortality, and this more complicated regimen is not widely used. The use of other adjunctive agents with full-dose fibrinolysis is being actively studied, with enoxaparin being compared with UFH in the EXTRACT-TIMI 25 trial, and clopidogrel being added to standard regimens versus placebo in the CLARITY-TIMI 28 trial.

Choice of reperfusion therapy

In summary, although thrombolysis is more widely available, is simple to administer, and produces results that are independent of operator experience, primary PCI in experienced hands is associated with less-recurrent infarction and ischemia; lower short-term mortality; and less stroke and intracranial hemorrhage than thrombolysis. PCI also results in higher early infarct-related artery patency rates and reduced residual stenosis compared with thrombolysis. The current ACC/AHA guidelines recommend invasive strategy with PCI if a timely intervention can be performed; that is, if door-to-balloon time is less than 90 minutes or if the delay to PCI compared with on-site thrombolysis is less than 1 hour. Primary PCI is also generally preferred for patients in cardiogenic shock, who have contra-indications to thrombolysis, and in whom thrombolysis is unlikely to produce meaningful benefit (eg, symptom onset more than 3 hours before presentation).

Summary

For patients who have ACS, risk stratification is key to initiating appropriate treatment. For STEMI, immediate reperfusion therapy is needed, and thus rapid identification of ST elevation on the ECG is critical. Having a standardized protocol for rapid treatment—with either primary PCI or thrombolysis—is critical. For UA/NSTEMI, one first has to identify the patients who have a higher likelihood of actually having an ACS as opposed to noncardiac chest pain. There are many modalities for this assessment, as reviewed in this issue. Among patients who have a moderate or high likelihood of ACS, stratification to high versus lower risk is needed to choose appropriate therapies. Thus, it is important for risk stratification to be a central part of all management of patients who have ACS.

References

[1] American Heart Association. Heart and stroke statistical update. American Heart Association, in press.

[2] The TIMI IIIA Investigators. Early effects of tissue-type plasminogen activator added to conventional therapy on the culprit lesion in patients presenting with ischemic cardiac pain at rest. Results of the Thrombolysis in Myocardial Ischemia (TIMI IIIA) Trial. Circulation 1993;87:38–52.

[3] Cannon CP, Weintraub WS, Demopoulos LA, et al. Comparison of early invasive and conservative strategies in patients with unstable coronary syndromes treated with the glycoprotein IIb/IIIa inhibitor tirofiban. N Engl J Med 2001;344(25):1879–87.

[4] Fox KA, Goodman SG, Klein W, et al. Management of acute coronary syndromes. Variations in practice and outcome; findings from the Global Registry of Acute Coronary Events (GRACE). Eur Heart J 2002;23(15):1177–89.

[5] Pope JH, Ruthazer R, Beshansky JR, et al. Clinical features of emergency department patients presenting with symptoms suggestive of acute cardia ischemia: a multicenter study. J Thromb Thrombolysis 1998;6:63–74.

[6] Kontos MC, Ornato JP, Tatum JL, et al. How many patients are eligible for treatment with GP IIb/IIIa inhibitors? Results from a clinical database. Circulation 1999;100(Suppl 1):1–775.

[7] Pozen MW, D'Agostino RB, Selker HP, et al. A predictive instrument to improve coronary-care-unit admission practices in acute ischemic heart disease. A prospective multicenter clinical trial. N Engl J Med 1984;310:1273–8.

[8] Tierney WM, Roth BJ, Psaty B, et al. Predictors of myocardial infarction in emergency room patients. Crit Care Med 1985;13:526–31.

[9] Goldman L, Cook EF, Brand DA, et al. A computer protocol to predict myocardial infarction in emergency department patients with chest pain. N Engl J Med 1988;318:797–803.

[10] Lee TH, Juarez G, Cook EF, et al. Ruling out acute myocardial infarction. A prospective multicenter validation of a 12-hour strategy for patients at low risk. N Engl J Med 1991;324:1239–46.

[11] Selker HP, Griffith JL, D'Agostino RB. A time-insensitive predictive instrument for acute myocardial infarction mortality: a multicenter study. Med Care 1991;29(12):1196–211.

[12] Sarasin FP, Reymond JM, Griffith JL, et al. Impact of the acute cardiac ischemia time-insensitive predictive instrument (ACI-TIPI) on th speed of triage decision making for emergency department patients presenting with chest pain: a controlled clinical trial. J Gen Intern Med 1994;9:187–94.

[13] Selker HP, Beshansky JR, Griffith JL, et al. Use of the acute cardiac ischemia time-insensitive predictive instrument (ACI-TIPI) to assist with triage of patients with chest pain or other symptoms suggestive of acute cardiac ischemia. A multicenter, controlled clinical trial. Ann Intern Med 1998;129(11):845–55.

[14] Goldman L, Cook EF, Johnson PA, et al. Prediction of the need for intensive care in patients who come to emergency departments with acute chest pain. N Engl J Med 1996;334(23):1498–504.

[15] Fox KA, Cokkinos DV, Deckers J, et al. The ENACT study: a pan-European survey of acute coronary syndromes. European Network for Acute Coronary Treatment. Eur Heart J 2000;21:1440–9.

[16] The Platelet Receptor Inhibition for Ischemic Syndrome Management in Patients Limited by Unstable Signs and Symptoms (PRISM-PLUS) Study Investigators. Inhibition of the platelet glycoprotein IIb/IIIa receptor with tirofiban in unstable angina and non-Q-wave myocardial infarction. N Engl J Med 1998;338:1488–97.

[17] The PURSUIT Trial Investigators. Inhibition of platelet glycoprotein IIb/IIIa with eptifibatide in patients with acute coronary syndromes. N Engl J Med 1998;339:436–43.

[18] Antman EM, McCabe CH, Gurfinkel EP, et al. Enoxaparin prevents death and cardiac ischemic events in unstable Angina/Non-Q-wave myocardial infarction: results of the Thrombolysis In Myocardial Infarction (TIMI) 11B trial. Circulation 1999;100(15):1593–601.

[19] The Global Use of Strategies to Open Occluded Coronary Arteries (GUSTO) IIb Investigators. A comparison of recombinant hirudin with heparin for the treatment of acute coronary syndromes. N Engl J Med 1996;335:775–82.

[20] Hochman JS, McCabe CH, Stone PH, et al. Outcome and profile of women and men presenting with acute coronary syndromes: a report from TIMI IIIB. J Am Coll Cardiol 1997;30:141–8.

[21] Hochman JS, Tamis JE, Thompson TD, et al. Sex, clinical presentation, and outcome in patients with acute coronary syndromes. Global Use of Strategies to Open Occluded Coronary Arteries in Acute Coronary Syndromes IIb Investigators. N Engl J Med 1999;341(4):226–32.

[22] Scirica BM, Cannon CP, Gibson CM, et al. Assessing the effect of publication of clinical guidelines on the management of unstable angina and non-ST-elevation myocardial infarction in the TIMI III (1990–93) and the GUARANTEE (1995–96) registries. Critical Pathways in Cardiology 2002;1:151–60.

[23] Cannon CP. Evidence-based risk stratification to target therapies in acute coronary syndromes. Circulation 2002;106(13):1588–91.

[24] Hamm CW, Heeschen C, Goldmann B, et al. Benefit of abciximab in patients with refractory unstable angina in relation to serum troponin T levels. N Engl J Med 1999;340(21):1623–9.

[25] Heeschen C, Hamm CW, Goldmann B, et al. Troponin concentrations for stratification of patients with acute coronary syndromes in relation to therapeutic efficacy of tirofiban. Lancet 1999;354(9192):1757–62.

[26] Morrow DA, Cannon CP, Rifai N, et al. Ability of minor elevations of troponin I and T to predict benefit from an early invasive strategy in patients with unstable angina and non-ST elevation myocardial infarction: results from a randomized trial. JAMA 2001;286:2405–12.

[27] Antithrombotic Trialists' Collaboration. Collaborative meta-analysis of randomised trials of antiplatelet therapy for prevention of death, myocardial infarction, and stroke in high risk patients. BMJ 2002;324(7329):71–86.

[28] Clopidogrel in Unstable Angina to Prevent Recurrent Events Trial Investigators. Effects of clopidogrel in addition to aspirin in patients with acute coronary syndromes without ST-segment elevation. N Engl J Med 2001;345:494–502.

[29] Budaj A, Yusuf S, Mehta SR, et al. Benefit of clopidogrel in patients with acute coronary syndromes without ST-segment elevation in various risk groups. Circulation 2002;106:1622–6.

[30] Boersma E, Pieper KS, Steyerberg EW, et al. Predictors of outcome in patients with acute coronary syndromes without persistent ST-segment elevation. Results from an international trial of 9461 patients. Circulation 2000;101:2557–67.

[31] Antman EM, Cohen M, Bernink PJ, et al. The TIMI risk score for unstable angina/non-ST elevation MI: A method for prognostication and therapeutic decision making. JAMA 2000;284:835–42.

[32] Morrow DA, Antman EM, Snapinn SM, et al. An integrated clinical approach to predicting the benefit of tirofiban in non-ST elevation acute coronary syndromes: application of the TIMI Risk Score for US/NSTEMI in PRISM-PLUS. Eur Heart J 2002;23(3):223–9.

[33] Braunwald E, Antman EM, Beasley JW, et al. ACC/AHA guidelines for the management of patients

with unstable angina and non-ST segment elevation myocardial infarction: a report of the American College of Cardiology/American Heart Association Task Force on Practice Guidelines (Committee on the Management of Unstable Angina and Non-ST Segment Elevation Myocardial Infarction). J Am Coll Cardiol 2000;36:970–1056.

[34] Theroux P, Ouimet H, McCans J, et al. Aspirin, heparin or both to treat unstable angina. N Engl J Med 1988;319:1105–11.

[35] Peters R, Zhao F, Lewis BS, et al. Aspirin dose and bleeding events in the CURE study. Eur Heart J 2002;4(Suppl):510.

[36] Yusuf S, Mehta SR, Zhao F, et al. Early and late effects of clopidogrel in patients with acute coronary syndromes. Circulation 2003;107(7):966–72.

[37] Steinhubl SR, Berger PB, Mann JT III, et al. Early and sustained dual oral antiplatelet therapy following percutaneous coronary intervention: a randomized controlled trial. JAMA 2002;288(19):2411–20.

[38] CAPRIE Steering Committee. A randomised, blinded, trial of clopidogrel versus aspirin in patients at risk of ischaemic events (CAPRIE). Lancet 1996; 348:1329–39.

[39] Boersma E, Harrington RA, Moliterno DJ, et al. Platelet glycoprotein IIb/IIIa inhibitors in acute coronary syndromes: a meta-analysis of all major randomised clinical trials. Lancet 2002;359:189–98.

[40] The GUSTO IV-ACS Investigators. Effect of glycoprotein IIb/IIIa receptor blocker abciximab on outcome in patients with acute coronary syndromes without early coronary revascularisation: the GUSTO IV-ACS randomised trial. Lancet 2001;357(9272):1915–24.

[41] Braunwald E, Antman EM, Beasley JW, et al. ACC/AHA guideline update for the management of patients with unstable angina and non-ST-segment elevation myocardial infarction-2002: summary article: a report of the American College of Cardiology/American Heart Association Task Force on Practice Guidelines (Committee on the Management of Patients with Unstable Angina). Circulation 2002; 106(14):1893–900.

[42] Oler A, Whooley MA, Oler J, et al. Adding heparin to aspirin reduces the incidence of myocardial infarction and death in patients with unstable angina. A meta-analysis. JAMA 1996;276:811–5.

[43] Antman EM, Cohen M, Radley D, et al. Assessment of the treatment effect of enoxaparin for unstable angina/non-Q-wave myocardial infarction: TIMI 11B-ESSENCE meta-analysis. Circulation 1999; 100:1602–8.

[44] Goodman SG, Fitchett D, Armstrong PW, et al. Randomized evaluation of the safety and efficacy of enoxaparin versus unfractionated heparin in high-risk patients with non-ST-segment elevation acute coronary syndromes receiving the glycoprotein IIb/IIIa inhibitor eptifibatide. Circulation 2003;107:238–44.

[45] Gruppo Italiano per lo Studio della Sopravvivenza nell'infarto Miocardico. GISSI-3: effects of lisinopril and transdermal glyceryl trinitrate singly and together on 6-week mortality and ventricular function after acute myocardial infarction. Lancet 1994;343:1115–22.

[46] ISIS-4 (Fourth International Study of Infarct Survival) Collaborative Group. ISIS-4: a randomized factorial trial assessing early oral captopril, oral mononitrate, and intravenous magnesium sulphate in 58,050 patients with suspected acute myocardial infarction. Lancet 1995;345:669–85.

[47] FRagmin and Fast Revascularisation during InStability in Coronary artery disease Investigators. Invasive compared with non-invasive treatment in unstable coronary-artery disease: FRISC II prospective randomised multicentre study. Lancet 1999; 354(9180):708–15.

[48] Neumann FJ, Kastrati A, Pogatsa-Murray G, et al. Evaluation of prolonged antithrombotic pretreatment ("cooling-off" strategy) before intervention in patients with unstable coronary syndromes: a randomized controlled trial. JAMA 2003;290:1593–9.

[49] Keeley EC, Boura JA, Grines CL. Primary angioplasty versus intravenous thrombolytic therapy for acute myocardial infarction: a quantitative review of 23 randomised trials. Lancet 2003;361(9351):13–20.

[50] Andersen HR, Nielsen TT, Rasmussen K, et al. A comparison of coronary angioplasty with fibrinolytic therapy in acute myocardial infarction. N Engl J Med 2003;349(8):733–42.

[51] Widimsky P, Budesinsky T, Vorac D, et al. Long distance transport for primary angioplasty vs immediate thrombolysis in acute myocardial infarction. Final results of the randomized national multicentre trial–PRAGUE-2. Eur Heart J 2003; 24(1):94–104.

[52] Grines CL, Westerhausen DR Jr, Grines LL, et al. A randomized trial of transfer for primary angioplasty versus on-site thrombolysis in patients with high-risk myocardial infarction: the Air Primary Angioplasty in Myocardial Infarction study. J Am Coll Cardiol 2002;39(11):1713–9.

[53] Fibrinolytic Therapy Trialists' (FTT) Collaborative Group. Indications for fibrinolytic therapy in suspected acute myocardial infarction: collaborative overview of early mortality and major morbidity results from all randomised trials of more than 1000 patients. Lancet 1994;343(8893):311–22.

[54] TIMI Study Group. The Thrombolysis in Myocardial Infarction (TIMI) Trial; Phase I findings. N Engl J Med 1985;312:932–6.

ELSEVIER
SAUNDERS

CARDIOLOGY
CLINICS

Cardiol Clin 23 (2005) 411–421

Chest Pain Unit Concept: Rationale and Diagnostic Strategies

Andra L. Blomkalns, MD*, W. Brian Gibler, MD

Department of Emergency Medicine, University of Cincinnati College of Medicine,
Mail Location 0769, 231 Albert Sabin Way, Cincinnati, OH 45267-0769, USA

Each year in the United States, over 8 million patients present to the emergency department (ED) with complaints of chest discomfort or other symptoms consistent with possible acute coronary syndrome (ACS). While over half of these patients are typically admitted for further diagnostic evaluation, fewer than 20% are diagnosed with ACS. With hospital beds and inpatient resources scarce, these admissions can be avoided by evaluating low- to moderate-risk patients in chest pain units (CPUs) [1–5].

This large, undifferentiated patient population represents a potential high-risk group for emergency physicians requiring a systematic approach and specific ED resources. This evaluation is required to appropriately determine if a patient is safe to be discharged home with outpatient follow-up versus requiring admission to the hospital for monitoring and further testing.

The concept of rapid diagnostic and treatment protocols for specific disease processes is not new. For instance, analogous approaches for trauma patients have been accepted widely for many years, resulting in decreased morbidity and improved survival for these patients. The same tenants of early evaluation, appropriate risk stratification, and intervention are appropriate for the patient presenting with possible ACS to the ED. Just as trauma centers have adopted strict protocols for diagnosis and treatment of the injured patient, CPUs should have basic principles for evaluation and treatment of patients who present with possible ACS. The evaluation of patients who exhibit symptoms consistent with ACS requires a protocol that includes testing for myocardial necrosis, rest ischemia, and exercise-induced ischemia.

Implementation

Implementation of a CPU approach in an emergency setting is nearly as challenging as evaluating the patients themselves. Several synergistic components are required to adequately, efficiently, and cost-effectively evaluate this patient population, including

1) Sufficient and dedicated space to evaluate and observe the patients
2) Nursing staff and other ED personnel that are knowledgeable and dedicated to this approach
3) Emergency physician staff that can be responsible for these patients
4) Collaboration of cardiologist colleagues on the protocols, testing, follow-up, and admission procedures
5) Availability of nuclear cardiology and radiology colleagues for the emergent performance and reading of nuclear imaging studies
6) Laboratory personnel to run serial cardiac biomarker measurements
7) Primary care physicians that understand the scope and limitations of a CPU evaluation for follow-up

Various physical models exist for CPUs. Several of these models are illustrated in Table 1 and Figs. 1 and 2. In Table 1, the Medical College of Virginia protocol integrates the use of radionuclide

* Corresponding author.
E-mail address: Andra.Blomkalns@uc.edu
(A.L. Blomkalns).

Table 1
Medical College of Virginia CPU protocol

Level	AMI risk	ACS risk	Strategy	Disposition
1	Very high	Very high	Fibrinolysis/PCI	CCU
2	High	High	ASA, heparin, NTG, GP IIb/IIIa	CCU
3	Moderate	Moderate	Markers + nuclear imaging	9-h observations
4	Low	Mod or low	Nuclear imaging	Home and OP stress test
5	Very low	Very low	As needed	Home

Abbreviation: AMI, acute myocardial infarction.

testing into a five-level risk stratification program. Figs. 1 and 2 demonstrate protocols for the University of Cincinnati and the Mayo Clinic, respectively. Both protocols integrate myocardial necrosis testing by cardiac biomarkers and functional exercise testing. Each model takes into account the specific patient population, cardiologist collaboration, nuclear imaging availability, and ED resources to design the optimal CPU for that hospital.

Most of these units are located in an area adjacent to, but separate from, the general emergency patient population. Often the CPU protocol patients are evaluated in conjunction with other observation unit (OU) protocols. As these patients are frequently in the ED for 6 hours or more, it is desirable to provide many of the in-hospital comforts generally not available in a traditional ED. These comforts may include hospital beds, meals, television sets, and telephones, which greatly improve patient satisfaction. This space allocation and additional patient resources may be prohibitive for some hospital physicians, nurses, and administrations considering the start-up of a new CPU and, thus, some of these protocols are performed within the regular department using basic ED resources. This alternative can be suboptimal as the increased time required for CPU protocols can hamper ED patient throughput, lowering patient satisfaction.

A successful CPU also requires a nursing staff dedicated to the care of these patients with special needs. These patients require frequent assessment, close monitoring, noninvasive testing, and serial cardiac biomarker testing and ECG acquisition. These tasks are generally in excess of those expected for a typical emergency patient and may require additional training and staffing as appropriate for the individual institution and ED. The overall success of the unit depends on adherence to the systematic evaluation protocol by nursing personnel.

Although most of these patients are placed on CPU protocols that do not require constant

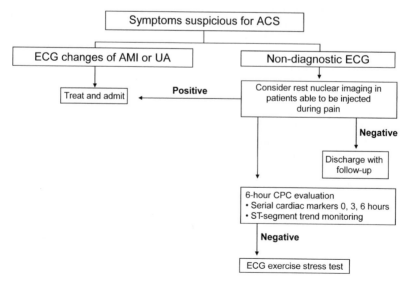

Fig. 1. University of Cincinnati "Heart ER" strategy. *Data from* [5] Gibler et al, Ann Emerg Med 1995;25:1–8 and [17] Storrow et al, Circulation 1998;98:I-425.

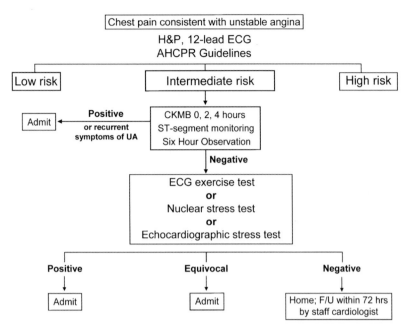

Fig. 2. Mayo Clinic Strategy.

emergency physician interaction, they must be continually re-evaluated and re-assessed while in the CPU. ACS is a dynamic process and can easily progress over the course of the patient's stay in the CPU. Symptom changes, cardiac biomarker positivity, and ECG ST-segment variation should prompt immediate therapy and potential intervention in the cardiac catheterization laboratory. The emergency physician must stay integrally involved with the patient to provide this increased level of therapy. A successful CPU requires the cooperation of many health care professionals in the ED and around the participating institution. An absolutely critical component of successful CPU operation is the collaboration and cooperation of cardiologists and radiologists. Cardiology involvement in CPU protocols is necessary for many reasons. Formulation, knowledge, and acceptance of CPU protocols particular for each institution requires active participation and expertise of the cardiologists. In addition, many CPU protocols successfully use provocative testing with radionuclide echocardiography, or standard graded exercise testing, and these tests generally require the interpretation of a cardiologist [5–10].

While collaboration between emergency medicine and cardiology is intuitive, integration with nuclear cardiologists and radiologists is also pivotally important to the success of every CPU.

Radionuclide perfusion imaging has emerged as an important tool in many centers for assessing patients who present with and without known cardiovascular disease and also in evaluating the patient presenting to the ED with possible ACS. Technetium-99 (Tc-99) sestamibi tomographic imaging is the most common agent currently being used in patients presenting to the ED with suspected ACS [11,12]. Studies have shown that positive rest perfusion imaging accurately identifies patients at high risk for adverse cardiac events [13]. Radionuclide perfusion imaging has thus become a cornerstone of evaluation for many units [14,15].

The diagnostic sensitivity of myocardial perfusion imaging is, in part, dependent on the timing of injection in relation to the cessation of chest pain. The major obstacles for radionuclide studies have traditionally included cost and accessibility. The perfusion agents have a 6- to 12-hour shelf life and, thus, have to be prepared several times a day to be available for acute imaging. Collaboration with nuclear cardiology and radiology colleagues is paramount for this reason. Timely evaluation of these patients requires immediate access to these studies and timely reading and reporting of the results by expert readers.

The laboratory must also be supportive of a CPU. Ideally, bedside point-of-care testing for cardiac biomarkers provides rapid data collection for these patients as creatine-kinase myocardial band (CK-MB) and, in particular, the troponins I (TnI) and T (TnT) allow risk stratification to be performed expeditiously [16]. A collaborative relationship between emergency physicians and laboratorians can ensure a consistent and effective evaluation of patients in the CPU.

Finally, primary care physicians must be supportive of the CPU and willing to have patients evaluated in this protocol-driven process. Communication between emergency physicians and the patient's primary care physician can then assure careful follow-up and patient compliance with lifestyle changes and treatment recommendations after evaluation.

Examples of chest pain units

Over the years, several manifestations of CPUs have evolved. Each of these models has been successfully adopted by specific institutions for its patient populations. An individual institution should carefully evaluate their patient population, physician expertise, physical structure, staffing model, and hospital environment to most adequately determine their optimal CPU protocol.

For instance, the University of Cincinnati Center for Emergency Care "Heart ER," established in October 1991, was one of the first ED-based CPUs. Patients at low to moderate risk for ACS are admitted to the Heart ER for a protocol-driven evaluation of their chest discomfort. The serial cardiac biomarkers CK-MB and troponin T levels are drawn at 0, 3, and 6 hours after presentation to the ED. The original protocol used continuous ST-segment trend monitoring, which has since been discontinued. Graded exercise testing or Tc-99 sestamibi radionuclide scanning is now performed depending on patient's functional status and test availability. Patients having negative evaluations in the Heart ER are released to home with careful follow-up as an outpatient [5].

In the first 2131 consecutive patients evaluated over a 6-year period, 309 (14.5%) required admission and 1822 (85.5%) were released to home from the ED. Of admitted patients, 94 (30%) were found to have a cardiac cause for their chest pain. Follow-up of 1696 patients discharged from the Heart ER to home yielded 9 cardiac events (0.53%, confidence interval [CI], 0.24%–1.01%; 7 percutaneous transluminal coronary angioplasty, 1 coronary artery bypass grafting, 1 death) [17]. These data suggest that the Heart ER program provides a safe and effective means for evaluating low- to moderate-risk patients who present with possible ACS to the ED.

Other institutions also have developed effective chest pain center strategies. The Medical College of Virginia has an elegant protocol that triages chest pain patients into five distinct levels (see Table 1) [14,18]. Level 1 patients have ECG criteria for acute myocardial infarction (AMI) while level 5 patients have clearly noncardiac chest discomfort. The triage level dictates further diagnostic measures and treatment. Intermediate level patients (levels 2 and 3) include individuals with variable probability of unstable angina. These patients are admitted to the CCU for diagnostic testing for ACS while less acute patients (level 4) undergo serial cardiac biomarker determination and Tc-99 sestamibi radionuclide imaging from the ED.

The University of California at Davis protocol uses a novel use of immediate exercise treadmill testing without serial cardiac biomarker determination. In a recent study of 1000 patients, 13% were positive and 64% were negative for ischemia. The remaining 23% of the patients had nondiagnostic tests. No adverse effects exist from exercise testing and no mortality occurred in either of the patient evaluation groups at 30-day follow-up. The authors concluded that immediate exercise testing of low-risk patients is safe and accurate for the determination of which patients can be safely discharged from the ED [6]. A careful history is required to ensure that only low- to moderate-risk patients for ACS are exercised acutely in the ED.

The Mayo Clinic separates patients into low-, intermediate-, and high-risk categories according to Agency for Health Care Policy Research (AHCPR) guidelines. Intermediate-risk patients are evaluated with CK-MB levels at 0, 2, and 4 hours while undergoing continuous ST-segment monitoring and 6-hour observation. If this evaluation is negative, an ECG exercise test, a nuclear stress test, or an echocardiographic stress test is performed. Patients with positive or equivocal evaluations are admitted, whereas patients having negative evaluations are discharged to home with a 72-hour follow-up [19].

Lastly, Brigham and Women's Hospital divides patients into three groups: unstable angina or AMI, possible ischemia, and nonischemic. Patients with unstable angina or AMI are admitted, whereas nonischemic chest pain patients are discharged from the CPU. The intermediate, or "possible ischemia," group either undergoes exercise treadmill testing with a 6-hour period of observation or a 12-hour period of observation. At the end of the observation period, stable patients are discharged to home. Nichol and colleagues [20] evaluated the impact of this pathway approach in a retrospective cohort of 4585 patients and found that a 17% reduction in admissions and an 11% reduction in length of stay would occur if even fewer than 50% of eligible patients for observation and exercise testing had participated.

Each institution has constructed its CPU protocols to suit its patient population, physician expertise, and resource availability to optimize chest pain evaluation. Each hospital and patient population represents a unique environment with specific needs and resources that must be reflected in the ultimate CPU design and implementation.

Once the patient "passes" the CPU protocol and apparently does not have ACS, the individual can be discharged safely to home and appropriate follow-up arranged. Adequate attention must be given to the cause of the patient's discomfort even if it is determined not to be cardiac in nature. Testing for other noncardiac chest pain, including gastrointestinal or psychiatric disease, must then be performed. Patients also require outpatient provocative testing, if not received in the CPU protocol, to further delineate their cardiac risk caused by fixed coronary artery lesions. These tests must be followed and acted on by a primary care physician.

Efficacy

The protocols developed for CPUs must provide testing to evaluate every patient who presents with potential ACS for three possibilities: myocardial necrosis, rest ischemia, and exercise-induced ischemia. Numerous studies in several different hospital environments have validated the use of the CPU. Even early CPUs without the benefits of cardiac troponins and immediate nuclear imaging were successful in safely evaluating patients who are at low probability for AMI [21].

Early myocardial necrosis "rule-out" protocols challenged the traditional notion of a 24-hour period required to detect AMI. Lee and colleagues' [22] multicenter trial validated a 12-hour algorithm using CK and CK-MB in patients identified as "low-risk" through assessment of clinical characteristics in the ED. "Low-risk" was defined as the probability of AMI less than

7%. Patients who have CK-MB levels lower than 5% of the total CK without recurrent chest pain after 12 hours had a 0.5% missed AMI rate while identifying 94% of AMI patients [22]. Farkouh and colleagues [19] demonstrated the use of a CPU protocol and CK-MB measurements for patients identified as intermediate risk for adverse cardiac events. In this study, patients underwent 6 hours of observation followed by provocative testing. This protocol identified all patients who experienced short and long term cardiac events while using fewer resources over a 6-month period [19].

Symptom onset to patient presentation is a crucial factor in the use of cardiac biomarker protocols. Marker release kinetics vary with time and as time to ED presentation may be as short as 90 minutes or as long as several days, no single biomarker determination is suitable for adequately "ruling-out" myocardial necrosis [5,23,24]. In one of the first studies with CPU protocols, Gibler and colleagues [5] used a 9-hour protocol with serial CK-MB levels performed at 0, 3, 6, and 9 hours along with continuous 12-lead ECG monitoring, echocardiography, and graded exercise testing. The authors found that serial cardiac biomarkers alone had a sensitivity and specificity for AMI of 100% and 98%, respectively [5,23,24]. Serial cardiac biomarker determinations are now recommended to increase sensitivity for detecting necrosis rather than a single determination on ED presentation.

Several other studies have examined the value of cardiac biomarkers in the risk stratification of heterogenous patients who present to the ED with chest pain. In a multicenter study of over 5000 patients in 53 EDs, the relative risk for ischemic complications and death for ED patients who have positive CK-MB at 0 or 2 hours was 16.1 and 25.4, respectively [25]. Serial CK-MB results also have proved to be sensitive in AMI detection when collected at 0 and 3 hours after ED presentation. Young and colleagues [26] found a 93% and 95% sensitivity and specificity when combining 0, 3, and net change in CK-MB levels. As expected, the sensitivity improved with increased time from symptom onset [26]. Serial cardiac biomarker measurements and comparison of biomarker elevation over 3 to 6 hours also improved sensitivity for MI [27–29]. Even minor elevations of CK-MB as small as twice the upper limit of normal are associated with an increased 6-month mortality when compared with those with normal levels [30].

Serial CK/CK-MB protocols have become the diagnostic standard for AMI in the CPU setting. Most all of studied protocols use a specific threshold above which is diagnostic for AMI. Fesmire and colleagues [29] studied a promising new approach that included the change in CK-MB levels within the normal range over the course of ED evaluation. In his population of 710 CPU patients, a CK-MB increase or delta of 1.6 ng/mL over 2 hours was more sensitive for AMI than a second CK-MB drawn 2 hours after patient arrival (93.8% versus 75.2%) [29]. Validation of these and other novel protocols will add further to the use of biomarkers in the CPU setting.

The beneficial attributes of myoglobin have made it a commonly used biomarker in CPU protocols. The diagnostic strength of myoglobin lies in its early release kinetics and sensitivity, whereas its primary weakness is a lack of specificity. Davis and colleagues [31] showed that serial myoglobin levels were 93% sensitive and 79% specific in detecting AMI in patients within 2 hours of arrival. Similarly, Tucker and colleagues [32] showed a myoglobin sensitivity of 89% in patients who had nondiagnostic ECGs within 2 hours of ED presentation. Myoglobin seems to achieve maximal diagnostic accuracy within 5 hours after symptom onset [33].

Therefore, it is reasonable and recommended that myoglobin should be combined with other more specific cardiac biomarkers when used in CPU protocols. Brogan and colleagues [34] found that a combination of carbonic anhydrase III and serum myoglobin was more sensitive and equally specific as CK-MB in patients presenting early, within 3 hours of symptom onset. In contrast, Kontos and colleagues [3] reported less encouraging results from a study of 2093 patients combining CK, CK-MB, and myoglobin obtained at 0, 3, 6, and 8 hours. A CK-MB level greater than 8.0 ng/mL at three hours was 93% sensitive and 98% specific for AMI; adding myoglobin decreased the specificity to 86% with no significant increase in sensitivity.

Much like the other cardiac biomarkers, myoglobin levels become increasingly useful when drawn in a serial fashion. In a study of 133 consecutive admitted chest pain patients, myoglobin levels were obtained at 2, 3, 4, and 6 hours after symptom onset. This regimen was found to be 86% sensitive for AMI at 6 hours. The negative predictive value (NPV) in patients who have negative myoglobin levels during 6 hours of evaluation, and without doubling over any 2-hour period, was 97% [32]. As CPUs continue to evolve, aggressive and innovative biomarker strategies have been developed. McCord and colleagues [35] found that AMI can be excluded 90 minutes after patient presentation using point-of-care myoglobin and cardiac troponin I.

Data from protocols using myoglobin measurements in patients who have a lower risk for AMI are sometimes conflicting. In a study of 3075 low-risk CPU patients with AMI prevalence of 1.4%, a 4-hour serial myoglobin protocol was reported as 100% sensitive for AMI [9]. Conversely, in a study of 368 patients whose AMI prevalence was 11%, the sensitivity and specificity of myoglobin at 0 and 2 to 3 hours was only 61% and 68%. Myoglobin change or increase did not improve diagnostic performance either [28].

Myoglobin in the CPU setting is probably best used in a serial fashion along with another biomarker of necrosis such as troponin which is highly specific for cardiac injury. It is most valuable when used in patients presenting early in the time course of symptoms and less so for remote events, as the myoglobin elevation can be normalized within 12 hours after symptom onset through renal clearance.

TnI and TnT have revolutionized the risk stratification of chest pain patients in CPU protocols and now are a cornerstone of serial evaluation. They have proved extremely valuable and sensitive in the diagnosis of myocardial necrosis [36,37]. In addition to diagnosis of myocardial necrosis in ACS, the troponins are valuable in risk stratification of low- and high-risk patient populations. Troponin release kinetics mimic CK-MB, but elevated levels persist for up to 12 days after AMI as a result of the breakdown of the contractile apparatus over this period.

The main two issues surrounding the cardiac troponins are: (1) cutoff values for TnI and TnT and (2) appropriately defining the time of chest pain onset in the context of the ED presentation. Most large studies and analyses have determined that TnI and TnT can identify patients at risk for adverse cardiac events [36–39].

Cardiac TnT is detected at slightly lower serum levels than most TnI assays and has proved valuable in the emergency setting for early identification of myocardial necrosis. The GUSTO-II Investigators compared TnI and TnT in short-term risk stratification of ACS patients. This model compared troponins collected within 3.5 hours of ischemic symptoms. Ohman and colleagues found that TnT showed a greater association with 30-day mortality ($Chi^2 = 18.0$, $P < .0001$) than TnI ($Chi^2 = 12.5$, $P = .0002$) [40]. These authors concluded that TnT is a strong, independent predictor of short-term outcome in ACS patients, and serial levels were useful in determining the risk for adverse cardiac events [41].

As with all new cardiac biomarkers, initial studies on troponin risk stratification were performed initially on patients who have known ACS. Studies using TnI in ACS patients showed a statistically significant increase in mortality among those patients who have levels greater than 0.4 ng/mL [42]. TnT was an extremely effective test for risk stratification of patients who have ACS in a large trial [43]. Stubbs and colleagues [44] showed that patients who have elevated baseline TnT levels had up to 4 times higher mortality than ACS patients with normal values.

While the increased risk for troponin positive patients is well-established, the degree of risk varies greatly between studies and patient populations. Meta-analyses have helped consolidate conclusions and clinically useful parameters when using troponins for the evaluation of patients. One such analysis in high-risk patients performed by Wu [45] demonstrated a cumulative odds ratio of a positive TnT for the development of AMI or death from hospital discharge to 34 months was 4.3 (2.8–6.8 95% CI). The cumulative odds ratio of a positive TnT for predicting need for cardiac revascularization within the same period was 4.4 (3.0–6.5 95% CI). Another analysis involving greater than 18,000 patients in 21 ACS studies found that troponin positive patients had an odds ratio of 3.44 for death or MI at 30 days. Troponin positive patients with no ST-segment elevation and patients with unstable angina carried odds ratios of 4.93 and 9.39 for adverse cardiac outcomes [39].

Benamer and colleagues [46] compared the prognostic value of TnI combined with C-reactive protein (CRP) in patients who present with unstable angina. They found that while 23% of patients with elevated TnI had major in-hospital cardiac events, there was no such prognostic significance associated with CRP [46].

Troponin applications in low- to moderate-risk patients presenting to EDs have shown similar encouraging results. Tucker and colleagues [47] used a comprehensive marker strategy including myoglobin, CK-MB, TnI, and TnT in ED patients over 24 hours after arrival. As expected within the first 2 hours of presentation, CK-MB and myoglobin maintained better sensitivity. The troponins were useful only when measured 6 or more hours after arrival, exhibiting sensitivities and specificities of 82% and 97% for TnI, and 89% and 84% for TnT [47]. Troponin use seems to be more beneficial in later or delayed patient presentations. In a study of 425 patients using serial TnI and CK-MB over 16 hours, Brogan and colleagues [48] showed no increase in sensitivity or specificity between troponin and CK-MB in patients with symptoms less than 24 hours. However, in patients presenting with greater than 24 hours of symptoms, TnI had a sensitivity of 100% compared with CK-MB (56.5%) [48].

Sayre and colleagues showed that patients who exhibited a TnT level of 0.2ng/L or greater were 3.5 times more likely to have a cardiac complication within 60 days of ED presentation [49]. In a CPU population, Newby and colleagues [50] determined that TnT positive patients had angiographically significant lesions (89% versus 49%) and positive stress testing (46% versus 14%) more frequently than TnT negative patients. Long-term mortality was also higher in TnT positive patients (27% versus 7%) [50]. Johnson and colleagues [37] studied a heterogeneous patient population admitted from an urban teaching hospital and found that TnT was elevated in 31% of patients who presented without AMI and who had major short-term complications as compared with CK-MB activity and mass [37].

Other investigators have found that while patients with troponin positivity are at higher risk for adverse cardiac events, the test in isolation lacks sensitivity. Kontos and colleagues [51] found that while TnI positive patients were more likely to have significant complications (43% vs 12%), the sensitivity for these end points was low (14%). Similarly, Polanczyk and colleagues [52] demonstrated that peak TnI greater than 0.4 ng/mL was associated with only a 47% sensitivity and 80% specificity for a major cardiac event within 72 hours of presentation.

The recent publication of the "redefinition" of MI has brought troponin to the forefront of diagnosis and risk stratification in this patient population [53]. In a re-analysis of the data from PARAGON B, GUSTO IIa, and CHECKMATE studies, patients with baseline troponin elevation without CK-MB elevation were found to be at increased risk for early and short term adverse outcomes [43,54–56]. McCord and colleagues [57] found that troponin and myoglobin measurement over a 9-hour period was most predictive of adverse events in their CPU population.

CPUs likely will incorporate a multimarker approach that includes some combination of myoglobin, CK-MB, and troponin, and an inflammatory marker such as CRP [46,58–60]. Additional biomarkers, such as brain natriuretic peptide (BNP), myeloperoxidase, and albumin cobalt binding assays, have been investigated and also show promising results [59–64].

The evaluation of patients for rest ischemia is also extremely important in the CPU setting. Rapid perfusion imaging using radionuclide testing has been a revolutionary step for CPUs. Perfusion imaging with agents, such as sestamibi, has been used in various CPU settings and protocols with great success [11–15]. Tatum and colleagues [14] found that patients with normal imaging findings had a 1-year event rate of 3% no MI or death compared with 42% with 11% experiencing MI and 8% cardiac death. Obtaining multiple 12-lead ECGs can also be an effective method for detecting rest ischemia in patients who present with possible ACS [5,65]. Other imaging modalities, such as computed tomography and MRI, may also improve diagnostic performance in the emergency setting [66,67]. In an ED in Rio de Janeiro, Brazil, a neural diagnostic tree offered an innovative approach to the evaluation of ACS in 566 patients, achieving sensitivities of 99% and 93% for ACS and AMI respectively, with a negative predictive value of 98% for both [68].

Finally, a CPU program must ultimately evaluate patients for exercise-induced ischemia. Fixed coronary artery atherosclerotic lesions may make a patient symptomatic only with exercise. Standard graded exercise testing is extremely useful for these patients [5–7,9]. Many programs use treadmill or chemical stress testing with radionuclide imaging or echocardiography to identify exercise-induced ischemia [3,10–15].

One frequently overlooked advantage of the CPU, is the potential to educate patients about atherosclerosis risk factors during their evaluation. For many patients, coming to the ED represents a key "interventional moment" where education about coronary artery disease and risk modification may be particularly effective [69].

Cost effectiveness

Continued economic constraints and scarce inpatient resources discourage unnecessary inpatient admissions, making CPU protocols more prevalent and important for effectively managing the large number of patients presenting to the ED with chest discomfort. "Rule-out MI" is no longer an acceptable diagnosis to assign for low and moderate risk patients with chest pain on admission. Increased financial pressures exerted by federal and private insurers on physicians and hospitals have indicated the need for more such units. Emergency physicians, in particular, have been challenged to develop more efficient and cost-effective strategies to evaluate these patients [70,71].

Admissions for ultimately diagnosed "noncardiac" chest pain cost our society billions of dollars annually [72]. The CPU has allowed physicians to condense a hospital admission into a 6- to 12-hour evaluation, risk stratification, and observation period. Even CPUs of a decade ago proved to have significant economic advantages over hospital admission [9,73,74]. Roberts and colleagues [75] determined that accelerated diagnostic protocols for low-risk patients with chest pain saved total hospital costs while reducing hospitalization rates and patient length of stay. Each CPU must be formulated and evaluated based on the target patient population, hospital occupancy and resources, and reimbursement patterns. Initial critics of CPUs contend that this evaluation is expensive and cost prohibitive in some studies [76]. These conclusions were largely based on previously immature protocols. CPUs, by their innovative nature, constantly must undergo a continuous evolution toward optimal patient care and cost savings.

In general, protocol and guideline driven medicine is effective for the evaluation of multiple disease processes in the ED, chest discomfort included. Continuous quality improvement should be an integral part of the continued assessment of every CPU. The 2002 ACC/AHA guidelines for non-ST-segment elevation MI and unstable angina should be reflected in every CPU protocol's diagnostic and treatment strategies [77].

Finally, it should be mentioned that CPUs are intended for the evaluation of low- to moderate-risk patients, and not "no-risk" patients. Evaluating all patients presenting with chest discomfort in a CPU would indeed be an inefficient use of ED and hospital resources. Continuous assessment of alternative, more effective, and possibly less expensive protocols will improve care standards for these units over time. Already, the last decade has seen a remarkable evolution of cardiac biomarker regimens and diagnostic and prognostic testing for the evaluation of patients who present with possible ACS. As more and more reports of successful CPUs are published and evidence expands for cost-effectiveness, likely it will be an expectation, rather than an exception, that EDs and hospitals have such units.

References

[1] Pope JH, Aufderheide TP, Ruthazer R, et al. Missed diagnoses of acute cardiac ischemia in the emergency department. N Engl J Med 2000;342:1163–70.

[2] Nourjah P. National hospital ambulatory medical care survey: 1997 emergency department summary. Advance data from vital and health statistics. Hyattsville (MD): National Center for Health Statistics; 2001.

[3] Kontos MC, Anderson FP, Schmidt KA, et al. Early diagnosis of acute myocardial infarction in patients without ST- segment elevation. Am J Cardiol 1999; 83:155–8.

[4] Graff LG, Dallara J, Ross MA, et al. Impact on the care of the emergency department chest pain patient from the chest pain evaluation registry (CHEPER) study. Am J Cardiol 1997;80:563–8.

[5] Gibler WB, Runyon JP, Levy RC, et al. A rapid diagnostic and treatment center for patients with chest pain in the emergency department. Ann Emerg Med 1995;25:1–8.

[6] Amsterdam EA, Kirk JD, Diercks DB, et al. Immediate exercise testing to evaluate low-risk patients presenting to the emergency department with chest pain. J Am Coll Cardiol 2002;40:251–6.

[7] Amsterdam EA, Kirk JD, Diercks DB. Early Exercise testing for risk stratification of low-risk patients in chest pain centers. Crit Path Cardiol 2004;3: 114–20.

[8] Sanchez CD, Newby LK, Hasselblad V, et al. Comparison of 30-day outcome, resource use, and coronary artery disease with and without diabetes mellitus assigned to chest pain units. Am J Cardiol 2003;91:1228–30.

[9] Mikhail MG, Smith FA, Gray M, et al. Cost-effectiveness of mandatory stress testing in chest pain center patients. Ann Emerg Med 1997;29:88–98.

[10] Levitt MA, Promes SB, Bullock S, et al. Combined cardiac marker approach with adjunct two-dimensional echocardiography to diagnose acute myocardial infarction in the emergency department [see comments]. Ann Emerg Med 1996;27:1–7.

[11] Hilton TC, Thompson RC, Williams HJ, et al. Technetium-99m sestamibi myocardial perfusion imaging in the emergency room evaluation of chest pain. J Am Coll Cardiol 1994;23:1016–22.

[12] Gersh BJ. Noninvasive imaging in acute coronary disease. A clinical perspective. Circulation 1991;84: I140–7.

[13] Kontos MC, Anderson FP, Hanbury CM, et al. Use of the combination of myoglobin and CK-MB mass for the rapid diagnosis of acute myocardial infarction. Am J Emerg Med 1997;15:14–9.

[14] Tatum JL, Jesse RL, Kontos MC, et al. Comprehensive strategy for the evaluation and triage of the chest pain patient. Ann Emerg Med 1997;29: 116–25.

[15] Abbott BG, Thwackers FJ. Emergency department chest pain units and the role of radionuclide imaging. J Nucl Cardiol 1998;5:73–9.

[16] Lee-Lewandrowski E, Corboy D, Lewandrowski K, et al. Implementation of a point-of-care satellite laboratory in the emergency department of an academic medical center. Impact on test turnaround time and patient emergency department length of stay. Arch Pathol Lab Med 2003;127:456–60.

[17] Storrow AB, Gibler WB, Walsh RA. An emergency department chest pain rapid diagnosis and treatment unit: results from a six year experience. Circulation 1999;98:I-425.

[18] Jesse RL, Kontos MC. Evaluation of chest pain in the emergency department. Curr Probl Cardiol 1997;22:149–236.

[19] Farkouh ME, Smars PA, Reeder GS, et al. A clinical trial of a chest-pain observation unit for patients with unstable angina. Chest Pain Evaluation in the Emergency Room (CHEER) Investigators. N Engl J Med 1998;339:1882–8.

[20] Nichol G, Walls R, Goldman L, et al. A critical pathway for management of patients with acute chest pain who are at low risk for myocardial ischemia: recommendations and potential impact. Ann Intern Med 1997;127:996–1005.

[21] Gaspoz JM, Lee TH, Cook EF, et al. Outcome of patients who were admitted to a new short-stay unit to "rule-out" myocardial infarction. Am J Cardiol 1991;68:145–9.

[22] Lee TH, Juarez G, Cook EF, et al. Ruling out acute myocardial infarction. A prospective multicenter validation of a 12-hour strategy for patients at low risk. N Engl J Med 1991;324:1239–46.

[23] Lambrew CT, Bowlby LJ, Rogers WJ, et al. Factors influencing the time to thrombolysis in acute myocardial infarction. Time to thrombolysis substudy of the National Registry of Myocardial Infarction-1. Arch Intern Med 1997;157:2577–82.

[24] Newby LK, Rutsch WR, Califf RM, et al. Time from symptom onset to treatment and outcomes after thrombolytic therapy. GUSTO-1 Investigators. J Am Coll Cardiol 1996;27:1646–55.

[25] Hoekstra JW, Hedges JR, Gibler WB, et al. Emergency department CK-MB: a predictor of ischemic complications. National cooperative CK-MB project group. Acad Emerg Med 1994;1:17–27.

[26] Young GP, Gibler WB, Hedges JR, et al. Serial creatine kinase-MB results are a sensitive indicator of acute myocardial infarction in chest pain patients with nondiagnostic electrocardiograms:

the second Emergency Medicine Cardiac Research Group Study. Acad Emerg Med 1997;4:869–77.

[27] Gibler WB, Young GP, Hedges JR, et al. Acute myocardial infarction in chest pain patients with nondiagnostic ECGs: serial CK-MB sampling in the emergency department. The Emergency Medicine Cardiac Research Group. Ann Emerg Med 1992;21:504–12.

[28] Polanczyk CA, Lee TH, Cook EF, et al. Value of additional two-hour myoglobin for the diagnosis of myocardial infarction in the emergency department. Am J Cardiol 1999;83:525–9.

[29] Fesmire FM, Percy RF, Bardoner JB, et al. Serial creatine kinase (CK) MB testing during the emergency department evaluation of chest pain: utility of a 2-hour delta CK-MB of + 1.6ng/ml. Am Heart J 1998;136:237–44.

[30] Alexander JH, Sparapani RA, Mahaffey KW, et al. Association between minor elevations of creatine kinase-MB level and mortality in patients with acute coronary syndromes without ST-segment elevation. PURSUIT Steering Committee. Platelet glycoprotein IIb/IIIa in unstable angina: receptor suppression using integrilin therapy. JAMA 2000;283:347–53.

[31] Davis CP, Barrett K, Torre P, et al. Serial myoglobin levels for patients with possible myocardial infarction. Acad Emerg Med 1996;3:590–7.

[32] Tucker JF, Collins RA, Anderson AJ, et al. Value of serial myoglobin levels in the early diagnosis of patients admitted for acute myocardial infarction. Ann Emerg Med 1994;24:704–8.

[33] Sallach SM, Nowak R, Hudson MP, et al. A Change in serum myoglobin to detect acute myocardial infarction in patients with normal troponin I levels. Am J Cardiol 2004;94:864–7.

[34] Brogan GX Jr, Vuori J, Friedman S, et al. Improved specificity of myoglobin plus carbonic anhydrase assay versus that of creatine kinase-MB for early diagnosis of acute myocardial infarction. Ann Emerg Med 1996;27:22–8.

[35] McCord J, Nowak RM, McCullough PA, et al. Ninety-minute exclusion of acute myocardial infarction by use of quantitative point-of-care testing of myoglobin and troponin I. Circulation 2001;104:1483–8.

[36] Falahati A, Sharkey SW, Christensen D, et al. Implementation of serum cardiac troponin I as marker for detection of acute myocardial infarction. Am Heart J 1999;137:332–7.

[37] Johnson PA, Goldman L, Sacks DB, et al. Cardiac troponin T as a marker for myocardial ischemia in patients seen at the emergency department for acute chest pain. Am Heart J 1999;137:1137–44.

[38] Ottani F, Galvani M, Ferrini D, et al. Direct comparison of early elevations of cardiac troponin T and I in patients with clinical unstable angina. Am Heart J 1999;137:284–91.

[39] Ottani F, Galvani M, Nicolini FA, et al. Elevated cardiac troponin levels predict the risk of adverse outcome in patients with acute coronary syndromes. Am Heart J 2000;140:917–27.

[40] Christenson RH, Duh SH, Newby LK, et al. Cardiac troponin T and cardiac troponin I: relative values in short- term risk stratification of patients with acute coronary syndromes. GUSTO-IIa Investigators. Clin Chem 1998;44:494–501.

[41] Newby LK, Christenson RH, Ohman EM, et al. Value of serial troponin T measures for early and late risk stratification in patients with acute coronary syndromes. The GUSTO-IIa Investigators. Circulation 1998;98:1853–9.

[42] Antman EM, Tanasijevic MJ, Thompson B, et al. Cardiac-specific troponin I levels to predict the risk of mortality in patients with acute coronary syndromes. N Engl J Med 1996;335:1342–9.

[43] Ohman EM, Armstrong PW, Christenson RH, et al. Cardiac troponin T levels for risk stratification in acute myocardial ischemia. GUSTO IIA Investigators. N Engl J Med 1996;335:1333–41.

[44] Stubbs P, Collinson P, Moseley D, et al. Prognostic significance of admission troponin T concentrations in patients with myocardial infarction. Circulation 1996;94:1291–7.

[45] Wu AH, Lane PL. Metaanalysis in clinical chemistry: validation of cardiac troponin T as a marker for ischemic heart diseases. Clin Chem 1995;41:1228–33.

[46] Benamer H, Steg PG, Benessiano J, et al. Comparison of the prognostic value of C-reactive protein and troponin I in patients with unstable angina pectoris. Am J Cardiol 1998;82:845–50.

[47] Tucker JF, Collins RA, Anderson AJ, et al. Early diagnostic efficiency of cardiac troponin I and Troponin T for acute myocardial infarction. Acad Emerg Med 1997;4:13–21.

[48] Brogan GX Jr, Hollander JE, McCuskey CF, et al. Evaluation of a new assay for cardiac troponin I vs creatine kinase-MB for the diagnosis of acute myocardial infarction. Biochemical Markers for Acute Myocardial Ischemia (BAMI) Study Group. Acad Emerg Med 1997;4:6–12.

[49] Sayre MR, Kaufmann KH, Chen IW, et al. Measurement of cardiac troponin T is an effective method for predicting complications among emergency department patients with chest pain. Ann Emerg Med 1998;31:539–49.

[50] Newby LK, Kaplan AL, Granger BB, et al. Comparison of cardiac troponin T versus creatine kinase-MB for risk stratification in a chest pain evaluation unit. Am J Cardiol 2000;85:801–5.

[51] Kontos MC, Anderson FP, Alimard R, et al. Ability of troponin I to predict cardiac events in patients admitted from the emergency department. J Am Coll Cardiol 2000;36:1818–23.

[52] Polanczyk CA, Lee TH, Cook EF, et al. Cardiac troponin I as a predictor of major cardiac events in

emergency department patients with acute chest pain. J Am Coll Cardiol 1998;32:8–14.

[53] Myocardial infarction redefined–a consensus document of The Joint European Society of Cardiology/American College of Cardiology Committee for the redefinition of myocardial infarction. J Am Coll Cardiol 2000;36:959–69.

[54] Rao SV, Ohman EM, Granger CB, et al. Prognostic value of isolated troponin elevation across the spectrum of chest pain syndromes. Am J Cardiol 2003;91:936–40.

[55] Newby LK, Storrow AB, Gibler WB, et al. Bedside multimarker testing for risk stratification in chest pain units: the Chest Pain Evaluation by Creatine Kinase-MB, Myoglobin, and Troponin I (CHECKMATE) Study. Circulation 2001;103:1832–7.

[56] Newby LK, Ohman EM, Christenson RH, et al. Benefit of glycoprotein IIb/IIIa inhibition in patients with acute coronary syndromes and troponin t-positive status: the paragon-B troponin T substudy. Circulation 2001;103:2891–6.

[57] McCord J, Nowak RM, Hudson MP, et al. The prognostic significance of serial myoglobin, troponin I, and creatine kinase-MB measurements in patients evaluated in the emergency department for acute coronary syndrome. Ann Emerg Med 2003;42:343–50.

[58] Pai JK, Pischon T, Ma J, et al. Inflammatory markers and the risk of coronary heart disease in men and women. N Engl J Med 2004;351:2599–610.

[59] Sabatine MS, Morrow DA, de Lemos JA, et al. Multimarker approach to risk stratification in non-ST elevation acute coronary syndromes: simultaneous assessment of troponin I, C-reactive protein, and B-type natriuretic peptide. Circulation 2002;105:1760–3.

[60] Gibler WB, Blomkalns AL, Collins SP. Evaluation of chest pain and heart failure in the emergency department: impact of multimarker strategies and B-type natriuretic peptide. Rev Cardiovasc Med 2003;4(Suppl 4):S47–55.

[61] Brennan ML, Penn MS, Van Lente F, et al. Prognostic value of myeloperoxidase in patients with chest pain. N Engl J Med 2003;349:1595–604.

[62] Apple FS, Murakami MM, Pearee LA, et al. Multibiomarker risk stratification of N-terminal pro-B-type natriuretic peptide, high-sensitivity C-reactive protein, and cardiac troponin T and I in end-stage renal disease for all-cause death. Clin Chem 2004;50:2279–85.

[63] Baldus S, Heeschen C, Meinertz T, et al. Myeloperoxidase serum levels predict risk in patients with acute coronary syndromes. Circulation 2003;108:1440–5.

[64] Bhagavan NV, Lai EM, Rios PA, et al. Evaluation of human serum albumin cobalt binding assay for the assessment of myocardial ischemia and myocardial infarction. Clin Chem 2003;49:581–5.

[65] Decker WW, Prina CD, Smars PA, et al. Continuous 12-lead electrocardiography monitoring in an emergency department chest pain unit: an assessment of potential clinical effect. Ann Emerg Med 2003;41:342–51.

[66] Achenback S, Ropers D, Pohle F-K, et al. The use of CTA in the chest pain center: a perspective. Crit Path Cardiol 2004;3:87–93.

[67] Kwong RY, Arai AE. Detecting patients with acute coronary syndrome in the chest pain center of the emergency department with cardiac magnetic resonance imaging. Crit Path Cardiol 2004;3:25–31.

[68] Bassan R, Pimenta L, Scofano M, et al. on behalf of the Chest Pain Project Investigators. Accuracy of a neural diagnostic tree for the identification of acute coronary syndrome in patients with chest pain and no ST-segment elevation. Crit Path Cardiol 2004;3:72–8.

[69] Bahr RD. The changing paradigm of acute heart attack prevention in the emergency department: a futuristic viewpoint? Ann Emerg Med 1995;25:95–6.

[70] National Heart Attack Alert Program issues report on how to shorten intervention time. Am Fam Physician 1994;50:1569–76.

[71] Emergency department. rapid identification and treatment of patients with acute myocardial infarction. National Heart Attack Alert Program Coordinating Committee, 60 Minutes to Treatment Working Group. Ann Emerg Med 1994;23:311–29.

[72] Weingarten SR, Ermann B, Riedinger MS, et al. Selecting the best triage rule for patients hospitalized with chest pain. Am J Med 1989;87:494–500.

[73] Gomez MA, Anderson JL, Karagounis LA, et al. An emergency department-based protocol for rapidly ruling out myocardial ischemia reduces hospital time and expense: results of a randomized study (ROMIO). J Am Coll Cardiol 1996;28:25–33.

[74] Lee TH. Emergency department observation units: has the time come? J Thromb Thrombolysis 1996;3:257–61.

[75] Roberts RR, Zalenski RJ, Mensah EK, et al. Costs of an emergency department-based accelerated diagnostic protocol vs hospitalization in patients with chest pain: a randomized controlled trial. JAMA 1997;278:1670–6.

[76] Shesser R, Smith M. The chest pain emergency department and the outpatient chest pain evaluation center: revolution or evolution? Ann Emerg Med 1994;23:334–41.

[77] Braunwald E, Antman EM, Beasley JW, et al. ACC/AHA 2002 guideline update for the management of patients with unstable angina and non-st-segment elevation myocardial infarction: a report of the american college of cardiology/american heart association task force on practice guidelines. J Am Coll Cardiol 2002;40(7):1366–74.

ELSEVIER
SAUNDERS

Cardiol Clin 23 (2005) 423–451

CARDIOLOGY
CLINICS

Acute Coronary Syndromes in the Emergency Department: Diagnostic Characteristics, Tests, and Challenges

J. Hector Pope, MD[a,b,c,*], Harry P. Selker, MD, MSPH[b,c]

[a]Baystate Medical Center, 759 Chestnut Street, Springfield, MA 01199, USA
[b]New England Medical Center, 750 Washington Street, #63 Boston, MA 02111, USA
[c]Tufts University School of Medicine, Boston, MA 02111, USA

Failure to diagnose patients who have acute coronary syndromes (ACSs)—either acute myocardial infarction (AMI) or unstable angina pectoris (UAP)—who present to the emergency department (ED) remains a serious public health issue. AMI is the leading cause of death for men and women in the United States, with as many as 1.2 million patients having myocardial infarctions (MIs) annually [1] and about half of whom come to EDs for their initial care. In addition, nearly twice as many patients come to EDs having UAP. However, only 25% of patients who present to the ED with symptoms suggestive of an ACS, either AMI or UAP, will have a confirmed diagnosis of the same on discharge [2]. The missed diagnosis rate for AMI and UAP in this setting is about 2% each [3]. Thus clinicians have the unenviable task on the one hand of identifying, treating, and hospitalizing (in the appropriate unit) those patients who have a true ACS and on the other hand of avoid filling hospital telemetry, step-down units, and coronary care units (CCUs) mostly with patients who have symptoms suggestive of an ACS but who in fact do not have one of these syndromes.

For many years, the diagnosis of ACSs was of more prognostic than therapeutic importance. Over the past 3 decades, physicians' diagnostic and triage decisions for patients who have suspected cardiac ischemia have reflected two tendencies. First, as the number of acute interventions for

treating dysrhythmias and preventing or limiting the size of AMI has grown, clinicians have tended to admit all patients who have even a low suspicion of acute ischemia. As a result, clinicians have generally admitted nearly all (92% to 98%) patients presenting with AMI [4–9] and nearly 90% of those presenting with ACSs (including those who have AMI and those who have UAP) [6,7,10]. The conscious strategy of maintaining a high diagnostic sensitivity (ie, that any error be toward overdiagnosis) has the intended effect: among patients who have AMI who seek attention in EDs, the diagnosis is generally missed in 2% [3]. High diagnostic sensitivity has been achieved at the cost of admitting many patients who do not have ACSs (low diagnostic specificity). Only 18% to 42% (typically about 30%) of the 1.5 million patients admitted annually to CCUs [11] actually experience AMI [7,12–16], and only 50% to 60% have acute cardiac ischemia (ACI) [6,7,10,12].

Investigating the causes, progression, and treatment of ACSs continues to be a national research priority, and this research continues to produce substantial progress in the areas of prevention, diagnosis, and treatment of ACI and in advances in understanding its molecular and cellular aspects. Over the past decade, there has been a virtual revolution in our understanding of the pathophysiology and management of coronary artery disease (CAD) [17]. The conversion of a stable atherosclerotic lesion into a ruptured plaque with thrombosis has provided a unifying hypothesis for the cause of ACSs. The understanding of ACSs has evolved from this thesis. Thus, UAP (eg, rest angina, new-onset angina, increasing

---

* Corresponding author. Tufts University School of Medicine, Boston, MA 02111.
E-mail address: jameshpope@aol.com (J.H. Pope).

angina) and AMI are now well appreciated as parts of a continuum of myocardial ischemia. The overarching diagnosis of ACS has provided a framework for understanding the pathogenesis, clinical features, treatment, and outcome of patients across the spectrum of myocardial ischemia. For emergency triage, the diagnosis of ACS better identifies patients for CCU or telemetry/step-down unit admission than does the diagnosis of AMI alone. This fact is partly because of the difficulty in differentiating unstable angina from infarction, and partly because of intent, as it helps to reverse ischemia and prevent frank infarction. For patients who have ACSs and prolonged chest pain without infarction, the medium- and long-term mortality may be as poor or worse than for those who actually have AMI [3,18]. In clinical medicine, much research has been focused on the early diagnosis and treatment of ACSs. This research has shown that early diagnosis and treatment of UAP is beneficial and may prevent AMI.

For clinical reasons, to promote the optimal use of a limited resource, and to reduce unnecessary expenditure, research has focused on improving physician's diagnostic and triage accuracy. However, there remains a need for improved methods of diagnosis that can reduce unnecessary hospitalization for patients incorrectly presumed to have acute ischemia without increasing the number of patients who have acute ischemia who are sent home inappropriately [19]. To this end, and as mandated by Congress, in 1991 the National Heart, Lung, and Blood Institute of the National Institutes of Health instituted the National Heart Attack Alert Program to focus on issues related to the rapid recognition and response to patients who have symptoms and signs of ACSs in emergency settings, and made reports in 1997 [20] and 2000 [21] on technologies for identifying ACI in such settings.

For as many as 50% of women and a small percentage of men who have a suspected ACSs, other mechanisms of illness are at work, including vasospastic angina, microvascular endothelial dysfunction, transient left ventricular apical ballooning syndrome, and mitral valve prolapse. The accurate identification of these syndromes in the ED or other acute care settings challenges the skill of even the most seasoned clinician. Clinical features, patient demographics, physical examination findings, and a firm understanding the strengths and limitations of the standard ECG can greatly assist with the identification of patients who have ACSs. Biochemical markers, cardiac imaging, myocardial performance indices, and computer-based decision aids remain under-evaluated adjuncts to, but not substitutes for, clinicians' judgment regarding diagnosis and triage of patients who have symptoms suggestive of ACSs. However, despite 2 decades of focused research and without compelling evidence for a noncardiac cause, there remains no single way to discriminate perfectly between those who should be admitted to exclude ACSs and those who could be managed safely without admission. In essence, for the continuum of patient risk for ACSs, the investigators have developed a matched continuum of triage options for each patient, from short-stay chest pain evaluation units to multiday admissions for more intensive evaluations. This article reviews the state of the art regarding the diagnosis of ACSs in the emergency setting and suggests reasons why missed diagnosis continues to occur, albeit infrequently, and outlines strategies to deal with the remaining "continuum of risk" for patients who have suspected ACSs.

Methodologic Issues

Consideration of the specific methods used in studies of patients who have ACSs is vital when critically reviewing studies of the diagnosis/misdiagnosis and triage of patients in the ED who have suspected cardiac ischemia. The key methodologic issues for applicability of study results are:

- Representative patient sample
- Representative prevalence of ischemic heart disease
- Broad patient inclusion criteria, not just chest pain
- Study setting includes a range of settings
- Diagnostic end point includes unstable angina and acute infarction
- Completeness of follow-up
- Follow-up data appropriate and significant
- Validation of findings in generalizable trials

Central to any study is whether the patient sample studied is representative of patients in the ED who are seen in actual practice. Also, the positive predictive value (ie, the proportion of patients that actually has ACSs among all those who have a positive test or attribute) of a symptom, sign, or test result depends on the prevalence of ischemic heart disease in the study population [22]. Thus, the proportion of patients who have false-positive results will be higher (and positive predictive value lower) in a population that has a low prevalence of ischemia (all patients in the ED) compared with a population that has a high prevalence (patients in the CCU). Even studies performed in EDs may not be comparable when ACSs prevalence is significantly different. Inclusion criteria can limit studies of patients in the ED if, for example, only patients who have chest pain are studied [23–25], compared with the use of broad entry criteria, including multiple symptoms that could be anginal equivalents such as any chest discomfort, epigastric pain, arm pain, shortness of breath, dizziness, or palpitations [26]. Study setting (eg, urban versus rural hospital, teaching versus community hospital) can also affect the applicability of any findings to various practice settings.

Aside from the study sample, other methodologic issues warrant attention, including the appropriateness of the measured diagnostic end point. Some past ED studies have focused on identifying or predicting only AMI, but identifying UAP is also important for monitoring and early therapy, especially considering that approximately 9% of patients admitted with new-onset angina or UAP progress to infarction [27,28]. Completeness of follow-up must be considered. Studies with substantial numbers of patients lost to follow-up may have ascertainment bias, especially when the participation rate among eligible patients is not high. Also important is the type of follow-up data collection; for example, the occurrence of AMI will be underestimated if follow-up evaluation does not include biomarker determination results.

Finally, validation of the findings of clinical studies is critical, especially for prediction rules and diagnostic aids; findings may be center- or data-dependent. The ideal validation study is a prospective trial of a finding's or prediction rule's effects on patient care in diverse settings [29].

Clinical presentation

The clinically obtained history must be concise, yet detailed enough to establish the probability of ACSs, and obtained expeditiously so as not to delay implementation of therapy.

Chest discomfort

Of all the symptoms for which patients seek emergency medical care, chest pain or discomfort is one of the most common and complex, accounting for about 5.6 million ED visits annually [1]. It is important to keep in mind that many patients will not admit having chest "pain," but will acknowledge the presence of chest "discomfort" because of their definition of pain. Published reports suggest that up to 5% of visits to the ED involve complaints relating to chest discomfort [30]. The complaint of chest discomfort encompasses many varying conditions, ranging from insignificant to high-risk in terms of threat to the patient's life, including, but not limited to, acute coronary syndromes (AMI and UAP), thromboembolic disease (pulmonary embolism), aortic dissection, pneumothorax, pneumonia, myocarditis, and pericarditis. Chest discomfort may be perceived as pain with descriptions such as crushing, vice-like constriction; a feeling equivalent to an "elephant sitting on the chest"; tightness; pressure; heartburn; or indigestion, or as discomfort most noticeable for its radiation to an adjacent area of the body such as the neck, jaw, interscapular area, upper extremities, or epigastrium. Elderly patients or those who have diabetes may have altered ability to specifically localize discomfort [31]. Individuals of each gender and different cultural groups vary in their expression of pain and ability to communicate with health professionals, so that presentation may range from merely bothersome to cataclysmic for conditions that seem nearly equivalent when objective criteria are matched. The level of discomfort does not necessarily correlate with the severity of illness, making identification of potentially life-threatening conditions difficult in certain patients. Because of the serious nature of many conditions presenting with chest discomfort and the potential for significant reduction in morbidity and mortality with early diagnosis and treatment, clinical policies have been developed to guide clinicians with their initial evaluation of chest discomfort, emphasizing prompt triage, assessment, and initiation of therapy [32]. This article only reviews the policies that apply to ACSs.

It is sometimes difficult to distinguish cardiac from noncardiac chest discomfort, even though chest pain is the hallmark of ACSs. Taking the time to elicit the exact character of the sensation (without prompting the patient, if possible) and any pattern of radiation (if present) is most helpful. Typically, the chest discomfort of acute ischemia has a deep visceral character, preventing the patient from localizing the discomfort to a specific region of the chest. It is often described as a pressure-like or heavy weight on the chest, a tightness, a constriction about the throat, or an aching sensation that is not affected by respiration, position, or movement and that comes on gradually, reaches its maximum intensity over a period of 2 to 3 minutes, lasts longer than 30 minutes rather than seconds, may wax and wane, and may be remitting. It may be described as indigestion and occasionally may be relieved by belching. In a large study of patients in the ED who had suspected ACSs, Pope and colleagues [2] found that the 76% of patients who presented with the complaint of chest pain or discomfort (including arm, jaw, or equivalent discomfort) had a 29% incidence of ACSs at final diagnosis (10% AMI, 19% UAP). In 69% of patients, chest pain or discomfort was the chief complaint, and this group had a 31% incidence of ACSs (10% AMI, 21% UAP). In 21% of patients, it was the only complaint, and this group had a 32% incidence of ACSs (9% AMI, 23% UAP). Furthermore, chest pain or discomfort as the chief complaint or presenting symptom was more frequently associated with a final diagnosis of ACS (88% ACS versus 62% non-ACS and 92% ACS versus 71% non-ACS, respectively; $P = .001$). Sharp, stabbing, or positional pain is less likely to represent ischemia [33] but does not exclude it. Lee and colleagues [34] found that among patients in the ED who had sharp or stabbing pain, 22% had acute ischemia (5% AMI, 17% UAP). Among those who had partially pleuritic pain, 13% had acute ischemia (6% AMI, 7% UAP), and among the group that had fully pleuritic pain, none was shown to have acute ischemia. Of the patients whose pain was fully reproduced by palpation, 7% nonetheless had acute ischemia (5% AMI, 2% UAP), and 24% had pain partially reproduced with palpation had ischemia (6% AMI, 18% UAP). Patients who describe their discomfort as similar to previous episodes of cardiac ischemia are more likely to have ACSs [16,35], but any chest discomfort carries a higher risk than no discomfort [6,26,36].

Combinations of variables improved discrimination in these patients [24]. In patients who had sharp or stabbing pain that was also pleuritic, positional, or reproducible by palpation, 3% had UAP and none had AMI. Furthermore, if these same patients had no history of ischemic heart disease, none had acute ischemia. The "partially" and "fully" groups were subjective and small in number.

Exact location of chest pain is not significantly different in patients who have or do not have AMI [37], but chest pain that radiates to the arms or neck does increase the likelihood [38–40]. In the study by Sawe [37] that looked at admitted patients who had AMI, 71% had pain radiation to arms or necks, whereas 39% of admitted patients who experienced pain radiation did not have AMI. Consistent with the classical description, 33% of patients who proved to have infarction had radiation to both arms, 29% had pain radiating to the left arm only, and 2% to the right arm only [37].

Some investigators believe that a significant number of patients who have cardiac ischemia can present with abdominal pain as their chief complaint [23,24]. However, Pope and colleagues [2] found that 14% of study patients had this complaint. This group had a 15% incidence of ACSs at final diagnosis (6% AMI, 9% UAP), but less than 1% of these patients complained of abdominal pain as their chief or only complaint and had a 4% incidence of ACI (2% AMI, 2% UAP). Abdominal pain as a chief complaint or presenting symptom was associated with a higher incidence of a non-ACS final diagnosis (0.6% non-ACS versus 0.1% ACS; 16% non-ACS versus 9% ACS, respectively; $P = .001–.002$). Esophageal reflux and motility disorders are common masqueraders of ACS. In a study of all patients discharged from a CCU with undetermined causes of chest pain, over half had esophageal dysfunction [41]. When these patients' presenting complaints were compared with those of patients who did not have ACSs, those who had esophageal disorders were more likely to complain of a lump in their throat, acid taste, overfullness after eating, a hacking cough, and chest pain that caused awaking at night, and they were less likely to report effort-related chest pain, a history of nitroglycerin use, or reliable chest pain relief with its use.

Anginal pain equivalents

Dyspnea, present in about one third of patients who have infarction in some series [24,38,42], is the most important angina equivalent. In their multicenter ED trial, Pope and colleagues [2] found that 16% of patients who had suspected ACSs presented with a chief complaint of shortness of breath and had an 11% incidence of ASCs at final diagnosis (6% AMI, 5% UAP); in 8%, this was the only complaint, with a 10% incidence of ACS (5% AMI, 5% UAP). However, a final diagnosis of ACSs was not more frequent in patients who had a presenting symptom of shortness of breath (56% ACS versus 56% non-ACS; $P = .5$); as a chief complaint, shortness of breath was more commonly associated with a final diagnosis of non-ACS (18% non-ACS versus 7% ACS; $P = .001$), possibly reflecting a high prevalence of patients who have lung disease in the study population. Yet, because 4% to 14% of patients who have AMI [23,24,26] and 5% of patients who have UAP present only with sudden difficulty breathing [2], ACSs should be considered as a cause of unexplained shortness of breath.

Diaphoresis and vomiting, when associated with chest pain, increase the likelihood of infarction [15,29,38]. Diaphoresis occurs in 20% to 50% of patients who have AMI [39,43]. One study showed that the presence of nausea without vomiting did not discriminate, but vomiting was significantly more frequent in patients who "ruled in" [38]. Pope and colleagues [2] found nausea in 28% of patients who had suspected ACSs. Patients who had nausea as a presenting symptom had a 26% incidence of ACSs at final diagnosis (10% AMI, 16% UAP); patients who had nausea or vomiting as chief complaint (2%) had a 15% incidence of ACSs (11% AMI, 4% UAP); and less than 1% of patients had nausea or vomiting as their only symptom. The same study found vomiting present in 10% of patients. Patients who had vomiting as a presenting symptom had a 23% incidence of ACSs (13% AMI, 10% UAP) and patients who had vomiting as the chief or only complaint had less than 1% incidence. Furthermore, investigators showed that a chief complaint of nausea or vomiting was more frequently associated with a final diagnosis of non-ACS (0.5% non-ACS versus 0.3% ACS; $P = .15$), yet a presenting complaint of nausea was more commonly associated with a final diagnosis of ACSs (30% ACS versus 27% non-ACS; $P = .004$); a presenting complaint of vomiting did not show this association (10% ACS versus 10% non-ACS; $P = .7$). In a CCU study, 43% of patients who had Q-wave infarction and only 4% of patients who had non–Q-wave infarctions or prolonged angina had vomiting [44].

So-called "soft clinical features," such as fatigue, weakness, malaise, dizziness, and "clouding of the mind," are surprisingly frequent, occurring in 11% to 40% of patients who have AMI [29,37,38,42]. Prodromal symptoms (those occurring in the preceding days or weeks) are also frequent: 40% report unusual fatigue or weakness, 20% to 39% dyspnea, 14% to 20% "emotional changes," 20% a change in appearance (ie, "looked pale"), and 8% to 10% dizziness [24,42]. Pope and colleagues [2] found that 28% of patients who had suspected ACSs presented to the ED with dizziness and had a 16% incidence of ACSs (5% AMI, 11% UAP). Dizziness was the primary complaint in 5% of study patients, with a 4% incidence of ACSs (2% AMI, 2% UAP), and it was the only symptom in 1% of patients (2% AMI, 0% UAP). In the same study, dizziness or fainting as a chief complaint were more commonly associated with a final diagnosis of non-ACS (7% non-ACI versus 1% ACS, $P = .001$). Similarly, dizziness or fainting as a presenting symptom was more frequently associated with final diagnoses of non-ACS (31% non-ACS versus 19% ACS; 8% non-ACS versus 2% ACS; respectively; $P = .001$). ECG evaluation is helpful in low-prevalence patients who have these vague complaints.

Atypical presentations

Few studies address what proportion of patients in the ED who have ACSs present with atypical symptoms—a group for which the diagnostic/triage decision is often most problematic. Among hospitalized patients who have AMI, 13% to 26% had no chest pain or had chief complaints other than chest pain (eg, dyspnea, extreme fatigue, abdominal discomfort, nausea, syncope) [23,24]. In a large ED study of patients presenting with a wide range of clinical symptoms, Pope and colleagues [2] found that 31% of patients who had suspected ACSs presented without chest pain, with a 26% incidence of ACSs at final diagnosis (18% infarction, 8% unstable angina), and had chief complaints other than chest pain (eg, shortness of breath, abdominal pain, nausea, vomiting, dizziness, fainting). Subanalysis of this same data by Coronado and colleagues [31] found pain to be absent in 6.2% of patients who had acute ischemia and 9.8% of patients who had AMI. These investigators found that age and heart failure were independently associated with painless ACSs, in addition to diabetes mellitus among those who had AMI, and that lack of pain predicted increased hospital mortality. Finally, in a large group of patients on Medicare who were hospitalized with confirmed UAP, Canto and colleagues [45] found over half of these patients had atypical presentations. Independent predictors of atypical presentation for patients who had UAP were older age, history of dementia, and absence of prior MI, hypercholesterolemia, or family history of heart disease. Patients who had atypical presentation received aspirin, heparin, and beta-blocker therapy less aggressively, but there was no difference in mortality.

Among patients in the ED, no single atypical symptom is of overwhelming diagnostic importance, although combinations of symptoms can identify high-risk patients who should be admitted regardless of ECG findings. Pope and colleagues [2] ranked atypical presenting symptoms in decreasing order of association with ACI at final diagnosis as follows: nausea (26%), shortness of breath (24%), vomiting (23%), dizziness (16%), abdominal pain (15%), and fainting (65%). Canto and colleagues [45], in their study of patients who had UAP, found the most frequent symptoms to be dyspnea (69%), nausea (38%), diaphoresis (25%), syncope (11%), and pain in the arms (12%), epigastrium (8%), shoulder (7%), or neck (6%).

Data from community-based epidemiologic studies [25,46–48] suggest that 25% to 30% of all Q-wave infarctions go clinically unrecognized. Of these, half were truly silent and half were associated with atypical symptoms in retrospect [25,46]. Because Q waves often resolve (in the Framingham Study)—10% of patients were discharged after anterior infarction and 25% of those discharged after inferior infarction lost their Q waves within 2 years—the true incidence was underestimated [49].

The rate of erroneous discharge from the ED of patients who have AMI may be a marker for atypical cases, but such studies are limited by inclusion criteria, small numbers, and lack of complete follow-up. Rates of 2% [50], 4% [9], and as high as 8% [8] have been reported. In a large ED series [3], patients who had suspected ACSs reported rates of erroneous discharge of 2% (2.1% AMI, 2.3% UAP). The early mortality (30-day) for these missed AMIs may be as high as 10% to 33% [3,8,9].

Finally, in a large ED study of patients who had UAP, Pope and colleagues [3] found that 2.3% were not hospitalized. Over three fourths of the patients were evaluated by an attending physician, and more than one fourth by a consulting cardiologist. Although there was disagreement over the interpretation of 16% of the ECGs on subsequent review by an experienced cardiologist, this was not believed to be clinically significant in any of the cases. Given that most of the patients who were not hospitalized had Canadian Cardiovascular Society class 3 angina with new symptoms or symptoms that changed within 3 days before presentation, inaccuracies in the clinician assessment of the dynamic nature of anginal symptoms may have contributed to the failure to hospitalize patients who had UAP.

Past medical history

In addition to the presenting clinical features, the presence of a CAD risk factor has traditionally been considered diagnostically helpful in the ED setting. In a large ED series [2] an association was shown between patients having a past history of diabetes mellitus (31% ACS versus 18% non-ACS; $P = .001$), MI (45% ACS versus 20% non-ACS; $P = .001$), or angina pectoris (63% ACS versus 29% non-ACS; $P = .001$), and a final diagnosis of ACSs; however, these findings require careful interpretation. From the Framingham Study, it is well known that the risk for developing ischemic heart disease is increased over decades by male gender, advancing age, a smoking habit, hypertension, hypercholesterolemia, glucose intolerance, ECG abnormalities, a type A personality, a sedentary lifestyle, and a family history of early CAD [24,51,52]. Clinicians customarily assess these factors when providing preventive care because they predict the incidence of future coronary disease. However, coronary risk factors were established to provide an estimate of risk over years. Thus, the Framingham Study showed that hypertension increases the risk for ischemic heart disease twofold over 4 years [25], but only a very small portion of this risk applies to the few hours of acute illness that the patient in the ED experiences. A patient's report of coronary risk factors is also subject to biases and inaccuracies. This history is presumably less reliable than the methods used to assign risk in longitudinal studies.

In a multicenter study, Jayes and colleagues [53] found that most of the classic coronary risk factors have little predictive value for ACSs when used in the ED setting. Except for diabetes and a positive family history in men, no coronary risk factor significantly increased the likelihood that a patient had acute ischemia. Diabetes and family history each confer only about a twofold relative risk for acute ischemia in men, whereas chest discomfort, ST-segment abnormalities, and T-wave abnormalities confer relative risks of about 12-, 9-, and 5-fold, respectively. Because these results run counter to the prevailing clinical wisdom, it is possible that physicians who give risk factor history great weight may inappropriately diagnose/triage patients in the ED, which is an issue that deserves further attention and investigation.

Finally, a past history of medication use for coronary disease increases the likelihood that the current chest pain is an ACS. In the Boston City Hospital and the multicenter predictive instrument trials, a history of nitroglycerin use was found to be one of the most powerful predictors of ACSs [6]. Although nitrates are an accepted mainstay in treating acute and chronic coronary disease, the diagnostic and prognostic value of chest pain relief with nitroglycerin has been poorly studied. In the largest study to date, Henrikson and colleagues [54] found that chest pain relief with nitroglycerin did not accurately predict active CAD or subsequent outcomes in a general population presenting to an ED. Nitrates can cause dramatic relief of chest pain from esophageal spasms [55], thus further questioning their diagnostic ability in ischemic heart disease.

Physical examination

The physical examination is generally not helpful in diagnosing ACSs when compared with the value of historical data and ECG findings, except when it points to an alternate process. On the other hand, clinicians must not be lulled into a sense of security by chest pain that is partially or fully reproduced by palpation, because 11% may have infarction or UAP [26]. Pope and colleagues [2] found the pulse rate to be lower in patients who had a final diagnosis of ACSs versus those who had a final diagnosis of non-ACS ($P = .02$), but this difference was not considered clinically significant.

Pulse rate observation in isolation appeared to be generally not helpful in ACSs identification. First, the patient's pulse rate could be slowed by the presence of β-blockers as part of a prior treatment regime, coincident vagal stimulation from ACSs (eg, reflex bradycardia and vasodepressor effects associated with inferoposterior wall AMI), or diagnostic/therapeutic procedures in the ED (eg, phlebotomy, intravenous access). Second, the patient's pulse may be increased by adrenergic excess from just having to come to the ED and everything that accompanies such a visit, in addition to the adrenergic excess (eg, tachycardia and increased peripheral vascular resistance) associated with possible ongoing ACSs.

In a large series of patients in the ED who had suspected ACS, median first and highest systolic blood pressures (SBPs) were higher in patients who had a final diagnosis of ACSs [2]. This finding suggests that the adrenergic excess associated with ACSs might be greater than that associated with non-ACS diagnoses. However, to use this hypothesis as a predictive factor, clinicians must have some idea of their patient's baseline blood pressure, which is not the case in most ED evaluations. Thus, the usefulness of this observation may be limited.

In the same series [2], in addition to the effect of adrenergic release during acute ischemia, the higher initial and highest pulse pressures found in patients who had a final diagnosis of ACSs may also reflect the lower compliance of the ischemic left ventricle. Of relevance to those who are candidates for thrombolytic therapy, excess pulse blood pressure (the extent to which a patient's pulse pressure exceeded 40 mmHg for patients who had an SBP of more than 120 mmHg) places these patients at increased risk for thrombolysis-related intracranial hemorrhage [29].

Pope and colleagues [3] found that median first, median highest, and median lowest SBPs of patients who had AMI and were subsequently classified as Killip class 4 (cardiogenic shock) were above the threshold of this classification (SBP ≤90 mmHg) for these three blood pressure observations. This finding suggests that the adrenergic excess associated with ACSs may be greater than that associated with non-ACS diagnoses. Although the number of such patients in this analysis was small, it did suggest that patients who have ACSs can present with apparently normal blood pressures and can go on to develop cardiogenic shock.

Abnormal vital signs and certain combinations of these have been shown to be critical observations in clinical outcome prediction. The reported probability of infarction decreases with a normal respiratory rate [38] and increases with diaphoresis [15], but other signs mainly help identify high-risk patients who have infarction [56]. In the predictive instrument for AMI mortality proposed by Selker and colleagues [36], blood pressure, pulse, and their interaction figured prominently in three of the six clinical variables used to develop the prediction instrument.

Finally, rales (of any degree), but not S3 gallops, have been more frequently seen in patients who have a final diagnosis of ACSs [2]. This finding is not surprising, as several clinical syndromes of pump failure can complicate ACSs. The investigators' failure to find association between an S3 gallop rhythm and ACSs at final diagnosis is surprising, but it may have to do with a failure to document this finding consistently in the medical record on the part of the physicians in the EDs at study sites.

ECG

Standard 12-lead ECG

A complete summary of evidence related to the diagnostic usefulness of the standard ECG was recently published [20,57], and this background will not be repeated in this article. However, the National Heart Attack Alert Program (NHAAP) Working Group on "Evaluation of Technologies for Identifying Acute Cardiac Syndrome" [57] found that most studies evaluate the accuracy of the technologies and only a few evaluate the clinical impact of routine use. Furthermore, the group concluded that although the standard ECG is a safe, readily available, and inexpensive technology with a high sensitivity for AMI, it is not highly sensitive or specific for ACSs. However, the ECG findings remain an integral, if not the most important, part of the evaluation of patients who have chest pain, and the Working Group recommended that they remain the standard of care for evaluating patients who have chest pain in the ED.

The ECG provides essential information when the diagnosis is not obvious by symptoms alone [58], despite one study noting that the results of the ECG infrequently changed triage decision based on initial clinical impressions [59]. The generally dominant weights given to ECG variables in mathematic models for predicting ACSs substantiate this impression [6,7,10,15,16]. Moreover, the initial ECG is increasingly important in intrahospital triage because of its value in predicting complications of AMI [60–62].

The fundamental limitations in the standard ECG include:

- Single brief sample
- Lack of perfect detection
- Confounding baseline patterns
- Interpretation
- Clinical context
- Imperfect sensitivity and specificity

First, it is a single brief sample of the whole picture of the changing supply-and-demand characteristics of unstable ischemic syndromes. If a patient who has UAP is temporarily pain-free when the ECG is obtained, the resulting tracing may poorly represent the patient's ischemic myocardium.

Second, 12-lead ECG is limited by its lack of perfect detection [63]. Small areas of ischemia or infarction may not be detected; conventional leads do not examine satisfactorily the right ventricle [64] or posterior basal or lateral walls (eg, AMIs in the distribution of the circumflex artery) [65,66].

Third, some ECG baseline patterns make interpretation difficult or impossible, including prior Q waves, early repolarization variant, left ventricular hypertrophy, bundle branch block, and dysrhythmias [67]. Lee and colleagues [9] demonstrated that when the current ECG shows ischemic findings, availability of a prior comparison ECG improved triage.

Fourth, ECG waveforms are frequently difficult to interpret, causing disagreement among readers—so-called "missed ischemia." In a study of patients who had AMI and were sent home, ECGs tended to show ischemia or infarction not known to be old, with 23% of the missed diagnoses owing to misread ECGs [8]. Jayes and colleagues [53] compared ED physician readings of ECGs with formal interpretations by expert electrocardiographers, and calculated sensitivities of 0.59 and 0.64 and specificities of 0.86 and 0.83 for ST-segment and T-wave abnormalities, respectively. McCarthy and colleagues [18] and a review of litigation in missed AMI cases [68] emphasized this factor of incorrect ECG interpretation. In the largest study to date of ACSs in the ED, Pope and colleagues [3] found that although the rate of missed diagnoses of ACSs (2.1% AMI, 2.3% UAP) was low, there was a small but important incidence of failure by the ED clinician to detect ST-segment elevations of 1 to 2 mm in the ECGs of patients who had MI (11%). Correct ECG interpretation by ED physicians is doubly important today because of the need to use interventions such as thrombolytic agents and percutaneous coronary intervention appropriately in ACSs.

Fifth, the implications of the ECG findings must be interpreted in their clinical context, a process performed intuitively by clinicians and formally stated in Bayesian analysis. When symptoms alone strongly suggest ischemia, a normal or minimally abnormal ECG will not substantially decrease the probability of ischemia. Conversely, when the presentation is inconsistent with acute ischemia, an abnormal ECG (unless diagnostic abnormalities are present) will only modestly increase the likelihood of ischemia. Bayes' rule tells us that the ECG will have the greatest impact when symptoms are equivocal [69].

Finally, the ECG suffers from imperfect sensitivity and specificity for ACS. When interpreted according to liberal criteria for MI (ie, ECGs that show any of the following as positive for AMI: nonspecific ST-segment or T-wave changes abnormal but not diagnostic of ischemia; ischemia, strain, or infarction, but changes known to be old; ischemia or strain not known to be old; and probable AMI), the ECG operates with high (but not perfect) sensitivity (99%) for AMI, at the cost of low specificity (23%; positive predictive value 21%; negative predictive value 99%). Conversely, when interpreted according to stringent criteria for AMI (only ECGs that show probable AMI), sensitivity (61%) drops and specificity equals 95% (positive predictive value 73%; negative predictive value 92%) [20].

Despite its usefulness, the ECG is insufficiently sensitive to make the diagnosis of ACSs consistently. The ECG should not be relied on to make the diagnosis but rather should be included with history and physical examination characteristics to identify patients who appear to have a high risk for ACSs (ie, a supplement to, rather than a substitute for, physician judgment). In rule-out AMI patients, a negative ECG carries an improved short-term prognosis [60,70–73]. Providing the interpreter with old tracings would intuitively seem to be of value because baseline abnormalities make current evaluation difficult. However, Rubenstein and Greenfield [74], in a study of 236 patients presenting to EDs with the complaint of chest pain, found that only a small proportion might have benefited from having a previous baseline ECG available (5% might have avoided unnecessary admission). Furthermore, there was no patient for whom a baseline ECG would have aided in avoiding an inappropriate discharge. ECG sampling should be periodic, not just static. The pitfalls of not ordering ECGs in younger, atypical patients, and of misinterpretation should be anticipated. Finally, clinicians should not be reluctant to obtain a second opinion—by fax transmission if necessary—for difficult tracings.

ST-segment and T-wave abnormalities

ST-segment and T-wave abnormalities are the sine quo non of ECG diagnosis of ACSs. Numerous studies [63,73,75] have found that 65% to 85% of CCU patients who have ST-segment elevation alone will have had an infarction. Other investigators found that if Q waves and ST-segment elevation were present, 82% to 94% actually sustained AMI [63]. However, it must be remembered that ST-segment elevation can occur in the absence of ischemia (ie, "early repolarization" variant, pericarditis, left ventricular hypertrophy, and previous infarction even in the absence of a ventricular aneurysm) [76]. Conversely, Pope and colleagues [2] showed that a large percentage of patients who have ACS (20% AMI, 37% UAP) can present with initial normal ECGs.

In their study of patients in the ED who had suspected ACS, Pope and colleagues [2] found that ST-segment elevation of either 1 to 2 mm or more than 2 mm was more frequently associated with a final diagnosis of ACSs (9% ACS versus 7% non-ACS; 5% ACS versus 1% non-ACS, respectively; $P = .001$). A full 30% of patients who have ST-segment elevation of 1 mm or greater had a final diagnosis of AMI. In addition, in a study of missed diagnosis of ACSs in the ED, Pope and colleagues [2] found a small but important incidence of failure by the ED clinician to detect ST-segment elevations of 1 to 2 mm in the ECGs of patients who had AMI (11%). This incidence represents an important and potentially preventable contribution to the failure to admit such patients.

ST-segment depression usually indicates subendocardial ischemia. If these abnormalities are new, persistent, and marked, the likelihood of AMI increases. About 50% to 67% of admitted patients who have new or presumed new isolated ST-segment depression have infarctions [64,75]; even more patients have probable ischemia. Pope and colleagues [2] found that all degrees of ST-segment depression (0.5, 1, 1–2, and ≥2 mm) were more commonly associated with a final diagnosis of ACSs (12% ACS versus 7% non-ACS; 8% ACS versus 3% non-ACS; 2% ACS versus 0% non-ACS, respectively; $P = .001$). A full 19% of patients who had ST-segment depression of at least 0.5 mm or greater had a final diagnosis of AMI. Quantitative ST-segment depression and cardiac Troponin T status have been found to be complementary in assessing risk among ACS patients [77]. ST-segment depression may also occur in nonischemic settings, including patients who are hyperventilating, those taking digitalis, those who have hypokalemia, and those who have left ventricular strain (without voltage criteria) [76].

Inverted T waves may reflect acute ischemia. One study showed that isolated T-wave inversion occurred in 10% of CCU admissions, of whom 22% had AMI [78]. T-wave changes may reflect prior myocardial damage or left ventricular strain [76]. The study by Pope and colleagues [2] found that certain T-wave patterns (inverted 1–5 mm, inverted ≥ 5 mm, or elevated) were more frequently associated with a final diagnosis of ACS (32% ACS versus 17% non-ACS; 1% ACS versus 0% non-ACS; 4% ACS versus 1% non-ACS, respectively; $P = .001$). Flattened T waves did not have the same association with an ACS final diagnosis (18% ACS versus 20% non-ACS; $P = .001$). Furthermore, 39% of patients who had inverted T waves of at least 1 mm or greater had a final diagnosis of AMI.

Q waves

Q waves are diagnostic of MI, but what is the age of the Q wave? In the Multicenter Investigation of the Limitation of Infarct Size (MILIS) study of admitted patients in the CCU, isolated new or presumed-new inferior or anterior Q waves were associated with acute infarction in 51% and 77% of patients, respectively [63]. Other findings of the MILIS study that should be kept in mind are: 12% of healthy young men have inferior Q waves [76,78,79]; pathologic Q waves can be from a previously unrecognized infarction and can mask new same-territory ischemia; Q waves alone do not identify ACSs and are rarely the sole manifestation of AMI (6% in the MILIS study); and, finally, infarction can occur in the absence of Q waves [80,81]. The investigators' ED study [2] showed that Q waves were more commonly associated with a final diagnosis of ACS (25% ACS versus 11% non-ACS; $P = .001$) and that 29% of patients who had Q waves present on their ECGs had a final diagnosis of AMI.

"Nondiagnostic" ECG patterns

"Nondiagnostic" ST-segment and T-wave abnormalities may be defined as follows: not having 1 mm or greater (0.1 mV) ST-segment elevation or depression in two contiguous leads, not having new T-wave inversion in two contiguous leads, absence of significant Q-waves (>1 mm deep and 0.3 s duration) in two contiguous leads, not having second- or third-degree heart block, and not having a new conduction abnormality (eg, bundle branch block). These patterns are the most difficult to interpret and can result in

overdiagnosis (no comparison ECG available) and underdiagnosis (baseline abnormality obscuration of ischemia) [82]. Lee and colleagues [34] found that emergency patients who had chest pain and nondiagnostic ECG abnormalities had a low risk for AMI but a significant risk for ACSs. Pope and colleagues [3] found that 53% of patients in the ED who had a missed diagnosis of AMI had normal or nondiagnostic ECGs, as did 62% of patients who had a missed diagnosis of UAP.

Normal ECG

Among patients in the ED who had normal ECGs (ie, lacking Q waves; primary ST-segment and T-wave abnormalities; and criteria for nondiagnostic abnormalities), 1% [34] to 6% [82] had AMI. Among admitted patients who had normal ECGs, 6% to 21% had AMI [12,78,81–83]. Of patients discharged home with a normal ECG, only 1% had acute infarction [82]. Patients who have a normal ECG and a suggestive clinical presentation still have a significant risk for ACI, especially if the ECG was obtained when the patient was pain free. On the other hand, a truly normal ECG in a patient unlikely to have acute ischemia provides strong evidence against ACS [34].

In their series, Pope and colleagues [2] found that patients who had normal ST-segment and T waves and no Q waves more commonly had a final diagnosis of non-ACS, yet 20% of these patients had AMI and 37% had UAP at final diagnosis.

Prehospital 12-lead ECG

The NHAAP Working Group on Evaluation of Technologies for Identifying ACSs [57] found that the diagnostic accuracy of prehospital ECG for AMI and ACSs, as expected, is similar to that of the standard 12-lead ECG, which is the standard of care in the management of patients suspected of having ACS (Tables 1 and 2). The accumulation of evidence is substantial in the total sample size and quality, and the data have been gathered from patient populations with few exclusion criteria. The evidence shows that obtaining a prehospital ECG does not prolong time in the field or delay transport to the ED. In addition, prehospital ECG-guided thrombolytic therapy can be administered 45 minutes to 1 hour earlier than hospital-based thrombolytics. Prehospital thrombolysis has a modest but significant impact

Table 1
Summary of test performance studies of diagnostic technologies for acute cardiac ischemia in emergency departments

Technology	Condition studied	Number of studies (subjects)	Population category of studies[a]	Studies' prevalence range (%)	Sensitivity[b] (95% CI) (%)	Specificity[b] (95% CI) (%)	Diagnostic odds ratio[b] (95% CI)	Overall quality of evidence
Prehospital 12-lead ECG	ACI	5 (4311)	I/II	46–92	76 (54–89)	88 (67–96)	23 (6.3–85)	B
	AMI	10 (4481)	I/II	14–51	68 (59–76)	97 (89–92)	104 (48–224)	B
Continuous/serial ECG	ACI	2 (1271)	III/IV	4–40	21–25[c]	92–99[c]	3.8–45[c]	C
	AMI	1 (261)	III/IV	11	39[c]	88[c]	4.9[c]	B
Nonstandard lead ECG	ACI	1 (52)	IV	48	96[c]	41[c]	17[c]	B
	AMI	4 (897)	IV	22–65	59–83[c]	76–93[c]	10–19[c]	B
Exercise stress ECG	ACI	2 (312)	III	6–10	70–100[c]	82–93[c]	11–320[d]	B
CK (presentation)	AMI	10 (2885)	I/II/III	7–41	36 (29–44)	88 (80–93)	4.0 (2.6–6.2)	C
CK (serial)	AMI	2 (786)	I	26–43	69–99[c]	68–84[c]	12–222[c]	C
CK-MB (presentation)	ACI	1 (1042)	III	20	23[c]	96[c]	7.2[c]	C
	AMI	10 (2504)	I/II/III	6–42	44 (35–53)	96 (94–97)	23 (17–32)	B
CK-MB (serial)	ACI	1 (1042)	III	20	31[c]	95[c]	8.5[c]	C
	AMI	7 (3381)	I/II/III	1–53	87 (67–95)	96 (94–97)	171 (58–505)	B
Myoglobin (presentation)	AMI	10 (1395)	I/II/III	12–413	49 (41–57)	93 (88–96)	13 (7.9–21)	B
Myoglobin (serial)	AMI	5 (831)	I/II/III	23–37	90 (78–96)	90 (78–96)	140 (66–300)	C
Troponin I (presentation)	AMI	2 (874)	II/III	6–39	23–66[c]	89–95[c]	5.7–14[c]	A
Troponin I (serial)	AMI	1 (773)	III	6	100[c]	83[c]	—[d]	A
Troponin T (presentation)	AMI	5 (1171)	II/III	6–39	44 (32–56)	92 (88–95)	10 (5.9–18)	B
Troponin T (serial)	AMI	2 (1440)	II/III	5–6	80–93[c]	65–90[c]	35–120[c]	A/C
P-selectin	ACI	1 (263)	II	33	35[c]	79[c]	2.0[c]	B
	AMI	same study		8.4	45[c]	76[c]	2.6[c]	
Rest echocardiography	ACI[e]	2 (228)	III	3–30	70 (43–88)	87 (72–94)	20 (9–48)	C
	AMI	3 (397)	I/II	3–30	93 (81–91)	66 (43–83)	20 (7–62)	B
Stress echocardiography	AMI	1 (139)	III	4	90[c]	89[c]	68[c]	C
Sestamibi (rest)	ACI	3 (702)	III	9–17	81 (74–87)	73 (56–85)	18 (11–29)	B
	AMI	same studies		2–12	92 (78–98)	67 (52–79)	26 (6–113)	
ACI-TIPI	ACI	4 (5496)	I	17–34	86–95[c,e]	78–92[c,e]	61–69[c,e]	A
Goldman chest pain protocol	AMI	3 (5359)	I	(ACI 27–30) 12–21	88–91[c]	70–74[c]	20–23[c]	A
Algorithm/protocols		No data from prospective studies						
Computer-based decision aids	AMI	6 (3606)	I/II/III	7–42	52–98[c]	58–96[c]	4.4–9.04	A

Abbreviations: ACI-TIPI, acute cardiac ischemia time-insensitive predictive instrument; CK, creatine kinase; CK-MB, creatine kinase subunit.

[a] Population categories: I: all patients who have symptoms suggestive of ACI; II: chest pain; III: chest pain with nondiagnostic ECG; IV: selected subpopulation.

[b] Results from meta-analysis of several studies using random effects calculations unless otherwise indicated.

[c] Point estimate from single study or a range of reported values; meta-analysis not performed.

[d] Upper range cannot be estimated because of a study with 100% sensitivity.

[e] ACI-TIPI is not intended to provide sensitivity and specificity. The results reported incorporate physicians' triage decisions and are not reflective of diagnostic test performance only.

Table 2

Summary of clinical impact studies of diagnostic technologies for acute cardiac ischemia in emergency departments

Technologies	Condition studied	Number of studies (subjects)	Population category[a]	Prevalence (%)	Clinical outcomes studied	Clinical impact	Quality of evidence
Prehospital 12-lead ECG	ACI	~10 studies[b]	I/II	46–100	Time to thrombolysis, ejection fraction, mortality	++	A
	AMI	~8000 pts[b]		15–51			
Continuous/ serial ECG		No study	—		—	Not known	—
Nonstandard lead ECG		No study	—		—	Not known	—
Exercise stress ECG	ACI	3 (272)	III	0–6	Feasibility and safety	Not known	C
CK (single/serial)		No study	—		—	Not known	—
CK-MB (single)		No study	—		—	Not known	—
CK-MB (serial)	ACI	1 (1042)	III	20	Additional admissions or discharges of ACI and non-ACI patients	++	C
Myoglobin (single/serial)		No study	—		—	Not known	—
Troponin I or T		No study	—		—	Not known	—
Other biomarkers		No study	—		—	Not known	—
Rest echocardiography		No study	—		—	Not known	—
Stress echocardiography		No study	—		—	Not known	—
Sestamibi		No study	—		—	Not known	—
ACI-TIPI	ACI	5 (14450)	I	17–59	CCU admission rate, inappropriate discharge	(+++)	A
Goldman chest pain protocol	AMI	1 (1921)	III	6.6	Hospitalization rate, length of stay, estimated costs	(+)	A
Algorithm/ protocols	ACI	2 (602)	III	6–9	Length of stay, hospital charges, 30-day and 150-day mortality	Not known	B
Computer-based decision aids	ACI	1 (977)	III	48 (AMI 30)	30-day mortality	Not known	A

Clinical impact scores range from low (+) to high (+++).

Quality of evidence scores range from low (C) to high (A).

Abbreviations: ACI-TIPI, acute cardiac ischemia time-insensitive predictive instrument; CK, creatine kinase; CK-MB, creatine kinase subunit.

[a] Population categories: I: all patients who have symptoms suggestive of ACI; II: chest pain; III: chest pain with non-diagnostic ECG; IV: selected subpopulation.

[b] Different outcomes analyzed involved different number of studies and patients.

on early mortality, with approximately 60 patients requiring prehospital treatment compared with hospital thrombolysis to save one additional life in the short-term. Short-term, beneficial effects of thrombolysis on left ventricular ejection fraction have not been reported in randomized trials. The long-term survival benefits of prehospital thrombolysis remain uncertain. Although it has promise, the Working Group [57] believed that its best use would be in areas with long EMS transport times and perhaps in conjunction with prehospital thrombolytic therapy. Its routine use was not recommended.

Continuous ECG/Serial ECG

The Working Group [57] found that two studies evaluated the test performance of continuous/serial 12-lead ECG in the ED, but there was no clinical impact study (see Tables 1 and 2). One study by Gibler and colleagues [84] included a large retrospective population of 1010 participating in a 9-hour protocol. The serial ECG consisted of a 20-second interval between readings. The second study [85] included patients from a veterans' hospital in which two ECGs were taken 4 hours apart. The prevalences of ACSs in these studies were very different (4% and 40%, respectively) given the low-risk populations. The sensitivity for ACSs was low (21% and 25%, respectively) and the specificity was high (92% and 99%, respectively). With the limitations and the varied source of data, a conclusion about the usefulness of this technology cannot be drawn.

Non–standard-lead ECG

The data on the diagnostic performance of non–standard-lead ECG from the four studies reported vary too much to draw any conclusion [57]. The studies used 15, 18, 22, and 24 leads and were conducted with selected patients for admission (see Tables 1 and 2). The prevalence is reflective of this selective population: it ranged between 22% and 65% for AMI. There are no clinical impact studies on non-standard ECGs.

Exercise stress ECG

The data on the diagnostic performance of exercise stress testing to detect ACSs in the ED are limited to only two studies (see Tables 1 and 2) [86,87]. The overall data include a small sample size of a low-risk population. Although the

diagnostic performance is encouraging, it would be premature to make conclusions regarding this technology until additional high-quality studies are conducted.

There are also limited data on the clinical impact of exercise testing for ACSs. Two studies [88,89] had no cardiac events and included very small sample sizes: 28 and 35, respectively. Adding a third study [86], these investigations comprised only 272 subjects and are of low methodologic quality; the clinical impact of this technology is unclear.

Biochemical markers

Creatine kinase, single and serial measurements

There is a large amount of evidence on creatine kinase (CK) as a single test administered at presentation to patients in the ED (see Tables 1 and 2) [57]. The evidence suggests that the sensitivity of a single CK reading for AMI is low (36%), and specificity is modest (88%). Limited evidence suggests that the sensitivity of the test depends on the duration of the patient's symptoms; sensitivity increases with longer symptom duration. Test performance across studies did not appear to vary by type of hospital, inclusion criteria, AMI prevalence, or test threshold.

Only two studies have evaluated serial CK testing [90,91]. These studies used broad inclusion criteria but enrolled populations in which the prevalence of AMI was moderate to high. Test sensitivity was high (95%–99%) in serial tests performed over about 15 hours after presentation to the ED (or from the onset of symptoms), but was only modest (69%) in the one study that drew serial samples for 4 hours. Test specificity was modest in both studies (68% and 84%).

As a single test, CK is insensitive and only modestly specific for AMI. Serial testing appears to have higher sensitivity, although the specificity remains modest. However, the evidence is insufficient to evaluate serial CK measurements over a short time. Because high serum CK levels represent infarcted myocardium, CK has not been evaluated for diagnosing ACSs in the ED. There are no clinical impact studies for CK.

Creatine kinase subunit, single and serial measurements

As is the case with CK, the total sample size and number of studies on a single CK subunit (CK-MB) measurement at presentation to the ED are large (see Tables 1 and 2) [57]. The evidence suggests that the sensitivity of single CK-MB for AMI is low (47%), although specificity is high (96%). Studies reported a broad range of sensitivity for diagnosing AMI. Again, as is the case for CK, limited evidence suggests that the sensitivity of CK-MB depends on the duration of the patient's symptoms; sensitivity increases with longer symptom duration. In general, studies reported a narrow range (92%–99%) of test specificity. Test performance across studies did not appear to vary by type of hospital, inclusion criteria, AMI prevalence, or test threshold.

The total sample size and number of studies of serial tests for CK-MB in the ED setting are large. Overall, serial testing has a modest sensitivity (87%) and high specificity (96%) for AMI. However, test sensitivity is strongly related to the timing of serial testing. All studies that performed serial testing for at least 4 hours after presentation to the ED (or until at least 8 hours after symptom onset) found test sensitivity to be greater than 90%. Conversely, all studies that performed serial testing to at most 3 hours found test sensitivity to be less than 90%. The pooled sensitivity for serial testing to at least 4 hours is 96%; pooled sensitivity for serial testing until 3 hours is only 81%. In general, test specificity was in a narrow range across studies and was above 90%. A recent report found that a 2-hour delta CK-MB level (sensitivity 93%; specificity 94%) outperformed a myoglobin level in the early identification of AMI when troponins are used as the criterion standard [92].

CK-MB as a single test is only modestly sensitive and specific for AMI; however, serial testing performed over 4 to 9 hours is highly sensitive and highly specific. Because serum CK-MB levels represent infarcted myocardium, CK-MB has not been tested for diagnosing ACS in the ED. There are no clinical impact studies for CK-MB.

Troponin T and troponin I

The cardiac troponins have expanded the spectrum of detectable myocardial injury and enhanced the clinician's ability to identify patients who have ACSs and are at higher risk for death or recurrent ischemic events even with low-level elevation of cardiac troponin T or I [93,94]. The notion that any reliably detected troponin elevation results from myocyte necrosis serves as the basis for the recent revision of diagnostic criteria for AMI. However, further research is necessary to conclusively refute the possibility that the release of cardiac troponins may also occur in the setting of reversible myocyte injury resulting from cellular ischemia [95]. Cardiac troponins offer extremely high tissue specificity but do not discriminate between ischemic and nonischemic mechanisms of myocardial injury; thus, presently the clinician must assess whether a patient's presenting symptoms are consistent with ACSs. In addition, renal failure does not appear to diminish the prognostic value of troponins among patients who have a high clinical probability of ACSs regardless of patient's creatinine clearance [96].

The evidence for the diagnostic performance of troponin T is substantial in diagnosing AMI but rather limited in diagnosing ACSs (see Tables 1 and 2) [57]. Data for troponin I are limited, but its performance is similar to that of troponin T. The sensitivity of presentation troponin T for diagnosing AMI in the ED is poor, but improves substantially if serial measurements are obtained for up to 6 hours after ED presentation. Most likely, the sensitivity is better for patients who have had symptoms for longer periods of time. The specificity of troponin T for AMI is in the range of 90%.

Myoglobin

The diagnostic performance of myoglobin has been well studied for diagnosing AMI, but not for diagnosing ACSs (see Tables 1 and 2) [57]. The sensitivity of myoglobin for diagnosing AMI in the ED is poor when a single initial measurement is obtained, but sensitivity improves greatly if a second measurement is obtained 2 to 4 hours after the first one. However, the sensitivity for patients only recently symptomatic is poor, and a second measurement in 2 to 4 hours may still not be sufficiently sensitive to be useful. Specificity is very good, but not excellent, depending on the extent to which other reasons for elevated myoglobin are excluded a priori. A doubling of myoglobin levels as soon as 1 to 2 hours after the initial measurement is almost perfectly sensitive for AMI.

The evidence suggests that a normal myoglobin value 2 hours after presentation may be used safely to rule out AMI. A doubling of myoglobin as early as 1 to 2 hours after the baseline measurement establishes a diagnosis of AMI. A small study [97] suggests that normal myoglobin and CK-MB values 2 hours after presentation completely rule out AMI. The incremental value of CK-MB compared with myoglobin alone cannot be evaluated given the small sample sizes. In a much larger study, Kontos and colleagues [98] found no advantage for myoglobin over baseline and 3-hour CK-MB values. In a subanalysis of patients who had non–ST-elevation ACS, serum myoglobin above the MI detection thresholds was associated with increased 6-month mortality and thus may be useful for early risk stratification.

Biomarkers of neurohumoral activation and inflammation

In addition to markers of myonecrosis, markers of neurohumoral activation and inflammation may provide important prognostic and possibly diagnostic information in ACS. Studies on P-selectin [99,100], malondialdehyde-modified low-density lipoprotein, high-sensitivity C-reactive protein (hsCRP) [101–104], B-type natriuretic peptide [105], pregnancy-associated plasma protein A (PAPP-A) [106], serum amyloid A (SAA) [107], soluble CD-40, myeloperoxidase [108], glutathione peroxidase 1 [109], placental growth factor (PlGF) [110], matrix metalloproteinases [111], and monocyte chemoattractant protein-1 (MCP-1) [112] are just beginning to appear.

P-selectin in platelets and endothelial cells mediates adhesion interaction with leukocytes to form thrombi. There is only one ED study of P-selectin that reported low sensitivity and low specificity for AMI. Traditionally, hsCRP has been thought of as a bystander marker of vascular inflammation, without playing a direct role in the cardiovascular disease. More recently, accumulating evidence suggests that hsCRP may have direct proinflammatory effects, which is associated with all stages of atherosclerosis, including plaque destabilization [104,107]. Laterza and colleagues [106] studied ED patients who had suspected ACSs and found pregnancy-associated protein A, a potential proatherosclerotic metalloproteinase, to be only a modest predictor of adverse events, with a sensitivity of 67% and a specificity of 51%. It is thought that cellular antioxidant enzymes such as glutathione peroxidase 1 and superoxide dismutase have a central role in the control of reactive oxygen species. In vitro data and studies in animal models suggest that these enzymes may protect against atherosclerosis, but little is known about their relevance to human disease. In a prospective study of patients who have suspected ACSs, Blankenberg and colleagues [109]

found that a low level of red-cell glutathione peroxidase 1 was independently associated with an increased risk for cardiovascular events. Experimental data suggest that PlGF, a member of the vascular endothelial growth factor family, acts as a primary inflammatory instigator of atherosclerotic plaque instability and thus may be useful as a risk-predicting biomarker in patients who have ACSs. In a subanalysis of data from the CAPTURE Trial, Heeschen and colleagues [110] found PlGF to be an independent marker of adverse outcome in patients who have suspected ACSs. Myeloperoxidase, an abundant leukocyte enzyme, is elevated in culprit lesions that have fissured or ruptured in patients who had sudden death from cardiac causes. Numerous lines of evidence suggest mechanistic links between myeloperoxidase and inflammation and cardiovascular disease. In a prospective assessment of patients in the ED who had suspected ACSs, Brennan and colleagues [108] found that a single initial measurement of plasma myeloperoxidase independently predicted the early risk for MI and the risk for major adverse cardiac events in the ensuing 30-day and 6-month periods.

In the future, tests for neurohormonal activation (B-type natriuretic peptide) and inflammation (C-reactive protein, PAPP-A, MCP-1, SAA) may augment the ability to identify patients who have ACSs and are at risk for adverse events. The use of these markers alone or in combination (a multimarker approach) could potentially augment the ability to reserve the most expensive and aggressive therapies for patients who have the highest risk [113].

Cardiac imaging

Echocardiography

The total sample size and the number of studies evaluating echocardiography for the diagnosis of ACSs are small (see Tables 1 and 2) [57]. Limited evidence suggests that resting echocardiography has high sensitivity (93%), although only modest specificity (66%) for AMI. The availability of previous echocardiograms for comparison may improve the specificity [114]. But even if this improved specificity were verified with additional studies, the need for previous echocardiography would limit its applicability in the general ED setting. In addition, the data pertain mostly to patients who have normal or nondiagnostic ECGs. The data for stress dobutamine

echocardiography are even more limited. One
study suggests that it may be the next diagnostic
step for patients who have a negative resting echocardiogram, normal ECG, and normal enzyme
levels. There is no clinical impact study for this
technology.

Technetium 99m sestamibi myocardial perfusion imaging

Data on the diagnostic accuracy of resting
technetium (Tc) 99m sestamibi imaging in the ED
are limited (see Tables 1 and 2). The test has been
used in selected patient populations that generally
have a low-to-moderate risk for an ACS, no history of MI, and a presenting ECG nondiagnostic
for an ACS. Thus, the generalizability of the current evidence is limited, and the test should be
reserved for these circumscribed populations. In
these patients, the test has excellent sensitivity
for AMI and very good, but not perfect, sensitivity for coronary disease in general. Specificity is
modest for AMI, and although it may be a little
better for ACSs, it is still far from excellent. In
a prospective ED trial, Udelson and colleagues
[115] showed that resting Tc 99m sestamibi imaging improved ED triage decision making for patients who had symptoms suggesting ACSs but
no obvious abnormalities on the initial ECG by
reducing unnecessary admissions without reducing appropriate admissions.

Myocardial performance index

Central aortic pressure

One index of myocardial contractility is the
rate of increase of intraventricular pressure during
isovolumetric contraction (left ventricular dP/dt;
arterial dP/dt). dP/dt represents the rate of change
of pressure during ejection [116–119]. It has been
shown previously that cardiac contractility and
dP/dt decrease during acute cardiac ischemia
[116,118]. Preliminary work by Gorenberg and
Marmor [120] suggests that a noninvasive device
that quantifies central aortic pressure through
brachial artery sensors may be a technique that
could be used in selected patient populations
that have a low-to-moderate risk for ACSs, no
history of MI, and a presenting ECG nondiagnostic for ACSs. However, the generalizability of the
current evidence is limited because of study size
and design.

Computer-based decision aids

Acute cardiac ischemia time-insensitive predictive instrument

The acute cardiac ischemia time-insensitive
predictive instrument (ACI-TIPI) [26] computes
a 0% to 100% probability that a given patient
has ACS (either acute MI or unstable angina pectoris) (see Tables 1 and 2). Applicable to any patient in the ED presenting with any symptom
suggestive of ACS, it is based on a logistic regression equation that uses presenting symptoms and
ECG variables. Originally in hand-held calculator
form, it is now incorporated into conventional
electrocardiographs so that the patient's ACI-
TIPI probability is printed with the standard
ECG header text. In large controlled interventional trials in a wide range of hospitals, its use
by ED physicians has been shown to reduce unnecessary admissions of patients who do not
have ACSs and patients who have stable angina,
while not reducing appropriate hospitalization
for patients who have ACSs. It has also been
shown to help the triage speed and accuracy of
less-trained and less-supervised residents. Although this decision aid is a widely available software option offered by all the major ECG
machines manufacturers in the United States, it
has not been widely used in clinical practice. The
greater dissemination and use of ACI-TIPI could
result in significant positive impact on the triage
of patients who have ACSs in the ED.

Thrombolytic predictive instrument

Correctly diagnosing STEMI for prompt use of
coronary reperfusion therapy can be lifesaving. In
EDs this can be difficult, especially for less obvious
candidates [121–123]. Efforts by physician leaders,
the NHAAP, health care organizations and monitoring entities, and pharmaceutical companies
[123–132], have helped increase use and promptness of reperfusion therapy [133]. Further improvement is needed [133,134], however,
particularly for other than anterior STEMI, the
category for which thrombolytic therapy first was
recognized as effective [121,122] and for women
who have received less coronary reperfusion therapy than men [134,135]. Also, a need remains for
ways to support prompt and accurate coronary reperfusion therapy decisions in hospitals and prehospital EMS settings where consultation with
off-site physicians is required.

Selker and colleagues [136] developed the thrombolytic predictive instrument (TPI), a collection of five component predictive instruments designed to accurately assess the patient-specific likely benefits and risks from the use of thrombolytic therapy for STEMI. The TPI helps clinicians identify patients for coronary reperfusion therapy based on their probabilities of benefits and complications and facilitates earliest possible use of reperfusion therapy [123,136]. In conventional computerized ECGs when significant ST segment elevation of STEMI is detected, the TPI predictions are automatically computed and printed on the ECG header: probabilities for acute (30-day) mortality either treated with thrombolytic therapy or untreated; 1-year mortality rates treated with thrombolytic therapy; cardiac arrest treated with thrombolytic therapy and untreated; thrombolytic therapy-related stroke and major bleeding requiring transfusion.

To test whether the ECG-based TPI improves ED selection of patients for coronary reperfusion therapy and promptness of treatment, the authors ran a 22-month randomized controlled clinical effectiveness trial of its impact on the use of thrombolytic therapy and overall coronary reperfusion therapy. The trial ran in EDs at 28 urban, suburban, and rural hospitals across the United States, from major cardiac centers to small community hospitals. Study endpoints were percentages of patients receiving (a) thrombolytic therapy; (b) thrombolytic therapy within 1 hour of ED presentation; and (c) all coronary reperfusion therapy, either by thrombolytic therapy or PTCA.

At participating hospitals, software generating TPI predictions was installed on their conventional computerized ECGs. When a significant ST elevation characteristic of STEMI was automatically detected, the ECG randomly assigned the patient to the control or intervention group. If assigned to the intervention group, the ECG automatically prompted the user to enter information needed to compute the TPI predictions: age, sex, history of hypertension or of diabetes, blood pressure, and time since ischemic symptom onset. The remaining variables, based on ECG waveform measurements, were automatically acquired by the ECG. Then the ECG was printed with TPI predictions on its header.

Among the 1197 patients who developed STEMI, the trial showed that the TPI increased use of thrombolytic therapy, use of thrombolytic therapy within 1 hour, and use of overall coronary reperfusion therapy by 11% to 12% for patients

who have developed inferior STEMI, 18% to 22% for women, and 30% to 34% for patients who have an off-site physician [137]. Although the TPI's effect was minimal on patients who had high baseline coronary reperfusion therapy rates, such as men who present with anterior STEMIs, for the groups needing the most improvement in their rates of recognition for coronary reperfusion, women and those with less obvious STEMIs, and where involved physicians were off-site, the TPI increased recognition of STEMI and use and timeliness of coronary reperfusion therapy. It is hoped that as TPI-capable ECGs become more widely available in ED and EMS settings, its use will facilitate the accuracy and speed of recognition and treatment of these patients.

Goldman Chest Pain Protocol

The Goldman Chest Pain Protocol [7] is based on a computer-derived model using recursive-partitioning analysis to predict MI in patients who have chest pain (see Tables 1 and 2). It has good sensitivity (about 90%) for AMI, but was not developed to also detect UAP. In a clinical impact study of "low-intensity, non-intrusive intervention" performed in the ED of a teaching hospital [16], no differences in hospitalization rate, length of stay, or estimated costs were demonstrated between the experimental group that used the protocol and the control group. Goldman and colleagues [35] eventually switched to predicting the need for intensive or other levels of care. They found that clinicians who had higher levels of training had a higher sensitivity for detecting AMI, but at the expense of decreased specificity [138]. Reilly and colleagues [139] developed a consensus to adapt the Goldman prediction rule and found a favorable impact on physicians' hospital triage decisions solely by different triage decisions for very low-risk patients. Unfortunately, any algorithm that incorporates only clinical elements and the ECG findings at presentation is likely to be suboptimal because of the substantial proportion of patients who present with atypical symptoms or with no or minimal ECG abnormalities.

Other computer-based decision aids

Several investigators have reported various computer-based decision aids to diagnose AMI (see Tables 1 and 2). The artificial neural network by Baxt and Skora [140] had high sensitivity and high specificity for AMI in a prospective study, but the clinical impact has not been demonstrated. A predictive model with automatic ECG interpretation has been shown to increase the use of fibrinolytic therapy for acute ST-segment elevation MI, especially in historically undertreated patients, such as those who have inferior AMI and women who have AMI [141].

Women

It is becoming apparent that one of the major contributing factors for the misdiagnosis of ischemic heart disease in women is pathophysiologic differences that appear to exist between men and women who have these syndromes and between the various ischemic syndromes themselves. Obstructive CAD continues to be a major public health problem in women and has represented the leading cause of death and disability for more than a decade [1,142,143]. In the United States alone, more than a quarter of a million women die of coronary heart disease (CHD) each year, translating into 1 death every 2 minutes [1]. Increased awareness of these statistics and a recent focus on women's health issues in general have resulted in renewed interest in trying to understand important gender differences in patients who have ACSs. Although women have a lower prevalence of obstructive CAD compared with men who have similar symptoms [144–146], women have a higher frequency of angina/chest pain than men partly because of the higher prevalence of the less common causes of ischemia, such as vasospastic angina and microvascular endothelial dysfunction; transient left ventricular apical ballooning syndrome (takotsubo cardiomyopathy) [147]; and syndromes of nonischemic chest pain, such as mitral valve prolapse [148]. Add to this the fact that young women who have obstructive CAD experience a significantly worse outcome with regard to prognosis after MI compared with men [149], and that older women who have obstructive CAD often have greater comorbidities that influence their outcome adversely after AMI or myocardial revascularization than do men [150–153]. Furthermore, women presenting with ACSs are less likely to receive effective acute diagnostic and treatment strategies than men [3,154,155]. When women develop obstructive CAD, they have a greater functional expression of their disease and disability compared with men. Most women who do not have obstructive CAD at angiography continue to have symptom-related disability and consume considerable health care resources [156–158], partly because the pathophysiology of ischemia in women is incompletely understood and gender-specific diagnostic and treatment strategies are underdeveloped [159]. Gender differences with regard to ischemic heart disease appear to exist in several areas, including established and novel risk factors; the metabolic syndrome; the physiology of endogenous reproductive hormones; the role of endothelial dysfunction in producing obstructive macrovascular CAD, myocardial ischemia, chronic chest pain syndromes, and ACS; genetic factors; proteomics; the menstrual cycle and reproductive status; pain threshold/perception; neurohumoral control; and behavioral/psychosocial factors.

The diagnostic evaluation of women who have suspected ACSs continues to be a major challenge. Knowing whether gender influences the likelihood that a given patient in the ED is having ACSs, and whether any specific presenting clinical features are differentially associated with ACSs in women compared with men, can aid clinicians in the accurate diagnosis of ACSs. The incidence of AMI in the general population has been shown to be higher in men than women [160–163], but until recently it has not been clear whether this gender difference holds among symptomatic patients who come to the ED. In addition, several studies have looked at gender differences in the presentation of patients who have AMI [157,164–167]. In a retrospective analysis of patients who have confirmed AMI, women had higher rates of atypical presentations, such as abdominal pain, paroxysmal dyspnea, or congestive heart failure [46,160,168–170]. In a group of patients in the ED who had typical presentations such as chest pain, the prevalence of AMI was lower in women [34,171]. However, in another study of patients in the ED who had chest pain, when adjustments were made for other presenting clinical features (specifically ECG), the gender difference was no longer significant [166]. From these results it is difficult to assess whether the gender-specific differences in AMI prevalence among symptomatic patients in the ED were the result of gender-specific biology or limitations in a particular study's patient selection.

One reason for such challenges is that chest pain in women is neither sensitive nor specific in predicting the presence of underlying CHD. The highest sensitivity is found in women presenting with symptoms of typical angina pectoris, whereas the highest specificity is found in women presenting with nonspecific symptoms. In fact, although women who have ACSs may present with symptom patterns that differ from men (ie, atypical symptoms), for most women, typical symptoms are the strongest symptom predictors of ACSs [172–174]. A further challenge is gender differences in reporting pain, including but not limited to chest pain. Gender differences in endogenous pain-modulating systems may contribute to differences in pain perception. Regarding biomarkers, there is a suggestion that women who have obstructive CHD may have a different pattern of presenting biomarkers compared with men. In a TACTICS-TIMI 18 subanalysis examining patients who have UA/NSTEMI, there was a different pattern of presenting biomarkers between the sexes: men were more likely to have elevated CK-MB and troponins, whereas women were more likely to have elevated C-reactive protein and brain natriuretic peptide, suggesting that a multimarker approach to diagnosis may improve triage in the ED. Lastly, the Women's Ischemic Syndrome Evaluation Study Group and others have suggested that those women who have chest pain without flow-limiting lesions by angiography may have associated microvascular endothelial dysfunction (cardiac syndrome X) [175] and impaired coronary flow reserve [176,177]. Preliminary data suggest that coronary microvascular dysfunction is associated with an increased rate of hospitalization for chest pain, poor quality of life, and ongoing health care costs. Newer technologies, such as MR spectroscopy and gadolinium cardiac MRI, may allow for the identification of abnormalities in vascular function and structure not identifiable by coronary angiogram that can cause or contribute to development of myocardial ischemia, and may aid in the initial risk assessment of UA/NSTEMI, especially in women [178].

Finally, numerous studies have found that women have poorer outcomes than men after a diagnosis of ACSs. Explanations have included gender differences in pathophysiology and response to treatment; prehospital delays in symptom recognition and action; and gender differences regarding evaluation and treatment in emergency medical services. Recent reports of similar or better outcomes in women who have ACSs compared with men suggest that pathophysiologic differences can be overcome with early, aggressive therapy [153,179]. The diagnosis of ischemia influences prognosis differently in various clinical ischemic syndromes. In unstable angina the detection of ischemia indicates the likelihood of persistence or recurrence of plaque instability and hence carries much more severe prognostic implications than in chronic stable angina, whereas although angina in patients who have normal coronary angiograms is not associated with increased short-term risk of infarction or sudden death, these patients may be crippled by pain. Inconsistent response to nitrates and antianginal drugs indicates the need for research on the various potential causes of coronary vascular dysfunction that burden women disproportionately, to facilitate development of rational forms of therapy.

Race

Blacks have high levels of risk factors for CAD, but how this finding influences diagnosis in patients presenting to the ED with symptoms suggesting ACSs is not well understood [180,181]. Studies that have included only patients who have chest pain and not other symptoms suggestive of ACSs have found no significant differences in presentation, natural history, or final diagnosis of AMI between black and white patients [182]. Evaluating chest pain and establishing the diagnosis of CAD in blacks is often difficult given the presence of excess hypertension and left ventricular hypertrophy and the increased occurrence of out-of-hospital cardiac arrest in blacks [183–186]. Furthermore, the paradoxical finding of severe chest pain without significant angiographic CAD that can be seen in 30% to 40% of men [187] complicates diagnosis and treatment of blacks who have symptoms suggestive of ACSs [180,183]. In subanalysis of the ACI-TIPI Trial data, Maynard and colleagues [188] found that black patients were 8 to 10 years younger and that a higher percentage were women than was the case among white patients, which may partially explain why physicians might be less inclined to suspect the presence of ACSs in black patients. Finally, Pope and colleagues [3] found that among patients who have ACSs, the adjusted risk for being sent home was more than two times as high among nonwhite as whites. Among those who had AMI, the risk was more than four times as high among nonwhites as whites. In this study, 5.8% of the black patients who had AMI were not hospitalized, as compared with 1.2% of the white patients who had infarction.

Outcomes

Each year in the United States, over 6 million patients who have chest pain or other symptoms suggesting ACSs (eg, IMIR Study inclusion symptoms) [23] present to EDs [4]. These patients can have various clinical outcomes ranging from discharge home to hospital admission after thrombolytic therapy or percutaneous coronary intervention. Table 3 shows the final diagnosis for the ACI-TIPI Trial [2] control subjects by ED triage disposition. These data were employed to develop a flowchart (Fig. 1) to represent the diagnoses and triage dispositions of patients in the ED presenting with chest pain or other symptoms suggestive of ACSs. Although these data are not recent and the triage and intervention options have expanded over the last decade, the proportions have remained remarkable similar.

The flowchart (see Fig. 1) demonstrates that of all such patients, only 23% of patients (hospital range 12%–34%) had ACSs at final diagnosis, of which 94% were hospitalized and 6% were sent home. Conversely, 77% did not have ACSs at final diagnosis, of which 59% were hospitalized and 41% were sent home. In the ACSs group of patients, 36% of patients had AMI and 64% had UAP, which represented 8% and 15%, respectively, of the overall group. In the AMI group, 97% were hospitalized and 3% were sent home; in the UAP group, 92% were hospitalized and 8% were sent home.

The authors' work with Pozen and colleagues [6] from 1979 to 1981 at the same hospitals as the present report demonstrated a 7% ED discharge rate for patients who had a final diagnosis of ACSs; McCarthy and colleagues [18] found that 2% of these subjects had AMI at final diagnosis. In the mid-1980s, Lee and colleagues [9] reported a 4% AMI discharge rate. The authors' study found a 6% discharge rate for ACSs and a 3% AMI discharge rate, demonstrating stability of these figures over the decade. The proportions of AMI and UAP in the authors' present study (36% AMI, 64% UAP) were essentially identical to those from their work with Pozen and

Table 3
Final diagnosis (%) for acute cardiac ischemia time-insensitive predictive instrument trial control subjects by emergency department triage disposition

Triage disposition	AMI (n = 496)	UAP (n = 898)	non-ACS (n = 4557)
Home	3	8	41
Ward	1	2	6
Telemetry	31	61	43
CCU	66	29	10

colleagues [6] in 1979 to 1981 (35% AMI, 65% UAP). Finally, in an analysis of the ACI-TIPI Trial data for failure to make the diagnosis of an ACS, the authors found that the missed diagnosis rate for ACSs was 2.2% (2.1% for AMI, 2.3% for UAP) [3].

Recent approaches to patient safety emphasize "systems thinking" rather than focusing on individual cognitive mistakes. The goal is to prevent human errors, which are commonly made by competent clinicians [189,190]. Suggested approaches include diagnostic protocols and pathways, decision aids, novel approaches to staffing, chest-pain units, and other systems changes.

Missed diagnosis of ACS

Several factors, listed in Box 1, have been associated with inappropriate discharge of patients who have symptoms suggestive of ACSs from EDs and other acute care settings. These factors include younger age (<55 years), female gender, nonwhite ethnicity, atypical symptoms, no previous MI, normal or nondiagnostic ECG findings, misinterpretation of the ECG (failure to recognize minimal ST-segment elevation), and failure to appreciate the dynamic nature of anginal symptoms, obtain multiple ECGs tracings over time, obtain previous ECG tracings for comparison, appreciate the dynamic nature of anginal symptoms, and appreciate nonobstructive cardiac ischemic syndromes [3].

Although women tend to develop obstructive CAD 10 years later than men, Pope and colleagues [3] found that women under the age of 55 years were at the highest risk for not being hospitalized with ACSs. Physicians must try not to pigeonhole patients into set categories, and remember that low risk for ACSs is not zero risk. Furthermore, because about 50% of women and a small percentage of men who have symptoms suggestive of ACSs have nonobstructive syndromes, it is important that this subset of patients not be overlooked as is has been previously, and that these patients are referred to cardiologists for definitive diagnosis and therapy. In addition, these researchers found that the risk for being sent home was twice as high for nonwhites and whites, citing younger age and higher percentage of women as possible reasons for lowering clinical suspicions about ACSs. Although most patients, including women who have ACSs, present in a typical fashion, many can present in an atypical fashion with complaints of shortness of breath [191].

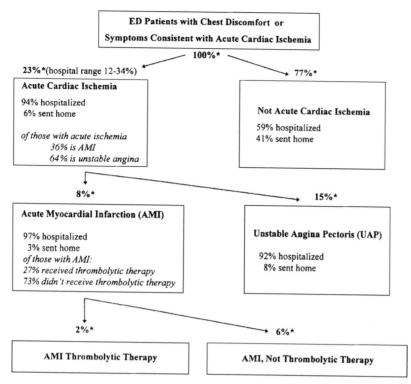

Fig. 1. Flowchart illustrating diagnoses and triage dispositions of patients presenting to the ED with chest pain or other symptoms suggesting ACI. *Percentage of ED patients in the control group who have chest pain or symptoms consistent with ACI.

Because about 25% of patients who are mistakenly discharged are sent home after an error in interpretation in their ECG [192], improving the analysis and interpretation of ECGs could improve decision making. Finally, some investigators have

suggested that as many as 3% of patients who have suspected noncardiac chest pain will go on to experience a adverse cardiac event within 30 days of that assessment [193], and suggest that features such as male gender, hypercholesteremia, advanced age, CHD, heart failure, features that are not typically associated with noncardiac chest pain, and a higher calculated ACI-TIPI score. However, safe noncardiac chest pain criteria have yet to be derived and validated. Clinicians must at least consider the possibility of the diagnosis of ACSs in patients who have these factors, especially if a less serious cause for the patient's symptoms is not readily apparent.

Box 1. Factors contributing to the misdiagnosis of acute coronary syndromes

- Younger age (<55 years of age)
- Female sex
- Nonwhite ethnicity
- Atypical symptoms
- No previous MI
- Normal or nondiagnostic ECG findings
- Misinterpretation of the initial ECG
- Failure to obtain multiple ECGs and obtain previous tracings
- Failure to appreciate the dynamic nature of anginal symptoms
- Failure to appreciate nonobstructive cardiac ischemic syndromes

Summary

Failure to diagnose patients who have ACSs, either AMI or UAP, who present to the ED remains a serious public health issue. Better understanding of the pathophysiology of CAD has allowed the adoption of a unifying hypothesis for the cause of ACSs: the conversion of a stable atherosclerotic lesion to a plaque rupture with thrombosis. Thus, physicians have come to appreciate UAP and AMI as parts of a continuum of ACSs. However, for as many as 50% of women who have a suspected ACSs, other mechanisms of illness are at work, including vasospastic angina, microvascular endothelial dysfunction, transient left ventricular apical ballooning syndrome, and mitral value prolapse. The accurate identification of these syndromes in the ED or other acute care settings challenges the skill of even the most seasoned clinician. Clinical features, patient demographics, physical examination findings, and a firm understanding the strengths and limitations of the standard ECG can greatly assist with the identification of patients who have ACSs. Biochemical markers, cardiac imaging, myocardial performance indices, and computer-based decision aids remain underevaluated adjuncts to, but not substitutes for, clinicians' judgment regarding diagnosis and triage of patients who have symptoms suggestive of ACSs. Several factors have been associated with inappropriate discharge of patients who have symptoms suggestive of ACSs from EDs and other acute care settings, including younger age (<55 years of age), female gender, nonwhite ethnicity, atypical symptoms, no previous MI, normal or nondiagnostic ECG findings, misinterpretation of the ECG, and failure to appreciate the dynamic nature of anginal symptoms. However, safe noncardiac chest pain criteria have yet to be derived and validated. Despite 2 decades of focused research and without compelling evidence for a noncardiac cause, there remains no single way to discriminate perfectly between those who should be admitted to exclude ACSs and those who could be managed safely without admission. For the continuum of patient risk for ACSs, there is a matched continuum of triage options for each patient, from short-stay chest pain evaluation units to multiday admissions for more intensive evaluations.

References

[1] American Heart Association. Heart Disease and Stroke Statistics–2005 Update. Dallas, TX: American Heart Association; 2004.

[2] Pope J, Ruthazer R, Beshansky J, et al. Clinical features of emergency department patients presenting with symptoms of acute cardiac ischemia: a multicenter study. J Thromb Thrombolysis 1998;6: 63–74.

[3] Pope J, Aufderheide T, Ruthazer R, et al. Missed diagnoses of acute cardiac ischemia in the emergency department. N Engl J Med 2000;342:1163–70.

[4] Van der Does E, Lubson J, Pool J, et al. Acute coronary events in a general practice: objectives and design of the Imminent Myocardial Infarction Rotterdam Study. Heart Bull 1976;7:91.

[5] McCaig L. National ambulatory care survey: 1992 emergency department summary. Adv Data 1994; 245:1–12.

[6] Pozen M, D'Agostino R, Selker H, et al. A predictive instrument to improve coronary care unit admission practices in acute ischemic heart disease: a prospective multicenter clinical trial. N Engl J Med 1984;310:1273–8.

[7] Goldman L, Weinberg M. A computer-derived protocol to aid in the diagnosis of emergency room patients with acute chest pain. N Engl J Med 1982;307:588–96.

[8] Schor S, Behar S, Modan B, et al. Disposition of presumed coronary patients from an emergency room; a follow-up study. JAMA 1976;236:941–3.

[9] Lee T, Rouan G, Weisberg M, et al. Clinical characteristics and natural history of patients with acute myocardial infarction sent home from the emergency room. Am J Cardiol 1987;60:219–24.

[10] Pozen M, D'Agostino R, Mitchell J, et al. The usefulness of a predictive instrument to reduce inappropriate admissions to the coronary care unit. Ann Intern Med 1980;92:238–42.

[11] Selker H, Pozen M, D'Agostino R. Optimal identification of the patient with acute myocardial ischemia in the emergency room. In: Calif R, Wagner G, editors. Acute coronary care: principles and practice. Boston: Martinus Nijhoff; 1985. p. 289–98.

[12] Bloom B, Peterson O. End results, costs, and productivity of coronary care units. N Engl J Med 1973;288:72–8.

[13] Eisenberg J, Horowitz L, Busch R, et al. Diagnosis of acute myocardial infarction in the emergency room: a prospective assessment of clinical decision making and usefulness of immediate cardiac enzyme determination. J Community Health 1979;4: 190–8.

[14] Fuchs R, Scheidt S. Improved criteria for admission to coronary care units. JAMA 1981;246:2037–41.

[15] Tierney W, Roth B, Psaty B, et al. Predictors of myocardial infarction in emergency room patients. Crit Care Med 1985;13:526–31.

[16] Goldman L, Cook E, Brand D, et al. A computer protocol to predict myocardial infarction in emergency department patients with chest pain. N Engl J Med 1988;318:707–803.

[17] Cannon CP. Management of coronary syndromes. In: Cannon CP, editor. Contemporary cardiology. Totowa (NJ): Humana Press; 1999. Chapter 1, p. 8.

[18] McCarthy B, Beshansky J, D'Agostino R, et al. Missed diagnoses of acute myocardial infarction in the emergency department: results from a multicenter study. Ann Emerg Med 1993;22:579–82.

[19] McCarthy B, Wong J, Selker H. Detecting acute cardiac ischemia in the emergency department: a

review of the literature. J Gen Intern Med 1990;5:
365–73.

[20] Selker HP, Zalenski RJ, Antman EM, et al. An
evaluation of technologies for identifying acute cardiac ischemia in the emergency department. Ann
Emerg Med 1997;29:1–87.

[21] Agency for Healthcare Research and Quality
(AHRQ) Evaluation of technologies for identifying
acute cardiac ischemia in emergency departments.
Technology assessment no. 26, prepared by Joseph
Lau, MD. AHRQ Pub no. 01-E006, May 2001.
103–5.

[22] Rifkin R, Hood WJ. Bayesian analysis of electrocardiographic exercise stress testing. N Engl J
Med 1979;297:681–6.

[23] Uretsky B, Farquhar D, Berezin A, et al. Symptomatic myocardial infarction without chest pain: prevalence and clinical course. Am J Cardiol 1977;40:
498–503.

[24] Kinlen L. Incidence and presentation of myocardial infarction in an English community. Br Heart
J 1973;35:616–22.

[25] Marglois J, Kannel W, Feinlieb M, et al. Clinical
features of unrecognized myocardial infarction-
silent and symptomatic. Am J Cardiol 1973;32:
1–6.

[26] Selker H, Beshansky J, Griffith J, et al. Use of the
Acute Cardiac Ischemia Time-Insensitive Predictive Instrument (ACI-TIPI) to assist with triage of
patients with chest pain or other symptoms suggestive of acute cardiac ischemia. Ann Intern Med
1998;129:845–55.

[27] Russell R. Unstable angina pectoris: National Cooperative Study Group to compare medical and
surgical therapy: IV. Results in patients with left
anterior descending coronary artery disease. Am J
Cardiol 1981;48:517–24.

[28] Krauss KR, Hutter AM Jr, DeSanctis RW. Acute
coronary insufficiency. Course and follow-up. Circulation 1972;45(Suppl 1):I66–71.

[29] Wasson J, Sox H, Neff R, et al. Clinical prediction
rules: applications and methodological standards.
N Engl J Med 1985;313:793–9.

[30] McCaig L, Burt C. National Hospital Ambulatory
Medical Care Survey: 2002 emergency department
summary. Adv Data 2004;340:1–34.

[31] Coronado BE, Pope JH, Griffith JL, et al. Clinical
features, triage, and outcome of patients presenting
to the ED with suspected acute coronary syndrome
but without pain: a multicenter study. Am J Emerg
Med 2004;22:568–74.

[32] American College of Emergency Physicians. Clinical policy for the initial approach to adults presenting with a chief complaint of chest pain with no
history of trauma. Ann Emerg Med 1995;25:
274–99.

[33] Short D. Diagnosis of slight and subacute coronary
attacks in the community. Br Heart J 1981;45:
299–310.

[34] Lee T, Cook E, Weisberg M, et al. Acute chest pain
in the emergency room: identification and examination of low-risk patients. Arch Intern Med 1985;
145:65–9.

[35] Goldman L, Cook E, Johnson P, et al. Prediction of
the need for intensive care in patients who come to
the emergency department with acute chest pain.
N Engl J Med 1996;334:1498–504.

[36] Selker H, Griffith J, D'Agostino R. A time-insensitive predictive instrument for acute myocardial infarction mortality: a multicenter study. Med Care
1991;29:1196–211.

[37] Sawe U. Pain in acute myocardial infarction. A
study of 137 patients in a coronary care unit.
Acta Med Scand 1971;190:79–81.

[38] Sawe U. Early diagnosis of acute myocardial infarction with special reference to the diagnosis of
the intermediate coronary syndrome: a clinical
study. Acta Med Scand 1972;520(Suppl):1–76.

[39] Levene D. Chest pain-prophet of doom or nagging
necrosis? Acta Med Scand 1981;644(Suppl):11–3.

[40] Sievers J. Myocardial infarction. Clinical features
and outcome in three thousand thirty-six cases.
Acta Med Scand 1964;406(Suppl 406):1–120.

[41] Areskog M, Tibbling L, Wranne B. Oesophageal
dysfunction in non-infarction coronary care unit
patients. Acta Med Scand 1979;205:279–82.

[42] Alonzo A, Simon A, Feilieb M. Prodromata of
myocardial infarction and sudden death. Circulation 1975;52:1056–62.

[43] Nattel S, Warnica J, Ogilivie R. Indications for
admission to a coronary care unit in patients
with unstable angina. Can Med Assoc J 1980;122:
180–4.

[44] Ingram D, Fulton R, Portal R, et al. Vomiting as
a diagnostic aid in acute ischemic cardiac pain.
BMJ 1980;281:636–7.

[45] Canto J, Fincher C, Kiefe C, et al. Atypical presentations among Medicare beneficiaries with unstable
angina pectoris. Am J Cardiol 2003;91:118–9.

[46] Kannel W, Abbott R. Incidence and prognosis of
unrecognized myocardial infarction: an update on
the Framingham Study. N Engl J Med 1984;311:
1144–7.

[47] Rosenman R, Friedman M, Jenkins C, et al. Clinically unrecognized myocardial infarction in the
Western Collaborative Group Study. Am J Cardiol
1967;19:776–82.

[48] Grimm R, Tillinghast S, Daniels K, et al. Unrecognized myocardial infarction; experience in the Multiple Risk Factor Intervention Trial (MRFIT).
Circulation 1987;75(Suppl 2):116–8.

[49] Kannel WB. Silent myocardial ischemia and infarction: insights from the Framingham study. Cardiol
Clin 1986;4:583–91.

[50] McCarthy B, Beshansky J, D'Agostino R, et al.
Can missed diagnoses of acute myocardial infarction in the emergency room be reduced? Clin Res
1989;37:779A.

[51] Gordon T, Sorlie P, Kannel W. Coronary heart disease, atherothrombotic brain infarction, intermittent claudication–a multivariate analysis of some factors related to their incidence: Framingham Study, 16-year follow-up. Washington (DC): US Government Printing Office; 1971.

[52] Truett J, Cornfield J, Kannel W. A multivariate analysis of the risk of coronary artery disease in Framingham. J Chronic Dis 1967;20:511–24.

[53] Jayes R, Larsen G, Beshansky J, et al. Physician electrocardiogram reading in the emergency department: accuracy and effect on triage decisions: findings from a multicenter study. J Gen Intern Med 1992;7:387–92.

[54] Henrikson C, Howell E, Bush D, et al. Chest pain relief by nitroglycerin does not predict active coronary artery disease. Ann Intern Med 2003;139: 979–86.

[55] Orlando R, Bozymski E. Clinical and manometric effects of nitroglycerin in diffuse esophageal spasm. N Engl J Med 1973;289:23–5.

[56] Killip T, Kimball J. Treatment of myocardial infarction in a coronary care unit. A two year experience with 250 patients. Am J Cardiol 1967;20: 457–64.

[57] Ornato JP, Selker HP, Zalenski RJ. NIH National Heart Attack Alert Program Working Group on Evaluation of Technologies for Identifying Acute Cardiac Ischemia in Emergency Departments Report. Ann Emerg Med 2001;37:450–94.

[58] Selker H. Electrocardiograms and decision aids in coronary care triage: the truth but not the whole truth. J Gen Intern Med 1987;2:67–70.

[59] Hoffman J, Igarashi E. Influence of electrocardiographic findings on admission decisions in patients with acute chest pain. Am J Med 1985;79: 699–707.

[60] Brush J, Brand D, Acampora D, et al. Use of the initial electrocardiogram to predict in-hospital complications of acute myocardial infarction. N Engl J Med 1985;312:1137–41.

[61] Slater D, Hlatky M, Mark D, et al. Outcome in suspected acute myocardial infarction with normal or minimally abnormal admission electrocardiographic findings. Am J Cardiol 1987;60:766–70.

[62] Stark M, Vacek J. The initial electrocardiogram during admission for myocardial infarction; use as a predictor of clinical course and facility utilization. Arch Intern Med 1987;147:843–6.

[63] Rude R, Poole W, Muller J, et al. Electrocardiographic and clinical criteria for recognition of acute myocardial infarction based on analysis of 3,697 patients. Am J Cardiol 1983;52:936–42.

[64] Lopez-Sendon J, Coma-Canella I, Alcasena S, et al. Electrocardiographic findings in acute right ventricular infarction: sensitivity and specificity of electrocardiographic alterations in right precordial leads V4R,V5R,V1,V2,V3. J Am Coll Cardiol 1985;19:1273–9.

[65] Wrenn K. Protocols in the emergency room evaluation of chest pain: do they fail to diagnose lateral wall myocardial infarction? J Gen Intern Med 1987;2:66–7.

[66] Nestico P, Hakki A, Iskandrian A, et al. Electrocardiographic diagnosis of posterior myocardial infarction revisited. J Electrocardiol 1986;19: 33–40.

[67] Fisch C. Electrocardiography, exercise stress testing, and ambulatory monitoring. In: Kelly W, editor. Textbook of internal medicine. Philadelphia: Lippincott; 1989. p. 305–16.

[68] Rusnak R, Stair T, Hansen K, et al. Litigation against the emergency physician: common features in cases of missed myocardial infarction. Ann Emerg Med 1989;18:1029–34.

[69] Griner P, Mayewski R, Mushlin A, et al. Selection and interpretation of diagnostic tests and procedures: principles and applications. Ann Intern Med 1981;94:557–92.

[70] Bell M, Montarello J, Steele P. Does the emergency room electrocardiogram identify patients with suspected myocardial infarction who are at low risk of acute complications? Aust N Z J Med 1990;20: 564–9.

[71] Zalenski R, Sloan E, Chen E, et al. The emergency department ECG and immediate life-threatening complications in initially uncomplicated suspected myocardial ischemia. Ann Emerg Med 1988;17: 221–6.

[72] Cohen M, Hawkins L, Geeenburg S, et al. Usefulness of ST-segment changes in ≥ 2 leads on the emergency room electrocardiogram in either unstable angina pectoris or non-Q-wave myocardial infarction in predicting outcome. Am J Cardiol 1991;67:1368–73.

[73] Fesmire F, Percy RF, Wears R, et al. Initial ECG in Q wave and non-Q wave myocardial infarction. Ann Emerg Med 1989;18:741–6.

[74] Rubenstein L, Greenfield S. The baseline ECG in the evaluation of acute cardiac complaints. JAMA 1980;244:2536–9.

[75] Miller DH, Kligfield P, Schreiber TL, et al. Relationship of prior myocardial infarction to false-positive electrocardiographic diagnosis of acute injury in patients with chest pain. Arch Intern Med 1987;147:257–61.

[76] Goldberger A. Myocardial infarction electrocardiographic differential diagnosis. St. Louis (MO): CV Mosby; 1979.

[77] Kaul P, Newby L, Fu Y, et al. Troponin T and quantitative ST-depression offer complementary prognostic information in the risk stratification of acute coronary syndrome patients. J Am Coll Cardiol 2003;41:371–80.

[78] Granborg J, Grande P, Pederson A. Diagnostic and prognostic significance of transient isolated negative T-waves in suspected acute myocardial infarction. Am J Cardiol 1986;57:203–7.

[79] Fisch C. Abnormal ECG in clinically normal individuals. JAMA 1983;250:1321–3.

[80] DeWood M, Stifer W, Simpson C, et al. Coronary arteriographic findings soon after non-Q-wave myocardial infarction. N Engl J Med 1986;315:417–23.

[81] Kennedy J. Non-Q-wave myocardial infarction. N Engl J Med 1977;315:451–3.

[82] Behar S, Schor S, Kariv I, et al. Evaluation of electrocardiogram in emergency room as a decision-making tool. Chest 1977;71:486–91.

[83] McGuinness J, Begg T, Semple T. First electrocardiogram in recent myocardial infarction. BMJ 1976;2:449–51.

[84] Gibler W, Runyon J, Levy R, et al. A rapid diagnostic and treatment center for patients with chest pain in the emergency department. Ann Emerg Med 1995;25:1–8.

[85] Hedges J, Young G, Henkel G, et al. Serial ECGs are less accurate than serial CK-MB results for emergency department diagnosis of myocardial infarction. Ann Emerg Med 1992;21:1445–50.

[86] Kirk J, Turnipseed S, Lewis W, et al. Evaluation of chest pain in low-risk patients presenting to the emergency department: the role of immediate exercise testing. Ann Emerg Med 1998;32:1–7.

[87] Lewis W, Amsterdam E, Turnipseed S. Immediate exercise testing of low-risk patients with known coronary artery disease presenting to the emergency department with chest pain. J Am Coll Cardiol 1999;33:1843–7.

[88] Tsakonis J, Shesser R, Rosenthal R, et al. Safety of immediate treadmill testing in selected emergency department patients with chest pain: a preliminary report. Am J Emerg Med 1991;9:557–9.

[89] Kerns J, Shaub T, Fontanarosa P. Emergency cardiac stress testing in the evaluation of emergency department patients with atypical chest pain. Ann Emerg Med 1993;22:794–8.

[90] Gerhardt W, Waldenstrom J, Horder M, et al. Creatine kinase and creatine kinase B-subunit activity in serum in cases of suspected myocardial infarction. Clin Chem 1982;28:277–83.

[91] Roxin L, Cullhed I, Groth T, et al. The value of serum myoglobin determinations in the early diagnosis of acute myocardial infarction. Acta Med Scand 1984;215:417–25.

[92] Fesmire F, Christenson R, Feintuch T. Delta creatinine kinase-MB outperforms myoglobin at two hours during emergency department identification and exclusion troponin positive non-ST-segment elevation acute coronary syndromes. Ann Emerg Med 2004;44:12–9.

[93] Morrow D, Cannon C, Rifai N, et al. Ability of minor elevations of troponins I and T to predict benefit from an early invasive strategy in patients with unstable angina or non-ST elevation myocardial infarction: results from a randomized trial. JAMA 2001;286:2405–12.

[94] Rao S, Ohman E, Granger C, et al. Prognostic value of isolated troponin elevation across the spectrum of chest pain syndromes. Am J Cardiol 2003;91:936–40.

[95] Morrow D. Troponins in patients with acute coronary syndromes: biologic, diagnostic, and therapeutic implications. Cardiovasc Toxicol 2001;1:105–10.

[96] Aviles R, Askari A, Lindahl B, et al. Troponin t levels in patients with acute coronary syndromes, with or without renal dysfunction. N Engl J Med 2002;346:2047–52.

[97] Montague C, Kircher T. Myoglobin in the early evaluation of acute chest pain. Am J Clin Pathol 1995;104:472–6.

[98] Kontos M, Anderson F, Schmidt K, et al. Early diagnosis of acute myocardial infarction in patients without ST-segment elevation. Am J Cardiol 1999;83:155–8.

[99] Ikeda H, Takajo Y, Ichiki K, et al. Increased soluble form of P-selectin in patients with unstable angina. Circulation 1995;92:1693–6.

[100] Itoh T, Nakai K, Ono M, et al. Can the risk for acute cardiac events in acute coronary syndromes be indicated by platelet membrane activation marker P-selectin? Coron Artery Dis 1995;6:645–50.

[101] Bassuk S, Rifai N, Ridker P. High-sensitivity C-reactive protein: clinical importance. Curr Probl Cardiol 2004;29:439–93.

[102] Oltrona L, Ottani F, Galvani M. Clinical significance of a single measurement of troponin-I and C-reactive protein at admission in 1773 consecutive patients with acute coronary syndromes. Am Heart J 2004;148:405–15.

[103] Avanzas P, Arroyo-Espliguero R, Cosin-Sales J, et al. Markers of inflammation and multiple complex stenoses (pancoronary plaque vulnerability) in patients with non-ST segment elevation acute coronary syndromes. Heart 2004;90:847–52.

[104] Pai J, Pischon T, Ma J, et al. Inflammatory markers and risk of coronary heart disease in men and women. N Engl J Med 2004;351:2599–610.

[105] de Lemos J, Morrow D, Bentley J, et al. The prognostic value of B-type natriuretic peptide in patients with acute coronary syndromes. N Engl J Med 2001;345:1014–21.

[106] Laterza O, Cameron S, Chappell D, et al. Evaluation of pregnancy-associated plasma protein A as a prognostic indicator in acute coronary syndrome patients. Clin Chim Acta 2004;348:163–9.

[107] Johnson B, Kip K, Marroquin O, et al. Serum amyloid A as a predictor of coronary artery disease and cardiovascular outcome in women: the National Heart, Lung, and Blood Institute-Sponsored Women's ischemia Syndrome Evaluation (WISE). Circulation 2004;109:726–32.

[108] Brennan M, Penn M, Van Lente F, et al. Prognostic value of myeloperoxidase in patients with chest pain. N Engl J Med 2003;349:1595–604.

[109] Blankenberg S, Rupprecht H, Bickel C, et al. Glutathione peroxidase 1 activity and cardiovascular events in patients with coronary artery disease. N Engl J Med 2003;349:1605–13.

[110] Heeschen C, Dimmeler S, Fichtlscherer S, et al. Prognostic value of placental growth factor in patients with acute chest pain. JAMA 2004;291: 435–41.

[111] Nomoto K, Oguchi S, Watanabe I, et al. Involvement of inflammation in acute coronary syndromes assessed by levels of high-sensitivity C-reactive protein, matrix metalloproteinase-9 and soluble vascular-cell adhesion molecule. J Cardiol 2003; 42:201–6.

[112] de Lemos J, Morrow D, Sabatine M, et al. Association between plasma levels of monocyte chemoattractant protein-1 and long-term clinical outcomes in patients with acute coronary syndromes. Circulation 2003;107:690–5.

[113] Sabatine MS, Morrow DA, de Lemos JA, et al. Multimarker approach to risk stratification in non-ST elevation acute coronary syndromes: simultaneous assessment of troponin I, C-reactive protein, and B-type natriuretic peptide. Circulation 2002;105:1760–3.

[114] Mohler ER III, Ryan T, Segar D, et al. Clinical utility of troponin T levels and echocardiography in the emergency department. Am Heart J 1998;135: 253–60.

[115] Udelson J, Beshansky J, Ballin D, et al. Myocardial perfusion imaging for evaluation and triage of patients with suspected acute cardiac ischemia. JAMA 2002;288:2693–700.

[116] Mohr R, Rath S, Meir O, et al. Changes in systemic vascular resistance detected by the arterial resistometer: preliminary report of a new method tested during percutaneous transluminal coronary angioplasty. Circulation 1986;74:780–5.

[117] Mohr R, Meir O, Smolinsky A, et al. A method for continuous on-line monitoring of systemic vascular resistance (COMS) after open heart procedures. J Cardiovasc Surg (Torino) 1987;28:558–65.

[118] Mohr R, Dinbar I, Bar-El Y, et al. Correlation between myocardial ischemia and changes in arterial resistance during coronary bypass surgery. J Cardiothorac Vasc Anesth 1992;6:33–41.

[119] Kantartzis M, Sunderdiek U, Bircks W, et al. Cardiac efficiency during coronary occlusion and during reperfusion after emergency revascularization under cardioprotection. Thorac Cardiovasc Surg 1996;44:20–6.

[120] Gorenberg M, Marmor A, Rotstein H. Detection of chest pain of non-cardiac origin at the emergency room by a new non-invasive device avoiding unnecessary admission to hospital. Emerg Med J 2005;22:486–9.

[121] Sarasin FP, Reymond JM, Griffith JL, et al. Impact of the acute cardiac ischemia time-insensitive predictive instrument (ACI-TIPI) on the speed of triage decision making for emergency department patients presenting with chest pain. J Gen Intern Med 1994;9:187–94.

[122] Gruppo Italiano per lo Studio Della Streptochinasi Nell'Infarcto Miocardico (GISSI). Effectiveness of intravenous thrombolytic therapy in acute myocardial infarction. Lancet 1986;1:397–401.

[123] Fibrinolytic Therapy Trialists' (FTT) Collaborative Group. Indications for fibrinolytic therapy in suspected acute myocardial infarction: collaborative overview of early mortality and major morbidity results from all randomized trials of more than 1000 patients. Lancet 1994;343: 311–22.

[124] Selker HP, Griffith JL, Beshansky JR, et al. The thrombolytic predictive instrument project: combining clinical study databases to take medical effectiveness research to the streets. Washington D.C.: AHCPR, DHHS; 1992:9–31.

[125] Cannon CP, Antman EM, Walls R, Braunwald E. Time as an adjunctive agent to thrombolytic therapy. J Thromb Thrombolysis 1994;1:27–34.

[126] National Heart Attack Alert Program Coordinating Committee. 60 Minutes to Treatment Working Group. Emergency department: rapid identification and treatment of patients with acute myocardial infarction. Ann Emerg Med 1994;23:311–29.

[127] National Heart Attack Alert Program Coordinating Committee Access to Care Subcommittee. Emergency medical dispatching: rapid identification and treatment of acute myocardial infarction. Am J Emerg Med 1995;13:67–73.

[128] National Heart Attack Alert Program Coordinating Committee Access to Care Subcommittee. 9–1–1: rapid identification and treatment of acute myocardial infarction. Am J Emerg Med 1995;13: 188–95.

[129] Rogers WJ, Bowlby LJ, Chandra NC, et al. Treatment of myocardial infarction in the United States (1990 to 1993) observations from the national registry of myocardial infarction. Circulation 1994;90: 2103–14.

[130] National Heart Attack Alert Program Coordinating Committee Access to Care Subcommittee. Access to timely and optimal care of patients with acute coronary syndromes—community planning considerations: a report by the National Heart Attack Alert Program. J Thromb Thrombolysis 1998; 6:19–36.

[131] National Heart Attack Alert Program Coordinating Committee Working Group on Educational Strategies to Prevent Prehospital Delay in Patients at High Risk for Acute Myocardial Infarction. Educational strategies to prevent prehospital delay in patients at high risk for acute myocardial infarction: a report by the National Heart Attack

Alert Program. J Thromb Thrombolysis 1998;6: 47–61.

[132] Sims RJ, Topol EJ, Holmes DR, et al. Link between the angiographic substudy and mortality outcomes in a large randomized trial of myocardial reperfusion: importance of early and complete infarct artery reperfusion. Circulation 1995;91: 1923–8.

[133] Ryan TJ, Antman EM, Brooks NH, et al. 1999 update: ACC/AHA guidelines for the management of patients with acute myocardial infarction: executive summary and recommendations: a report of the American College of Cardiology/ American Heart Association Task Force on Practice Guidelines (Committee on Management of Acute Myocardial Infarction). Circulation 1999; 100:1016–30.

[134] Rogers WJ, Canto JG, Lambrew CT, et al, for the Investigators in the National Registry of Myocardial Infarction 1, 2, and 3. Temporal trends in the treatment of over 1.5 million patients with myocardial infarction in the US from 1990 through 1999. J Am Coll Cardiol 2000;36:2056–63.

[135] Berger AK, Radford MJ, Krumholtz HM. Factors associated with delay in reperfusion therapy in elderly patients with acute myocardial infarction: analysis of the cooperative cardiovascular project. Am Heart J 2000;139:985–92.

[136] Selker HP, Beshansky JR, Griffith JL, for the TPI Trial Investigators. Use of the electrocardiograph-based thrombolytic predictive instrument to assist thrombolytic and reperfusion therapy for acute myocardial infarction: a multicenter randomized clinical effectiveness trial. Ann Intern Med 2002; 137:87–95.

[137] Barron HV, Bowlby LJ, Breen T, et al, for the National Registry of Myocardial Infarction 2 Investigators. Use of reperfusion therapy for acute myocardial infarction in the United States. Data from the National Registry of Myocardial Infarction 2. Circulation 1998;97:1150–6.

[138] Ting H, Lee T, Soukup J, et al. Impact of physician experience on triage of emergency room patients with acute chest pain at three teaching hospitals. Am J Med 1991;91:401–8.

[139] Reilly B, Evans A, Schaider J, et al. Impact of a clinical decision rule on hospital triage of patients with suspected acute cardiac ischemia in the emergency department. JAMA 2002;288:342–50.

[140] Baxt W, Skora J. Prospective validation of artificial neural network trained to identify acute myocardial infarction. Lancet 1996;347:12–5.

[141] Selker H, Beshansky J, Griffith J. Use of the electrocardiograph-based thrombolytic predictive instrument to assist thrombolytic and reperfusion therapy for acute myocardial infarction. Ann Intern Med 2002;137:87–95.

[142] Centers for Disease Control (CDC). Coronary heart disease incidence, by sex—United States,

1971–1987. MMWR Morb Mort Wkly Rep 1992; 41:526–9.

[143] Misra D. The women's health data book: a profile of women's health in the United States. 3rd edition. Washington (DC): Jacobs Institute of Women's Health. The Henry J. Kaiser Family Foundation; 2001. p. 69–73.

[144] Diamond G, Staniloff H, Forrester J, et al. Computer-assisted diagnosis in the noninvasive evaluation of patients with suspected coronary artery disease. J Am Coll Cardiol 1983;1:444–55.

[145] Merz C, Kelsey S, Pepine C, et al. The Women's Ischemia Syndrome Evaluation (WISE) study: protocol design, methodology and feasibility report. J Am Coll Cardiol 1999;33:1453–61.

[146] Kennedy J, Killip T, Fisher L, et al. The clinical spectrum of coronary artery disease and its surgical and medical management, 1974–1979. The Coronary Artery Surgery study. Circulation 1982;66: III16–23.

[147] Bybee K, Kara T, Prasad A, et al. Systemic review: transient left ventricular apical ballooning: a syndrome that mimics ST-segment elevation myocardial infarction. Ann Intern Med 2004; 141:858–65.

[148] Douglas P, Ginsburg G. The evaluation of chest pain in women. N Engl J Med 1996;334: 1311–5.

[149] Coronado B, Griffith J, Beshansky J, et al. Hospital mortality in women and men with acute cardiac ischemia: a prospective multicenter study. J Am Coll Cardiol 1997;29:1490–6.

[150] Vaccarino V, Parsons L, Every N, et al. Sex-based differences in early mortality after myocardial infarction. National Registry of Myocardial Infarction 2 participants. N Engl J Med 1999;341:217–25.

[151] Jacobs A, Kelsey S, Brooks M, et al. Better outcome for women compared with men undergoing coronary revascularization: a report from the Bypass Angioplasty Revascularization Investigation (BARI). Circulation 1998;98:1279–85.

[152] Edwards F, Carey J, Grover F, et al. Impact of gender on coronary bypass operative mortality. Ann Thorac Surg 1998;66:125–31.

[153] Mehilli J, Kastrati A, Dirschinger J, et al. Differences in prognostic factors and outcomes between women and men undergoing coronary artery stenting. JAMA 2000;284:1799–805.

[154] Maynard C, Beshansky J, Griffith J, et al. Influence of sex on the use of cardiac procedures in patients presenting to the emergency department: a prospective multicenter study. Circulation 1996;94:II93–8.

[155] Ayanian J, Epstein A. Differences in the use of procedures between women and men hospitalized for coronary heart disease. N Engl J Med 1991;325: 221–5.

[156] Romeo F, Rosano G, Martuscelli E, et al. Long-term follow-up of patients initially diagnosed as syndrome X. Am J Cardiol 1993;71:669–73.

[157] Sullivan A, Holdright D, Wright C, et al. Chest pain in women: clinical, investigative, and prognostic features. BMJ 1994;308:883–6.

[158] Kaski J, Rosano G, Collins P, et al. Cardiac syndrome X: clinical characteristics and left ventricular function. Long-term follow-up study. J Am Coll Cardiol 1995;25:807–14.

[159] Bairey Merz N, Bonow RO, Sopko G, et al. Women's Ischemic Syndrome Evaluation: current status and future research directions: report of the National heart, Lung and Blood Institute workshop. Circulation 2002;109:805–7.

[160] Lerner D, Kannel W. Patterns of coronary heart disease morbidity and mortality in the sexes: a 26-year follow-up of the Framingham population. Am Heart J 1986;111:383–90.

[161] Smith W, Kenicer M, Tunstall-Pedoe H, et al. Prevalence of coronary heart disease in Scotland: Scottish Heart Health Study. Br Heart J 1990; 64:295–8.

[162] Elveback L, Connolly D. Coronary heart disease in residents of Rochester, Minnesota, V: prognosis of patients with CAD based on initial manifestation. Mayo Clin Proc 1985;60:305–31.

[163] Seeman T, Mendes de Leon C, Berkman L, et al. Risk factors for coronary heart disease among older men and women: a prospective study of community-dwelling elderly. Am J Epidemiol 1993;138: 1037–49.

[164] Maynard C, Weaver W. Treatment of women with acute MI: new findings from the MITI Registry. J Myocard Ischemia 1992;4:27–37.

[165] Sharpe P, Clark N, Janz N. Differences in the impact and management of heart disease between older women and men. Women Health 1991;17: 25–34.

[166] Cunningham M, Lee T, Cook E, et al. The effect of gender on the probability of myocardial infarction among emergency department patients with acute chest pain. J Gen Intern Med 1989;4:392–8.

[167] Liao Y, Lui K, Dyer A, et al. Sex differential in the relationship of electrocardiographic ST-T abnormalities to risk of coronary death: 11.5 year follow-up findings of the Chicago heart association detection project in industry. Circulation 1987;75: 347–52.

[168] Lusiani L, Perrone A, Pesavento R, et al. Prevalence, clinical features, and acute course of atypical myocardial infarction. Angiology 1994;45:49–55.

[169] Fiebach N, Viscoli C, Horwitz R. Differences between women and men in survival after myocardial infarction: biology or methodology? JAMA 1990; 263:1092–6.

[170] Dittrich H, Gilpin E, Nicod P, et al. Acute myocardial infarction in women: influence of gender on mortality and prognostic variables. Am J Cardiol 1988;62:1–7.

[171] Murabito JM, Anderson KM, Kannel WB, et al. Risk of coronary heart disease in subjects with chest discomfort: the Framingham Heart Study. Am J Med 1990;89:297–302.

[172] Milner K, Funk M, Arnold A, et al. Typical symptoms are predictive of acute coronary syndromes in women. Am Heart J 2002;143:283–8.

[173] Milner K, Funk M, Richards S, et al. Gender differences in symptom presentation associated with coronary heart disease. Am J Cardiol 1999;84:396–9.

[174] Goldberg R, Goff D, Cooper L, et al. Age and sex differences in presentation of symptoms among patients with acute coronary disease: the REACT trial. Coron Artery Dis 2000;11:399–407.

[175] Maseri A, Crea F, Kaski J, et al. Mechanisms of angina pectoris in syndrome X. J Am Coll Cardiol 1991;17:499–506.

[176] Panting J, Gatehouse P, Yang G, et al. Abnormal subendocardial perfusion in cardiac syndrome X detected by cardiovascular magnetic resonance imaging. N Engl J Med 2002;346:1948–53.

[177] Quyyumi A. Endothelial function in health and disease: new insights into the genesis of cardiovascular disease. Am J Med 1998;105:32S–9S.

[178] Wiviott S, Cannon C, Morrow D, et al. Differential expression of cardiac biomarkers by gender in patients with unstable angina/non-ST-elevation myocardial infarction: a TACTICS-TIMI 18 substudy. Circulation 2004;109:580–6.

[179] Mueller C, Neumann F, Roskamm H, et al. Women do have an improved long-term outcome after non-ST-elevation acute coronary syndromes treated very early and predominantly with percutaneous coronary intervention: a prospective study in 1,450 consecutive patients. J Am Coll Cardiol 2002;40:245–50.

[180] Maynard C, Fisher L, Passamani E, et al. Blacks in the Coronary Artery Surgery Study (CASS): risk factors and coronary artery disease. Circulation 1986;74:64–71.

[181] Cooper R, Ford E. Comparability of risk factors for coronary artery disease among black and whites in the NHANES-I epidemiologic follow-up study. Ann Epidemiol 1992;2:637–45.

[182] Johnson P, Lee T, Cook E, et al. Effect of race on the presentation and management of patients with acute chest pain. Ann Intern Med 1993;118:593–601.

[183] Curry C, Lewis J. Cardiac anatomy and function in hypertensive blacks. In: Hall W, Sanders E, Shulman N, editors. Hypertension in blacks. Chicago (IL): Year Book Medical Publishers; 1985. p. 61–7.

[184] Lenfant C. Report of the NHLBI working group on research in coronary artery disease in blacks. Circulation 1994;90:1613–23.

[185] Becker L, Han B, Meyer P, et al. Racial differences in the incidence of cardiac arrest and subsequent survival. N Engl J Med 1993;329:600–6.

[186] Cowie M, Fahrenbruch C, Cobb L, et al. Out-of-hospital cardiac arrest: racial differences in outcome in Seattle. Am J Public Health 1993; 83:955–9.

[187] Maseri A. Women's Ischemic Syndrome Evaluation: current status and future research directions. Circulation 2004;109:e62–3.

[188] Maynard C, Beshansky J, Griffith J, et al. Causes of chest pain and symptoms suggestive of acute cardiac ischemia in African-American patients presenting to the emergency department: a multicenter study. J Natl Med Assoc 1997;89:665–71.

[189] Kohn L, Corrigan J, Donaldson N, editors. To err is human: building a safer health system. Washington (DC): National Academy Press; 2000.

[190] Leale L. Error in medicine. JAMA 1994;272: 1851–7.

[191] Zucker D, Griffith J, Beshansky JR, et al. Presentations of acute myocardial infarction in men and women. J Gen Intern Med 1997;12: 79–87.

[192] Jayes R, Beshansky J, D'Agostino R, et al. Do patients' coronary risk factor reports predict acute cardiac ischemia in the emergency department? A multicenter study. J Clin Epidemiol 1992;45: 621–6.

[193] Miller C, Lindsell C, Khandelwal S, et al. Is the initial diagnostic impression of "noncardiac chest pain" adequate to exclude cardiac disease? Ann Emerg Med 2004;44:565–74.

Use of Biomarkers in the Emergency Department and Chest Pain Unit

Allan S. Jaffe, MD

*Consultant in Cardiology and Laboratory Medicine Mayo Clinic and Mayo Medical School,
200 First Street SW, Rochester, MN 55905, USA*

The use of biomarkers of cardiac injury in the emergency department (ED) and observation unit settings has several nuances that are different and, therefore, worthy of its own set of use guidelines. The markers that are used, however, are the same. The primary marker of choice continues to be cardiac troponin (Tn). Other markers that have been advocated for use in the ED because of the need for rapid triage have been myoglobin and fatty acid binding protein. In addition, some centers still prefer less sensitive and less specific markers, such as creatine kinase myocardial band (CK-MB). More recently, a push has occurred to develop markers of ischemia, such as ischemia modified albumin (IMA), to determine which patients have ischemia, even in the absence of cardiac injury. As troponin assays become more sensitive and how to use them becomes better understood, the use of other markers are being relegated to lesser and lesser roles. Markers of ischemia would be useful but at present, despite some enthusiasm, they are not ready for routine use. Before describing the recommendations for clinical use of biomarkers in the ED, a basic understanding of some of the science and measurement issues related to these analytes is helpful.

Background

Troponin

The Tns are a complex of three proteins (I, C, and T) that regulate the calcium mediated

Dr. Jaffe receives research support and is a consultant for Dade, Beckman, and Roche. He has consulted for most major diagnostic companies over the years.

E-mail address: Jaffe.Allan@Mayo.edu

interaction of actin and myosin [1]. Tissue-specific isoforms of each troponin exist; however, the cardiac form of troponin C is shared by smooth muscle, so it lacks cardiac specificity [2,3]. For cardiac troponin I (cTnI), the cardiac isoform is structurally different due to the presence of a 32-amino acid posttranslational tail [4] and sequence dissimilarity with other isoforms [5]. Various monoclonal antibodies have been developed that are highly specific and have no cross-reactivity with other forms [6]. Since cTnI has not been found in any tissue outside of the heart, even in response to tissue injury, it has unique specificity for the heart [7,8].

Three different genes control the expression of cardiac troponin T. These genes and alternative mRNA splicing produce a series of isoforms with varying sequences [9]. Cardiac muscle contains four of these isoforms, but only one is characteristic of the normal adult heart, and that is the one against which antibodies have been made [10]. Some of the other cardiac troponin T (cTnT) isoforms are expressed in other tissues, including skeletal muscle in response to injury [11], and the initial assay for cTnT detected some of these and cross-reacting skeletal muscle TnT [12]. However, it has been established with immuno-histochemistry and PCR, that the antibodies used in the present iteration of the assay do not detect these forms [13,14]. Accordingly, cTnI and cTnT have high specificity for the heart.

In addition to having high specificity, these proteins have high sensitivity. Most of the troponin is complexed to the contractile apparatus. A small amount (3% for cTnI and 6% for cTnT) exists which is not structurally bound [15,16]. This "small amount" has been termed the "cytosolic pool," although its localization was not proved definitively. The relative amount of troponin in this pool is similar to that of CK-MB [15]. This pool is released acutely. Because it is of the same magnitude as CK-MB, troponin might be expected to have similar sensitively, but the sensitivity of the troponins is substantially better because a greater percentage of what is lost from the heart eventually resides in blood (ie, the so-called "release ratio" is higher) [17]. Subsequently, prolonged elevations of troponin occur as a result of degradation of the contractile pool in the area that has been injured. The cytosolic pool permits the early kinetics of release similar to that of CK-MB or even earlier with more sensitive assays. The persistence of elevation is due to release from the structural pool, since the half life of troponin in the circulation is short [18]. The degree of persistence varies tremendously and is somewhat longer for cTnT [19] than for some of the cTnI assays. For cTnI, the degree of persistence in part depends on which forms are measured and which epitopes the antibodies used in the assay are targeted toward. A 7- to 10-day time window during which elevations may be present, however, is a reasonable estimate. Accordingly, if the initial troponin in a patient who presents with chest pain is elevated, it may be from a prior event or from an acute event. In that situation, a rising pattern is helpful in determining if the event is acute.

The heterogeneity of assays indicated above is of particular importance. Different assays detect different forms, and various complex formations and protein modifications exist that can alter the relative sensitivity and specificity of one assay compared with another. The International Federation of Clinical Chemistry and Laboratory Medicine (IFCC) group has published quality specifications for troponin assays and an analysis of the presently available assays [20,21]. Clinicians must understand which assay is being used in their center to understand how to use the data optimally [22]. As lower values are used, such as the recommended value of the 99th percentile as recommended by the ESC/ACC Committee on the Redefinition of MI [23,24], the assays invariably perform with less precision. This puts clinicians and patients at risk for false-positive and false-negative results. Accordingly, a recommendation has been made that the 99th percentile be measured with a less than 10% coefficient of variability (CV). This measurement will eliminate many false-positive and false-negative values and has been recommended until all assays can achieve

detection of the 99th percentile of a normal reference population with that level of precision [21,25]. At present, only one assay meets that specification. In general, the 10% CV value is close to the 99th percentile but how close they are varies assay to assay (Table 1). Thus, clinicians must know the characteristics of the assay that they rely on. In addition, other analytic issues exist that can confound assays. Good laboratories should be able to help trouble-shoot potential problems. The most common problem is fibrin interference, which may on occasion require additional centrifugation of the sample to remove cross-reacting fibrin.

In addition, it should be appreciated that troponin elevations indicate cardiac injury but do not define the nature of the cardiac injury. In patients who present with chest pain, most troponin elevations likely are related to coronary artery disease. The astute clinician must be aware, however, that elevations in troponin can occur from acute pulmonary embolism, myocarditis, and congestive heart failure to name just a few common entities that can confound the diagnosis of acute myocardial infarction [26]. Thus, the idea that an elevated troponin is synonymous with

Table 1
Concentrations corresponding to 10% CV imprecision and 99th percentile reference limit for the evaluated troponin assays

Platform	99th percentile limit* ($\mu g/L$)	10% total CV concentration ($\mu g/L$)	Ratio of 10% CV concentration to 99th percentile limit
AxSYM	0.30	1.22	4.1
Centaur	0.10	0.33	3.3
Access	0.04	0.06	1.5
Vidas	0.10	0.36	3.6
Dimension RxL	0.07	0.26	3.7
Stratus CS	0.07	0.10	1.4
Alpha Dx	0.15	ND	
E170	0.01	0.04	4.0
AIA21	0.06	0.09	1.5

Abbreviations: CV, coefficient of variability; ND, not determined.

* Data obtained from manufacturer's package insert or through personal communications with manufacturers.

Data from Panteghini M, Pagani F, Yeo KT, et al. Evaluation of imprecision for cardiac troponin assays at low-range concentrations. Clin Chem 2004;50:327–32.

coronary artery disease can lead to missed diagnoses and suboptimal patient care.

Creatine kinase myocardial band

CK-MB [27] served us well for many years, and facile assays exist that are reasonably sensitive. The percentage of CK-MB depleted from the heart that ends up in the blood, however, is modest (15% in the absence of reperfusion and 30% with reperfusion), limiting its sensitivity compared with troponin. In addition, because there is CK-MB in skeletal muscle, individuals have a circulating constitutive level and CK-MB elevations can be diagnosed only when that broad normal range is exceeded. This further limits sensitivity, but it also has implications for specificity. Elevations can occur as a result of skeletal muscle damage in patients with renal failure and abnormalities in clearance associated with hypothyroidism. In addition, re-expression of the B-chain gene in skeletal muscle when damage to muscle occurs can increase the percentage of CK-MB and confound diagnosis. The use of the relative index, which relies on the percentage of CK-MB with respect to total CK, improves specificity, but because there is so much CK in skeletal muscle, it diminishes sensitivity in individuals who may have coronary and skeletal muscle diseases [28]. In addition, a multiplicity of assay issues for CK-MB exist that assay issues often are more complex than those related to troponin. The role of CK-MB in 2005 is unclear beyond its role in helping to evaluate the timing of events in patients who present with chest discomfort.

Myoglobin

Myoglobin [27] is a 17.8 kd protein that is released from all tissues ubiquitously. It is released rapidly and has a short persistence in the circulation (< 20 minutes in studies in which it has been injected) and, therefore, a pattern of increases and reductions are common. This protein responds rapidly and quickly to insults, and if the insults are sustained, elevations will persist. Because it has cleared renally, abnormalities in renal function can cause substantial elevations, and because it is ubiquitous, it lacks specificity for the heart. Myoglobin can and has been used as a nonspecific marker to screen for disease in patients who often have been poorly triaged. In addition, many studies have used high, rather then conventional,

troponin cutoff values in their studies, which amplifies the value of the testing [29,30]. As better troponin assays have been developed, the amount of time saved by a nonspecific marker like myoglobin has progressively diminished [31].

Fatty acid binding protein

Fatty acid binding protein [27] is similar to myoglobin in its release kinetics, but a much larger percentage exists in the heart relative to skeletal muscle. This increased percentage has led some to claim an increased degree of specificity for elevations. Again, with more sensitive assays for troponin, it is unclear how much time measuring fatty acid binding protein might save.

Markers of ischemia

The only test presently approved for detection of ischemia by the Federal Drug Administration (FDA) is IMA. Based on experimental data, it has been argued that ischemia injures the amino terminal end of albumin, which inhibits it from binding cobalt [32]. This fact has been taken advantage of in an assay that looks at the percentage of delivered cobalt that becomes bound. The argument is that this test can provide information concerning whether ischemia has occurred in the absence of necrosis. In response to ischemia, elevations of IMA do occur. They are short lived (roughly four hours), however, and then diminish [33]. These elevations, it is argued, can be used to define if ischemia has occurred and, thus, could be helpful in the triage of patients in the ED setting, especially in excluding ischemia. The problem with these studies is the lack of a clear gold standard. In addition, low levels of IMA seem protective and high levels seem to have some prognostic significance for eventual troponin elevations [34]. In the high pretest probability high-risk group, however, it is unclear whether this test is necessary to further define risk. In the low-risk group, a similar question can be posed. Most of the patients in whom clinicians are unsure, however, have values in the middle range and it is unclear how well they separate those with ischemia from those without ischemia. Furthermore, ischemia in other tissues also stimulates abnormalities in albumin binding also and assay issues exist related to the effect of lactate and pH [35]. These issues are why the FDA-approval was predicated on the fact that a negative test excludes ischemia. The argument, has been made, therefore, that if a test is performed and fails to show an elevation, that those patients are probably safe to be sent home without further testing. Various studies, some of which are commented on in later discussion, have attempted to prove that postulate. On the other hand, what should be done with a positive test is less clear. Obviously, if markers of cardiac injury subsequently show that necrosis exists, then the patient is triaged easily. Suppose, however, that no evidence of necrosis exists. Is there a reason, based on the fact that an ischemic bed exists somewhere, to do more work on that particular patient? Perhaps this is the group that requires stress testing? Do these patients require evaluation of other organ systems also? These questions require answers before advocacy for the widespread use of the test.

These markers of cardiac injury need to be intertwined within the overall risk assessment of patients who present to the ED.

Clinical use of troponin and other biomarkers in specific patient subsets seen in the emergency department or chest pain unit

The use of biomarkers is predicated in large part on the underlying nature of the patients being evaluated. The following suggestions are developed predicated on risk stratification.

Patients with ST elevation and myocardial infarction

Patients who present with ST elevation myocardial infarction (STEMI) do not need biomarker measurements before the initiation of therapy. Therapy should be started before the return of biomarker data to ensure the most rapid initiation of therapy, which is critical in this setting. Recent data suggests that troponin elevations identify patients at high risk for adverse events. Patients who have elevated troponins have a lower rate of coronary recanalization with thrombolysis [36] or in response to direct percutaneous coronary intervention (PCI) (Fig. 1) [37]. The largest part of this effect probably is related to the fact that it takes time for elevations of troponin to develop, and therefore, patients who present with elevated troponin, are patients who present later than those who do not manifest elevations. Time from the onset of symptoms to treatment is the most critical determinant of the success or failure of recanalization and limitation of infarction size, which is likely the largest reason why patients who present with

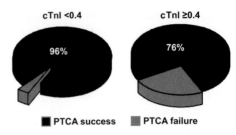

Fig. 1. Frequency of successful direct PCI when troponin is elevated (cTnI > .4 ng/ml) compared with when it is "normal" (< 0.4ng/ml). *From* Matetzky S, Sharir T, Domingo M, et al. Elevated troponin I level on admission is associated with adverse outcome of primary angioplasty in acute myocardial infarction. Circulation 2000;102:1611–6; with permission).

elevated troponins do poorly. In analyses where one attempts to correct for the time from the onset of infarction to presentation, however, a major adverse effect of having an elevated troponin still exists (Fig. 2) [38]. The ability to determine when the onset of symptoms has occurred may be inaccurate or it may be that other pathophysiology exists related to how infarction is initiated, which mediates this effect. Nonetheless, knowing that the troponin is elevated in patients who present with STEMI predicts a lower likelihood of recanalization, a lower TIMI flow grade with reperfusion [39], and an adverse short- and long-term prognosis. The therapeutic implications of this phenomenon are unclear at this time, but in one study, stenting seemed to have a positive impact [40]. No

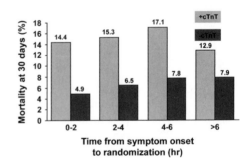

Fig. 2. Relationship between the time of onset of symptoms, troponin and mortality. Note at any given time from the onset of symptoms to randomization there is an increased risk associated with an elevated troponin. *From* Ohman EM, Armstrong PW, White HD, et al. Risk stratification with a point-of-care cardiac troponin T test in acute myocardial infarction. GUSTO III Investigators. Global use of strategies to open occluded coronary arteries. Am J Cardiol 1999;84:1281–6; with permission.

data exist about this issue with biomarkers other than troponin.

High-risk patients with acute coronary syndromes

The high-risk patient group that has been well represented in most of the major intervention trials. These patients are often elderly, have had chest discomfort at rest, have transient ST segment changes or bundle branch block, an increase in the tempo of their symptoms or signs, and can have evidence of hemodynamic instability or arrhythmias. This group often has a high frequency of elevated troponins in the range of 50% to 60% [41–44]. If so, they fulfill the definition of non-STEMI per the ESC/ACC [23,24].

In this patient subset, as with STEMI, an elevated troponin often is unnecessary for decisions concerning admission. Information suggests, however, that elevated troponin values define a subset at high risk [41–45] and provide important information with which to guide therapy. Patients who present with elevated troponins have adverse coronary anatomy as assessed angiographically with more thrombus, reduced TIMI grades of perfusion, more complex lesions, and more extensive disease (Fig. 3) [46]. Thus, they require and are more apt to benefit from the use of more sophisticated therapies. These patients have fewer ischemic events if treated with low molecular weight heparin rather than unfractionated heparin [47]. These studies do not show a mortality benefit. IIB/IIIA agents also have been found to markedly reduce death and recurrent MI in these patients, but, again, the benefit is almost

exclusively in the recurrent event category. The effects of IIB/IIIA agents are particularly strong in those patients who undergo percutaneous intervention [48]. Their use, then, is the present standard of care for patients who present with acute coronary syndromes and elevated troponins [49]. Patients who present without elevated troponins do not seem to benefit from the adjunctive use of low molecular weight heparin or IIB/IIIA agents in the setting of acute coronary syndromes. The recent accelerating use of clopidogrel has raised questions about whether the results of these previous studies would be the same if clopidogrel had been used adjunctively. Clopidogrel recapitulates the benefits of IIB/IIIA agents, it could be argued. Alternatively, it is possible that synergism exists between clopidogrel and IIB/IIIA agents and that patients would benefit even more from the combination. Until ongoing trials answer this key question, the standards and guidelines proposed by the American Heart Association/American Cardiac College would recommend that patients who present with an acute coronary syndrome and an elevated troponin receive IIB/IIIA agents [49]. In the CURE trial, clopidogrel seemed to benefit patients who presented with and without troponin elevations [50].

As might be expected, because short-term benefit is associated with the use of these agents so is long term benefit [51]. In addition, recent data has substantiated that the use of early invasive therapy, which in the United States means cardiac catheterization within the next 12 to 24 hours and interventional therapy (with stenting and a PCI or coronary artery bypass grafting),

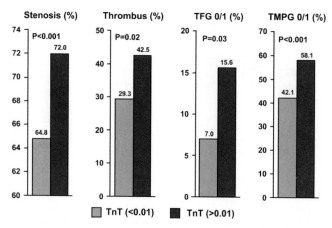

Fig. 3. Angiographic relationships with troponin in patients with acute coronary syndromes. *From* Scirica BM, Morrow DA. Troponins in acute coronary syndromes. Prog Cardiovasc Dis 2004;47:177–88; with permission.

leads to substantial benefit in patients who present with acute coronary syndromes and elevated troponins [52,53]. This benefit is not generally observed in patients who present without elevations. The one exception recently published is that women who more often present with normal values of troponin but elevated BNP or CRP may, nonetheless, benefit from an early aggressive invasive strategy (Fig. 4) [54]. Unfortunately, the data were based not on serial troponin data but on only the initial sample. Few other data exist at present to substantiate this claim.

Intermediate and low risk for the patient subsets

The intermediate and low-risk subsets of patients are the groups that usually are problematic in the ED or chest pain unit. The intermediate risk group often does not have rest pain or ongoing pain and lacks ECG changes, although this group may have a high pretest probability of having coronary artery disease. In contrast, the low-risk group usually has normal ECGs or only minimal T changes and often may not have impressive risk factors. Nonetheless, because of the need to diagnose as many patients as possible at risk for acute infarction given its morbidity and potential mortality, these patients need to be triaged and evaluated aggressively. In addition, this group is where a high percentage of malpractice dollars are lost. For these reasons, a conservative approach often is mandated. The downside of this approach is that it is costly to admit a large number of patients solely because of this concern.

In this setting, troponin markers are again the markers of choice. In a landmark study of 733 consecutive patients who presented with chest discomfort, Hamm and colleagues [55] demonstrated that almost all patients at short-term risk could be identified using troponin (Fig. 5). Several caveats existed that were important in that study. The first caveat was that at least one troponin value needed to have been obtained at least 6 hours after the onset of symptoms to make sure that there had been time for the marker to rise. Unless the onset of symptoms is totally clear, it is wise to start the clock at the time of presentation. A second important caveat was the troponin value used was the limit of detectablity (ie, a highly sensitive standard). Although the assays involved were less sensitive than contemporary assays, the concept probably is still correct. With modern assays, the use of the so-called 10% CV value is advocated [21,25]. When there is a high pretest probability of disease, as in the patients with overt acute coronary syndromes, the data are clear that using the lowest level of troponin detectable, (ie, the 99th percentile), provides greater predictive accuracy [56]. The pretest probability of a given elevation, being a true positive rather than a false positive, is high in the group with severe disease. When one deals with a patient population where the pretest probability of disease is somewhat less, severe disease is less likely. In that

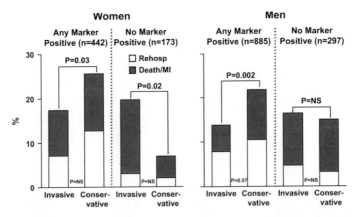

Fig. 4. Outcomes of therapy by gender. Note patients with any positive marker (troponin, BNP or CRP) benefited. Some suggestion of detriment exists in an invasive therapy in patients without an elevations in any marker. *From* Wiviott SD, Cannon CP, Morrow DA, et al. Differential expression of cardiac biomarkers by gender in patients with unstable angina/non-ST-elevation myocardial infarction: a TACTICS-TIMI 18 (Treat Angina with Aggrastat and determine Cost of Therapy with an Invasive or Conservative Strategy-Thrombolysis In Myocardial Infarction 18) substudy. Circulation 2004;109:580–6; with permission.

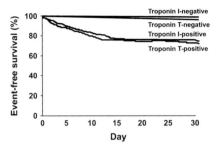

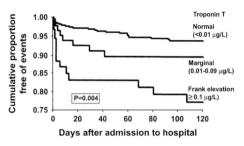

Fig. 5. Survival of patients evaluated to include or exclude acute myocardial infarction. *From* Hamm CW, Goldmann BU, Heeschen C, et al. Emergency room triage of patients with acute chest pain by means of rapid testing for TnT or troponin I. N Engl J Med 1997;337:1648–53; with permission.

Fig. 6. Events in patients with various troponin values. Note even what are called in this figure marginal elevations have prognostic significance. *From* Henrikson CA, Howell EE, Bush DE. et al. Prognostic usefulness of marginal troponin T elevation. Am J Cardiol 2004;93:275–9; with permission.

population, if one uses values where the assays are imprecise, the percentage of false-positive elevations is far greater. For that reason, in this population, it is important to use what is known as the 10% CV value rather than the 99th percentile, which is a level where few, if any, false-positive elevations are caused by imprecision. Most would advocate using the 10% CV level (which is usually close to the 99th percentile) in all patients with the recognition that in patients who are at high risk clinically even lower levels may have a prognostic and therapeutic significance. In the intermediate and lower-risk groups, however, if one uses the lower level (ie, the 99th percentile), an unacceptably high percentage of patients is apt to have false positives. The 99th percentile and the 10% CV values for present assays are shown in Table 1 [21]. Caution is advised because the assays themselves and, thus, the values, presented change frequently.

Many of the studies that have been done have used high cutoff values for troponin in evaluating ED patients. Recently, a study from Johns Hopkins [57] evaluated patients who had low levels and patients who had intermediate levels between the 99th percentile and what is known as the ROC determined cutoff value for MI, a level initially used when the assays were novel to match the sensitivity of CK-MB. As with almost every other study that has been done, a substantial short- and long-term adverse prognostic effect was observed with even minor elevations of troponin (Fig. 6). More of these studies are needed, but they were consonant with the vast body of clinical information that suggests the elevated troponin values usually have important prognostic significance.

Intermediate or low-risk patients who present with an elevated troponin may or may not have acute ischemic heart disease. Many etiologies exist for troponin elevations, and many of them may need to be evaluated as part of an evaluation in the ED or chest pain center. Two of the more common ones are pulmonary embolism [58,59] and congestive heart failure [60,61]; these can mimic the presentation of an acute coronary syndrome and both are associated with an adverse prognosis when troponin elevations occur. In general, the troponin elevations observed are modest. Elevations associated with pulmonary embolism resolve rapidly (by 40 hours) [62]. Elevations in patients who present with congestive heart failure persist for a longer period and are found in patients with and without coronary artery disease. Chest pain and elevated troponins in patients may be caused by some of these other etiologies for elevated troponins, but no overt coronary artery disease angiographically were at accentuated risk in the Tactics-TIMI-18 trial [63]. The coronary angiogram may not be, in every instance, totally reliable for the detection of acute coronary artery disease, especially when a delay exists between the onset of symptoms and implementation of the diagnostic procedure. Nonetheless, these data suggest that the due diligence of any good clinician seeing a patient who presents with an elevated troponin in these intermediate and lower-risk groups is not only to determine whether or not the patient is at risk for acute ischemic heart disease. The physician must also make sure that the elevations are not a result of other causes that may require different types of therapy (see later discussion).

Extensive evaluations of low risk patients have not been common. In an important study, however, the group from Galveston [64] evaluated a cohort of over 400 patients who presented with a low-risk history and normal or near normal ECG. They selected their inclusion criteria to be associated with a 5% to 7% incidence of MI. They then evaluated the frequency of coronary artery disease by offering angiography to all those patients with an elevated troponin and enrolling a control group that was selected from similar patients with chest pain but without elevated troponins as a comparison group. In that study, which used a higher troponin than has been advocated by this author, patients who presented with an elevated troponin had a 90% frequency of angiographic coronary artery disease. In two thirds, it was double or triple vessel disease. In addition, during follow up, these individuals had a 33% incidence of ischemic events caused by coronary heart disease (Fig. 7). These data demonstrate the importance of an elevated troponin in patients who present with chest pain, even those at low risk. Had the investigators used a lower cutoff value, the 10% CV value for example, it is possible there may well have been a larger number of patients with increases attributable to diseases other than acute ischemic heart disease. However, it is possible that the frequency of coronary artery disease seen in the control group of 23% would have been substantially diminished. Thus, it seems likely that the use of the low cutoff values may help to identify patients who are at risk when they present with chest discomfort.

No comparable data exist with any other markers in either risk group.

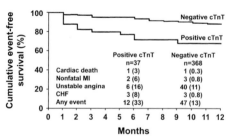

Fig. 7. Prognostic significance of troponin elevations in patients with normal or near normal electrocardiograms. *From* deFilippi CR, Tocchi M, Parmar RJ, et al. Cardiac troponin T in chest pain unit patients without ischemic electrocardiographic changes: angiographic correlates and long-term clinical outcomes. J Am Coll Cardiol 2000;35:1827–34; with permission.

Patients with renal failure

The most common cause of death in patients who present with renal failure is cardiovascular [65]. Coronary artery disease is common and events tend to occur during the period when patients have a longer interval between dialysis visits [65,66]. In patients who present with acute coronary syndromes, the interpretation of troponin elevations should not be altered by the presence of renal failure [67].

Other dialysis patients at risk who do not have acute coronary syndromes can often also be identified by having an elevated troponin [68,69]. These patients invariably have pathologic evidence of cardiac injury [70]. This group manifests differences in the frequency of elevations of cTnT and cTnI [68]. Many more elevations of cTnT occur than cTnI, and this has led some people to believe that the elevations of cTnT are false positives. With the initial iteration of the assay this might have been the case but is no longer a credible explanation. The present iteration of the assay has been shown not to cross-react with noncardiac isoforms of cTnT [10–14], nor does it detect the isoforms of cardiac cTnT that can be re-expressed in response to skeletal muscle injury. The epitopes for detection of cTnI may be lost in the milieu of renal failure. A substantial percentage of patients on dialysis, therefore, have elevations of troponin, especially cTnT, posing a difficult problem in the ED because the initial samples in these patients may indicate an elevation. Having a baseline cTnT is helpful. The FDA has approved the use of cTnT for risk stratification in patients who are on dialysis, and it is recommended that baseline values be available for comparison. If baseline values are not available, looking for a change in serial values is helpful. Patients who experience rising elevations are far more likely to have acute events than those whose values stay the same. This information does not imply that the latter are false positives only that they are less apt to be associated with an acute event. In a group, such as dialysis patients, where elevations in the absence of acute ischemic heart disease are common, this is a helpful approach to determine which patients require admission or urgent care and which do not. This same principle seems to be the case in patients who seem to be at risk for re-infarction [71]. Initial guidelines suggested the use of other markers to help in this area, but it is clear clinically, although extensive collaborating data have yet to be developed in the literature, that using rising values are an effective strategy. Thus, dialysis patients who present with rising values are those in need of aggressive care. Patients who present with more chronic elevations can be evaluated more electively assuming no other clinical signs exist pointing to acute disease. This evaluation can include considerations of all other entities capable of causing elevations in troponin, such as pulmonary embolism, congestive heart failure, and the like.

These caveats apply only to patients who are on dialysis. Although there are an increased number of elevations of troponin in patients who present with significant renal dysfunction, most seem to be caused by concomitant co-morbidities and are not synonymous with the chronic elevations seen in dialysis patients. Accordingly, the caveats above should be applied to dialysis patients only. The concept that elevations in troponin with milder forms of renal dysfunction can be attributed to this chronic process is at present unsupported by data. The potential etiologies of troponin elevations in dialysis patients likely are related to the metabolic milieu of dialysis, concomitant endothelial dysfunction, severe hypertension with LVH, acute ventricular stretch, and various other mechanisms that occur in patients who present with renal dysfunction. Delayed clearance of the troponin by way of the kidneys is an unlikely cause of the troponin elevations.

Other etiologies for elevated troponins

As indicated in earlier discussion and in Box 1, acute ischemic heart disease is only one reason for elevations. Many other reasons exist that need to be considered [26]:

1. Many of the entities listed involve some degree of ischemia but it is not ischemia necessarily caused by acute coronary abnormalities. For example, patients who present with left ventricular hypertrophy, whether caused by hypertension, aortic stenosis, or hypertrophic cardiomyopathy, and so forth, are known to have an underperfused subendocardium. Thus, patients may be at risk if rapid heart rates, hypotension, or hypertension for elevated troponins as a result of injury to the sub-endocardium. When patients have arrhythmias, a similar mechanism could be involved. This mechanism is probably the mechanism for elevations by

---

Box 1. Elevations of troponins without overt ischemic heart disease

- Trauma (including contusion; ablation; pacing; ICD firings, such as atrial defibrillators, cardioversion, endomyocardial biopsy, cardiac surgery, after-interventional–closure of ASDs)
- Congestive heart failure—acute and chronic
- Aortic valve disease and HOCM with significant LVH
- Hypertension
- Hypotension, often with arrhythmias
- Postoperative noncardiac surgery patients who seem to do well
- Renal failure
- Critically ill patients, especially with diabetes, respiratory failure
- Drug toxicity (eg, adriamycin, 5 FU, herceptin, snake venoms)
- Hypothyroidism
- Coronary vasospasm, including apical ballooning syndrome
- Inflammatory diseases (eg, myocarditis, including Parvovirus B19, Kawasaki disease, sarcoid, smallpox vaccination, or myocardial extension of BE)
- Post-PCI patients who seem to be uncomplicated
- Pulmonary embolism, severe pulmonary hypertension
- Sepsis
- Burns, especially if TBSA greater than 30%
- Infiltrative diseases, including amyloidosis, hemachromatosis, sarcoidosis, and scleroderma
- Acute neurologic disease, including CVA, subarchnoid bleeds
- Rhabdomyolysis with cardiac injury
- Transplant vasculopathy
- Vital exhaustion

---

which pulmonary embolism albeit in the right rather than the left ventricle, induces injury.

2. Cardiac toxicity as a result of drugs, snake bites, or other toxins in the environment are certainly capable of causing troponin

elevations. Heat shock protein or TNF are believed to participate in cardiac injury seen with sepsis.

3. Myocarditis, acute or chronic, can cause troponin elevations and a series of patients who might be confused with those suffering with STEMI has been published. The diagnosis should be considered in patients initially suspected of having acute coronary syndromes who have normal coronary arteries.

4. Cardiomyopathies, congestive or infiltrative, and congestive heart failure likely caused by wall stress and reduced subendocardial perfusion are also capable of leading to elevated troponins and have significant prognostic significance.

5. Critically ill patients. A large body of information suggests that elevations in troponin are common and highly prognostic in patients who are critically ill whether in the hospital or ED.

The use of other markers

Many studies previously done suggest that because increases in short-acting markers, such as myoglobin or fatty acid binding protein, or in the past, isoforms of CK increase more rapidly than troponin that they may save time in the ED

or chest pain clinic [27,29,30,72]. The value of this approach is predominantly to exclude infarction at an earlier point in time because these analytes lack cardiac specificity and often are falsely positive. Thus, what has been relied on is their negative predictive value, which is fairly high. A critical issue in this area has been that many of these studies done evaluating these analytes have used insensitive troponin assays or high cutoff values despite the use of sensitive assays. Recent data suggest that as one begins to use cutoff values, such as the 99th percentile and 10% CV that the difference in timing associated with these other laboratory tests becomes more modest than previously suggested (Fig. 8) [31]. A similar approach relying on the negative predictive value of nonelevated values has been taken with IMA [32–34], which is a marker of ischemia rather than necrosis. The influence of more sensitive troponin assays on the timing of elevations can also influence the amount of time saved with this analyte. The time saved which is now more modestly worthwhile compared with the cost and the confounds associated with the frequent false positives. The studies done with IMA have used more contemporary troponin assays and cutoff values [32–34] but continuing issues exist concerning the proper cutoff values for the test, analytic issues related to pH and lactate [35] and concern

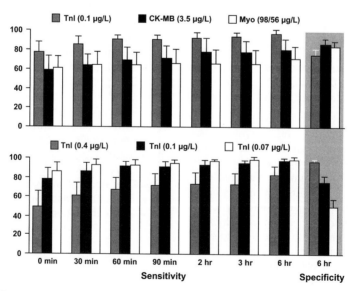

Fig. 8. Sensitivity of cTnI, CK-MB and myoglobin over time using modern prognostic cutoff values. Note that 0.7 ng/ml is the 99th percentile for the assay used. *From* Eggers KM, Oldgren J, Nordenskjold A, et al. Diagnostic value of serial measurement of cardiac markers in patients with chest pain: limited value of adding myoglobin to troponin I for exclusion of myocardial infarction. Am Heart J 2004;148:574–81;with permission.

about what should be done if a patient has an elevated IMA without an elevated troponin. Accordingly, a much simpler, more cost-effective paradigm would be to measure troponins on two occasions: (1) when the patient first presents and (2) 6 hours later or earlier if the onset of symptoms is totally clear. Additional data likely will shorten this time somewhat also. This paradigm would be a highly sensitive, highly specific, and cost-effective way of triage but requires thoughtful consideration of the etiologies of the potential troponin elevations, some clinical judgment, and a knowledge of the assays that are used locally.

References

[1] Takeda S, Yamashita A, Maeda K, et al. Structure of the core domain of human cardiac troponin in the Ca(2 +)-saturated form. Nature 2003;424:35–41.

[2] Dhoot GK, Gell PG, Perry SV. The localization of the different forms of troponin I in skeletal and cardiac muscle cells. Exp Cell Res 1978;117:357–70.

[3] Dhoot GK, Perry SV. Distribution of polymorphic forms of troponin components and tropomyosin in skeletal muscle. Nature 1979;278:714–8.

[4] Perry SV. Troponin I: inhibitor or facilitator. Mol Cell Biochem 1999;190:9–32.

[5] Katrukha A. Antibody selection strategies in cardiac troponin assay. In: Wu AHB, editor. Cardiac markers. 2nd edition. Totowa (NJ): Humana Press Inc.; 2003. p. 173–85.

[6] Larue C, Defacque-Lacquement H, Calzolari C, et al. New monoclonal antibodies as probes for human cardiac troponin I: epitopic analysis with synthetic peptides. Mol Immunol 1992;29:271–8.

[7] Toyota N, Shimada Y. Differentiation of troponin in cardiac and skeletal muscles in chicken embryos as studied by immunofluorescence microscopy. J Cell Biol 1981;91:497–504.

[8] Bodor GS, Porterfield D, Voss EM, et al. Cardiac troponin-I is not expressed in fetal and healthy or diseased adult human skeletal muscle tissue. Clin Chem 1995;41:1710–5.

[9] Perry SV. Troponin T genetics, properties and function. J Muscle Res Cell Motil 1998;19:575–602.

[10] Muller-Bardorff M, Hallermayer K, Schroder A, et al. Improved troponin T ELISA specific for cardiac troponin T isoform: assay development and analytical and clinical validation. Clin Chem 1997;43:458–66.

[11] Bodor GS, Survant L, Voss EM, et al. Cardiac troponin T composition in normal and regenerating human skeletal muscle. Clin Chem 1997;43:476–84.

[12] Katus HA, Looser S, Hallermayer K, et al. Development and in vitro characterization of a new immunoassay of cardiac troponin T. Clin Chem 1992;38:386–93.

[13] Ricchiuti V, Voss EM, Ney A, et al. Cardiac troponin T isoforms expressed in renal diseased skeletal muscle will not cause false-positive results by the second generation cardiac troponin T assay by Boehringer Mannheim. Clin Chem 1998;44:1919–24.

[14] Haller C, Zehelein J, Remppis A, et al. Cardiac troponin T in patients with end-stage renal disease: absence of expression in truncal skeletal muscle. Clin Chem 1998;44:930–8.

[15] Adams JE III, Schechtman KB, Landt Y, et al. Comparable detection of acute myocardial infarction by creatine kinase MB isoenzyme and cardiac troponin I. Clin Chem 1994;40:1291–5.

[16] Katus HA, Remppis A, Scheffold T, et al. Intracellular compartmentation of cardiac troponin T and its release kinetics in patients with reperfused and non-reperfused myocardial infarction. Am J Cardiol 1991;67:1360–7.

[17] Tanaka H, Abe S, Yamashita T, et al. Serum levels of cardiac troponin I and troponin T in estimating myocardial infarct size soon after reperfusion. Coron Artery Dis 1997;8:433–9.

[18] Jaffe AS, Landt Y, Parvin CA, et al. Comparative sensitivity of cardiac troponin I and lactate dehydrogenase isoenzymes for diagnosing acute myocardial infarction. Clin Chem 1996;42:1770–6.

[19] Katus HA, Remppis A, Looser S, et al. Enzyme linked immuno assay of cardiac troponin T for the detection of acute myocardial infarction in patients. J Mol Cell Cardiol 1989;21:1349–53.

[20] Panteghini M, Gerhardt W, Apple FS, et al. Quality specifications for cardiac troponin assays. Clin Chem Lab Med 2001;39:175–9.

[21] Panteghini M, Pagani F, Yeo KT, et al. Evaluation of imprecision for cardiac troponin assays at low-range concentrations. Clin Chem 2004;50:327–32.

[22] Jaffe A. Caveat emptor. Am J Med 2003;115:241–4.

[23] Alpert JS, Thygesen K, Antman E, et al. Myocardial infarction redefined–a consensus document of The Joint European Society of Cardiology/American College of Cardiology Committee for the redefinition of myocardial infarction. J Am Coll Cardiol 2000;36:959–69.

[24] Jaffe AS, Ravkilde J, Roberts R, et al. It's time for a change to a troponin standard. Circulation 2000;102:1216–20.

[25] Apple FS, Wu AH, Jaffe AS. European Society of Cardiology and American College of Cardiology guidelines for redefinition of myocardial infarction: how to use existing assays clinically and for clinical trials. Am Heart J 2002;144:981–6.

[26] Jaffe AS. Elevations in cardiac troponin measurements: false false-positives. Cardiovasc Toxicol 2001;1(2):87–92.

[27] Adams JE III, Abendschein DR, Jaffe AS. Biochemical markers of myocardial injury. In: MB creatine kinase the choice for the 1990s [review]? Circulation 1993;88:750–63.

[28] Adams JE III, Bodor GS, Davila-Roman VG, et al. Cardiac troponin I. A marker with high specificity for cardiac injury. Circulation 1993;88:101–6.

[29] Newby LK, Storrow AB, Gibler WB, et al. Bedside multimarker testing for risk stratification in chest pain units: the chest pain evaluation by creatine kinase-MB, myoglobin, and troponin I (CHECK-MATE) study. Circulation 2001;103:1832–7.

[30] McCord J, Nowak RM, McCullough PA, et al. Ninety-minute exclusion of acute myocardial infarction by use of quantitative point-of-care testing of myoglobin and troponin I. Circulation 2001;104: 1483–8.

[31] Eggers KM, Oldgren J, Nordenskjold A, et al. Diagnostic value of serial measurement of cardiac markers in patients with chest pain: limited value of adding myoglobin to troponin I for exclusion of myocardial infarction. Am Heart J 2004;148: 574–81.

[32] Bar-Or D, Lau E, Winkler JV. Novel assay for cobalt-albumin binding and its potential as a marker for myocardial ischemia-a preliminary report. J Emerg Med 2000;19:311–5.

[33] Sinha MK, Gaze DC, Tippins JR, et al. Ischemia modified albumin is a sensitive marker of myocardial ischemia after percutaneous coronary intervention. Circulation 2003;107:2403–5.

[34] Christenson RH, Duh SH, Sanhai WR, et al. Characteristics of an albumin cobalt binding test for assessment of acute coronary syndrome patients: a multicentric study. Clin Chem 2001;47:464–70.

[35] Zapico-Muniz E, Santalo-Bel M, Mercé-Muntanola J, et al. Ischemia-modified albumin during skeletal muscle ischemia. Clin Chem 2004;50:1063–5.

[36] Ohman EM, Armstrong PW, Christenson RH, et al. Cardiac troponin T levels for risk stratification in acute myocardial ischemia. GUSTO IIA Investigators. N Engl J Med 1996;335:1333–41.

[37] Matetzky S, Sharir T, Domingo M, et al. Elevated troponin I level on admission is associated with adverse outcome of primary angioplasty in acute myocardial infarction. Circulation 2000;102:1611–6.

[38] Ohman EM, Armstrong PW, White HD, et al. Risk stratification with a point-of-care cardiac troponin T test in acute myocardial infarction. GUSTO III Investigators. Global use of strategies to open occluded coronary arteries. Am J Cardiol 1999;84: 1281–6.

[39] Giannitsis E, Muller-Bardorff M, Lehrke S, et al. Admission troponin T level predicts clinical outcomes, TIMI flow, and myocardial tissue perfusion after primary percutaneous intervention for acute ST-segment elevation myocardial infarction. Circulation 2001;104:630–5.

[40] Giannitsis E, Lehrke S, Wiegand UK, et al. Risk stratification in patients with inferior acute myocardial infarction treated by percutaneous coronary interventions: the role of admission troponin T. Circulation 2000;102:2038–44.

[41] Hamm CW, Ravkilde J, Gerhardt W, et al. The prognostic value of serum troponin T in unstable angina. N Engl J Med 1992;327:146–50.

[42] Antman EM, Tanasijevic MJ, Thompson B, et al. Cardiac-specific troponin I levels to predict the risk of mortality in patients with acute coronary syndromes. N Engl J Med 1996;335:1342–9.

[43] Lindahl B, Venge P, Wallentin L. Relation between troponin T and the risk of subsequent cardiac events in unstable coronary artery disease. The FRISC study group. Circulation 1996;93:1651–7.

[44] Galvani M, Ottani F, Ferrini D, et al. Prognostic influence of elevated values of cardiac troponin I in patients with unstable angina. Circulation 1997;95: 2053–9.

[45] Ottani F, Galvani M, Nicolini FA, et al. Elevated cardiac troponin levels predict the risk of adverse outcome in patients with acute coronary syndromes. Am Heart J 2000;140:917–27.

[46] Heeschen C, van Den Brand MJ, Hamm CW, et al. Angiographic findings in patients with refractory unstable angina according to troponin T status. Circulation 1999;100:1509–14.

[47] Morrow DA, Antman EM, Tanasijevic M, et al. Cardiac troponin I for stratification of early outcomes and the efficacy of enoxaparin in unstable angina: a TIMI-11B substudy. J Am Coll Cardiol 2000;36:1812–7.

[48] Newby LK, Ohman EM, Christenson RH, et al. Benefit of glycoprotein IIb/IIIa inhibition in patients with acute coronary syndromes and troponin t-positive status: the paragon-B troponin T substudy. Circulation 2001;103:2891–6.

[49] Braunwald E, Antman EM, Beasley JW, et al. American College of Cardiology. American Heart Association. Committee on the Management of Patients With Unstable Angina. ACC/AHA 2002 guideline update for the management of patients with unstable angina and non-ST-segment elevation myocardial infarction summary article: a report of the American College of Cardiology/American Heart Association task force on practice guidelines (Committee on the Management of Patients With Unstable Angina). J Am Coll Cardiol 2002;40:1366–74.

[50] Yusuf S, Zhao F, Mehta SR, et al. Effects of clopidogrel in addition to aspirin in patients with acute coronary syndromes without ST-segment elevation. N Engl J Med 2001;345:494–502.

[51] Aviles RJ, Wright RS, Aviles JM, et al. Long-term prognosis of patients with clinical unstable angina pectoris without elevation of creatine kinase but with elevation of cardiac troponin I levels. Am J Cardiol 2002;90:875–8.

[52] Invasive compared with non-invasive treatment in unstable coronary-artery disease: FRISC II prospective randomised multicentre study. FRagmin and Fast Revascularisation during InStability in Coronary artery disease Investigators. Lancet 1999;354: 708–15.

[53] Morrow DA, Cannon CP, Rifai N, et al. Ability of minor elevations of troponins I and T to predict benefit from an early invasive strategy in patients with unstable angina and non-ST elevation myocardial infarction: results from a randomized trial. JAMA 2001;286:2405–12.

[54] Wiviott SD, Cannon CP, Morrow DA, et al. Differential expression of cardiac biomarkers by gender in patients with unstable angina/non-ST-elevation myocardial infarction: a TACTICS-TIMI 18 (Treat Angina with Aggrastat and determine Cost of Therapy with an Invasive or Conservative Strategy-Thrombolysis In Myocardial Infarction 18) substudy. Circulation 2004;109:580–6.

[55] Hamm CW, Goldmann BU, Heeschen C, et al. Emergency room triage of patients with acute chest pain by means of rapid testing for cardiac troponin T or troponin I. N Engl J Med 1997;337:1648–53.

[56] James S, Armstrong P, Califf R, et al. Troponin T levels and risk of 30-day outcomes in patients with the acute coronary syndrome: prospective verification in the GUSTO-IV trial. Am J Med 2003;115:178–84.

[57] Henrikson CA, Howell EE, Bush DE, et al. Prognostic usefulness of marginal troponin T elevation. Am J Cardiol 2004;93:275–9.

[58] Konstantinides S, Geibel A, Olschewski M, et al. Importance of cardiac troponins I and T in risk stratification of patients with acute pulmonary embolism. Circulation 2002;106:1263–8.

[59] La Vecchia L, Ottani F, Favero L, et al. Increased cardiac troponin I on admission predicts in-hospital mortality in acute pulmonary embolism. Heart 2004;90:633–7.

[60] Missov E, Calzolari C, Pau B. Circulating cardiac troponin I in severe congestive heart failure. Circulation 1997;96:2953–8.

[61] Horwich TB, Patel J, MacLellan WR, et al. Cardiac troponin I is associated with impaired hemodynamics, progressive left ventricular dysfunction, and increased mortality rates in advanced heart failure. Circulation 2003;108:833–8.

[62] Muller-Bardorff M, Weidtmann B, Giannitsis E, et al. Release kinetics of cardiac troponin T in survivors of confirmed severe pulmonary embolism. Clin Chem 2002;48:673–5.

[63] Dokainish H, Pillai M, Murphy SA, et al. TACTICS-TIMI-18 Investigators. Prognostic implications of elevated troponin in patients with suspected acute coronary syndrome but no critical epicardial coronary disease: a TACTICS-TIMI-18 substudy. J Am Coll Cardiol 2005;45:19–24.

[64] deFilippi CR, Tocchi M, Parmar RJ, et al. Cardiac troponin T in chest pain unit patients without ischemic electrocardiographic changes: angiographic correlates and long-term clinical outcomes. J Am Coll Cardiol 2000;35:1827–34.

[65] Herzog CA, Ma JZ, Collins AJ. Poor long-term survival after acute myocardial infarction among patients on long-term dialysis. N Engl J Med 1998;339:799–805.

[66] Bleyer AJ, Russell GB, Satko SG. Sudden and cardiac death rates in hemodialysis patients. Kidney Int 1999;55:1553–9.

[67] Aviles RJ, Askari AT, Lindahl B, et al. Troponin T levels in patients with acute coronary syndromes, with or without renal dysfunction. N Engl J Med 2002;346:2047–52.

[68] Apple FS, Murakami MM, Pearce LA, et al. Predictive value of cardiac troponin I and T for subsequent death in end-stage renal disease. Circulation 2002;106:2941–5.

[69] deFilippi C, Wasserman S, Rosanio S, et al. Cardiac troponin T and C-reactive protein for predicting prognosis, coronary atherosclerosis, and cardiomyopathy in patients undergoing long-term hemodialysis. JAMA 2003;290:353–9.

[70] Ooi DS, Isotalo PA, Veinot JP. Correlation of antemortem serum creatine kinase, creatine kinase-MB, troponin I, and troponin T with cardiac pathology. Clin Chem 2000;46:338–44.

[71] Apple FS, Murakami MM. Cardiac troponin and creatine kinase MB monitoring during in-hospital myocardial reinfarction. Clin Chem 2005;61:460–3.

[72] Tanaka T, Hirota Y, Sohmiya K-I, et al. Serum and urinary human heart fatty acid binding protein in acute myocardial infarction. Clin Biochem 1991;24:195–201.

ELSEVIER
SAUNDERS

Cardiol Clin 23 (2005) 467–490

CARDIOLOGY
CLINICS

Point-of-Care Testing and Cardiac Biomarkers: The Standard of Care and Vision for Chest Pain Centers

Gerald J. Kost, MD, PhD, MS, FACB[a,b,*], Nam K. Tran, BS[a]

[a]Point-of-Care Testing Center for Teaching and Research, Department of Pathology and Laboratory Medicine,
UCD Health System, School of Medicine, University of California, Davis, CA, USA
[b]Affiliate Faculty, Chulalongkorn University, Bangkok, Thailand

Point-of-care testing (POCT) is defined as testing at or near the site of patient care [1]. POCT decreases therapeutic turnaround time (TTAT), increases clinical efficiency, and improves medical and economic outcomes [2,3]. TTAT (Fig. 1) represents the time from test ordering to patient treatment [2]. POC technologies have become ubiquitous in the United States, and, therefore, so has the potential for speed, convenience, and satisfaction, strong advantages for physicians, nurses, and patients in chest pain centers. POCT is applied most beneficially through the collaborative teamwork of clinicians and laboratorians who use integrative strategies, performance maps, clinical algorithms, and care paths (critical pathways) [2–5]. For example, clinical investigators [6–9] have shown that on-site integration of testing for cardiac injury markers (myoglobin, creatinine kinase MB isoenzyme [CK-MB], and cardiac troponin I [cTnI]) in accelerated diagnostic algorithms produces effective screening, less hospitalization, and substantial savings. Chest pain centers [10], which now total over 150 accredited in the United States [11], incorporate similar types of protocol-driven performance enhancements. This optimization allows chest pain centers to improve patient evaluation, treatment, survival, and discharge [12]. This article focuses on cardiac biomarker POCT for chest pain centers and emergency medicine.

POC test clusters encompass electrolytes (eg, K^+, Ca^{++}), metabolites (glucose, lactate), function monitors (acid-base, hemostasis), and several biomarkers [2]. Hospital penetration of POC cardiac biomarker testing increased from 4% in 2001 to 12% in 2004, a threefold change [13,14]. Now, with a strong annual growth rate, cardiac biomarker POCT represents one of the most rapidly expanding areas in clinical diagnostics. The growth rate, estimated as 10% to 20% [13,15], could double use quickly. Sales are expected to grow from about $200 million in 2003 to around $400 to $500 million in 2008, an increase of over 100% in five years. The current market trend is driven by the following: (a) an evolving standard of care for the timeliness of evaluation and treatment in chest pain centers and EDs; (b) motivation to produce cost-effective medical solutions for acute coronary syndromes (ACS) and other cardiovascular conditions, such as congestive heart failure; (c) need to reduce medicolegal risk in emergency department (ED) settings where acute myocardial infarction (AMI) is missed too frequently; (d) physician and nurse demands for rapid response testing and consistently fast test results, day and night; (e) emphasis on the total value of diagnostic information (versus piecemeal costs of individual tests); (f) smaller, smarter, faster, and cheaper portable devices with improved technologies for POCT, such as critical care profiling, faster immunotesting, and integrated multimarker indexing; (g) a continuing paradigm shift to the "hybrid

---

* Corresponding author. 506 Citadel Drive, Davis, CA 95616.

E-mail address: gjkost@ucdavis.edu (G.J. Kost).

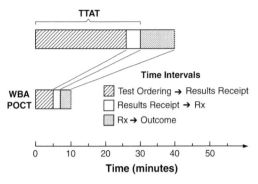

Fig. 1. Therapeutic turn around time (TTAT) is time from test ordering to appropriate treatment (Rx). If blood specimens are obtained first or before verbal orders are documented after, as may occur in critical situations, TTAT starts with collection. POCT and whole-blood analysis (WBA) shorten TTAT. The interval from Rx to outcome typically also decreases, thereby enhancing efficiency of patient care and usually improving medical and economic outcomes.

laboratory" [2] where laboratorians work more closely on-site with clinicians who perform bedside testing; (h) increasing penetration of POC cardiac biomarkers in a niche hospital market previously characterized by slow growth; and (i) physician expectations, patient empowerment, health consciousness, and early detection extending even to the home because too many patients succumb to AMI before reaching the hospital.

An important goal of this article is to help optimize the guidelines- and evidence-based clinical practice of POCT [16] in chest pain centers through systematic planning and implementing of POC cardiac biomarker testing. Themes include: (a) POCT should be applied broadly to reduce medical risk; (b) POCT for cardiac biomarkers is evolving into the standard of care; and (c) whole-blood analysis (WBA) time ultimately determines the minimum time interval for rapid response testing. This article delineates POC cardiac test clusters; describes clinical priorities for their application; summarizes handheld, portable, and transportable instruments and test kits; and identifies future needs that must be fulfilled to serve acute care patients efficiently and efficaciously. Current heavy investment in commercial development raises unique opportunities for creative interdigitation of POCT, bedside decision making, and evidence-based therapy in chest pain centers. Active leadership participation during this dynamic phase of expansion of cardiac

biomarker POCT will help maximize future benefits.

Status of cardiac biomarker point-of-care testing

In 2004, an Enterprise Analysis Corporation [13] telephone interview survey of 493 United States hospitals with bed size of at least 150 showed that cardiac biomarkers were evaluated for use more frequently but rejected more commonly than other types of POCT, which implies that devices offered fall short of meeting needs [14]. Of hospitals deciding not to install a new POCT system, 75% (82 of 110) evaluated cardiac biomarkers [13]. Reasons for not installing included: (a) lack of improved turnaround time (TAT), (b) high costs, (c) inaccuracy, (d) not user friendly for nonlaboratorians, and (e) laboratory unwillingness to relinquish test control. Nonetheless, as noted above, between 2001 and 2004, hospital penetration of POC cardiac marker testing by discipline trebled with smaller hospitals (150 to 299 beds) most frequently adopting POCT. Sites where hospitals used cardiac biomarker POCT included: (a) ED (56%), (b) core laboratory (52%), (c) outpatient area (8%), (d) stat laboratory (6%), (e) cardiac catheterization laboratory (3%), (f) intensive care unit (2%), and (g) operating room (2%)—sum of 129% because of multiple sites. Overall, Biosite Diagnostics (San Diego, CA) led the market in cardiac biomarkers with B-type natruiretic peptide (BNP) on the Triage Cardiac Panel platform. Note that EDs holding their own Clinical Laboratory Improvements Act licenses were not contacted in the survey; therefore, the frequency of distributed testing in EDs may exceed 56%.

According to the United States survey [13], cardiac biomarker tests performed included: (a) cardiac troponin (cTn) alone (24% of hospitals using cardiac biomarker POCT); (b) cTn, CK-MB, and myoglobin (67%); and (c) BNP (74%). Forty-five percent reported they would switch BNP to the main laboratory if possible. Average POC cTn test volume (5227) represented about twice that of BNP (2766), but all types constituted 20% or less of total cardiac biomarker test volume in 58% of institutions. Overall, hospitals streamlined the number of POCT systems (average about three) under pressures for training, quality control, maintenance, integration, and oversight. Of those hospitals projecting rapid or very rapid growth, speed and improved technology were cited most frequently. Thus, the survey showed that high accuracy, speed, improved technology, user friendliness, broad test menu, cost-effectiveness, quality control, and information integration, as well as faster quantitative analysis, represent key design specifications to be fulfilled by cardiac biomarker POC devices. Other important features include built-in data management and quality control, plus error alerting [17]. Use of POCT does not excuse inaccuracy or errors. Clinicians and laboratorians should insist on accuracy and reliability irrespective of where testing is performed.

Technologies for cardiac biomarker point-of-care testing

Instruments, decision levels, and applications

Handheld, portable, and transportable instruments and devices available for cardiac biomarker POCT are summarized in Table 1 [18–38]. Test clusters, methods, analysis times, sample types, and other pertinent information are shown. Disposable qualitative test kits are shown also. For additional details of POC analytic principles, see Tang and colleagues [39] and for an earlier analysis of technology, see the University HealthSystem Consortium report by Cummings and colleagues [40]. Note that several of the devices and test kits in Table 1 may be used in near-patient laboratories or at the bedside. Before implementation, operators should check with manufacturers regarding regulatory constraints, decision thresholds, and test classifications. Currently, none of the tests listed qualify for so-called waived status under federal statutes governing diagnostic testing [41]. Thus, testing must be performed by licensed, certified, and validated personnel in accredited facilities with attention to required daily quality control, and should be supervised by POC coordinators who assure high-quality, satisfy inspection requirements, and incorporate proficiency testing (objective external performance review). Nurses and POCT coordinators and, often, experienced medical technologists, have become indispensable partners stitching these aspects of POCT together and maintaining the fabric of excellence in testing irrespective of where it is performed [42,43]. Chest pain centers should not attempt to implement and manage POCT without the assistance of an experienced POCT coordinator who provides valuable liaison with laboratory medicine and essential continuity of POCT throughout the hospital.

Several areas for potential improvement in the POC cardiac biomarker repertoire are identified in Table 1. Miniaturized bedside immunochemistry has just passed its infancy and integrated multimarker test clusters have appeared only recently on portable and handheld devices. Despite over one decade of development [44], WBA times for immunochemistry remain prolonged, in the order of 15 minutes. Following the precedent set in other clinical applications, such as biosensor-based bedside glucose testing, analysis time should be reduced to just a few minutes while analytic sensitivity (minimum detection level) should be improved. These potentially conflicting goals may justify the use of novel nano- or microfluidics, microarray, or optical approaches heretofore not commonly present on POC devices. Complex manufacturing and funding hurdles stall efforts to combine cardiac biomarkers with other critical care analytes, such as electrolytes (eg, K^+ and Ca^{++}), blood gases, and pH. Currently, these analytes can be measured with exchangeable cartridge-based systems (eg, i-STAT) but should be fully integrated on other instruments for the evaluation, diagnosis, and monitoring of critically ill patients.

The inconsistency in qualitative and quantitative decision levels is emphasized in Table 2. In this phase of rapid growth, standardization of cardiac biomarker measurements and decision levels should occupy a position of high priority. Standardization, which demands consideration of subject reference levels and assay characteristics (eg, epitopes, antibodies, and matrices, all producing in the case of cTnI, varying specificities for different forms released), improves the consistency of diagnostic interpretation, reduces the potential for errors, and allows physicians to follow trends if different assays are used for testing after patients are admitted. Inadequate computer interfacing of devices and lack of critical results alerting represent two additional weaknesses. Full integration with hospital computerized systems is required for settings using an electronic medical record. As noted in later discussion of risk, missed diagnoses resulting from poor communication and other root causes can result in significant financial penalties. Examples of special situations where cardiac biomarker POCT is being developed or can help facilitate unusual clinical problem solving are presented in Table 3 [45–58]. Generally, per test cost for POCT exceeds that on larger mainframe chemistry analyzers found in clinical laboratories. Despite high costs, POCT can improve overall cost-effectiveness [3,6–9], discussed below.

Table 1
Cardiac Biomarker POCT

Test/Device name	Biomarker(s)	Device characteristics	Reference notes
Cardiac Reader • Cardiac T • Cardiac M • Cardiac D • NT-proBNP (Portable) Roche Diagnostics	cTnT Myoglobin D-dimer NT-proBNP[a]	Sample: 150 μL heparinized or EDTA WB Analysis time: 12 min, TnT; 8 min, myoglobin; and 8 min, D-dimer Method: Immunoassay and photosensor	Cardiac Reader interprets Cardiac T/M/D rapid assay strips. Comparison between the rapid test and a established laboratory-based method showed sufficient agreement of results with a correlation of r = 0.89 for troponin T and r = 0.912 for myoglobin [18]. The Cardiac T exhibited Sn = 100% and Sp = 76.2% for MI [19]. See also [20].
TropT sensitive (Handheld, disposable) Roche Diagnostics Indianapolis, IN www.roche.com	cTnT (QUAL)	Sample: 150 μL heparinized or EDTA WB Analysis time: 15 min Method: Immunoassay	Out of 34 patients who present with AMI, the TropT sensitive test showed positive quantitative results for 20 patients versus 29 patients when the Cardiac Reader was used [21]. At 3 hours after onset of symptoms for AMI, Sn = 50%, Sp = 96.3%, PPV = 80%, and NPV = 86.7% for AMI [22].
Cardiac STATus (Handheld, disposable) Spectral Diagnostics Toronto, Ontario, CAN www.spectraldx.com	Myo + cTnI Myo + cTnI + CK-MB (test clusters) cTnI CK-MB	Sample: 150 μL heparinized WB, heparinized plasma or serum Analysis time: 15 min Method: Lateral flow based immunoassay	Qualitative results from CK-MB and myoglobin test cards were comparable diagnostically to quantitative results from the Ciba Corning ACS-180 and Dade Stratus IIntellect [23]. cTnI tests showed 98% concordance with ELISA [24]. In comparison with Roche TropT, the Cardiac STATus proved more effective in early diagnosis of AMI [25]. The Cardiac STATus had a sensitivity of 96% for the detection of AMI within 3 hours of presentation [26].
i-Lynx (Handheld, portable) Spectral Diagnostics Toronto, Ontario, CAN www.spectraldx.com	NA	The system consists of two interfaced components; a handheld electronic device to capture and analyze an image from the current Cardiac STATus rapid test strip, and a local area network compatible docking station to automate data capture communication	The i-Lynx is a connectivity solution with full QC functionality in open architecture, including system maintenance, user ID, QC log, lockout, passcode protection, universal barcode, and connectivity by way of TCP-IP for POC Coordinators (Chris Wayne, Spectral Diagnostics, e-mail communication.)

Cholestech LDX (Portable) Cholestech Corp. Hayward, CA www.cholestech.com	CRP	Sample: 50 µL WB or 40–50 µL plasma Analysis time: 7 min Other analytes: Total cholesterol, HDL, triglycerides, ALT, and glucose. Method: Reflectance photometry, immunoassay	WB and plasma samples showed a concordance rate of 94% and 90%, respectively, with results from Dade Behring BN100 [27].
i-STAT 1 and PCA (Handheld) i-STAT East Windsor, NJ www.i-stat.com	cTnI	Sample: 16 mL heparinized WB or plasma Analysis time: 10 min, cTnI Other analytes: Na^+, K^+, Cl^-, Ca^{2+}, glucose, creatinine, lactate, BUN, Hct, Hb, pH, pCO_2, pO_2, ACT, and PT Method: ELISA	cTnI test performance proved insensitive to hematocrits between 0 to 65%, but higher hematocrits produced imprecision [28].
LifeSign MI (Handheld, disposable) PBM Princeton, NJ www.pbmc.com	cTnI + myo CK-MB + myo CK-MB + myo + cTnI (test clusters) MLC-1[b] NT-proBNP[b]	Sample: 120 µL WB, plasma, or serum Analysis time: 15 min Method: Chromatographic immunoassay	Each test cluster is equipped with a built in control for quality assurance [29].
NycoCard Reader II (Portable) Axis-Shield Oslo, Norway www.axis-shield.co.uk	CRP D-dimer	Sample: 5 µL heparinized/EDTA/ citrated WB or serum (dilution to 50 µL required) Analysis time: 3 min Other analytes: HbA1c, microalbumin Method: Reflectometric immunoassay	NycoCard Reader II interprets CRP and D-dimer test strips.
Nexus Dx (Handheld, disposable) Syn X Pharma Inc. Toronto, CAN www.synxpharma.com	cTnI + myo[a] cTnI + myo + CK-MB[a] (test clusters) cTnI[a] NT-proBNP[a,b]	Sample: 120 µL WB, plasma or serum for cTnI Analysis time: 15 min, cTnI Method: Chromatographic immunoassay	NT-proBNP test was approved in Europe mid-2004 and is pending FDA approval in the United States. Other tests are available only in Canada and Europe [30].
One-Step Marker Test (Handheld, disposable) ACON Labs San Diego, CA www.aconlabs.com	cTnI + myo + CK-MB[a] (test cluster)	Sample: 120 µL WB, plasma, or serum Analysis time: 15 min Method: Chromatographic immunoassay	Device is only available outside the United States. Quality controls are built into the test card.

(continued on next page)

Table 1 (*continued*)

Test/Device name	Biomarker(s)	Device characteristics	Reference notes
RAMP Reader (Portable) Response Biomedical British Columbia, CAN www.responsebio.com	Myoglobin CK-MB cTnI	Sample: 70 µL WB Analysis time: ~15 min Other analytes: WNV antigen Method: Fluorescence-based immunoassay	At 95% CI, Sn (cTnI) = 90%, Sp (cTnI) = 86%, Sn (CK-MB) = 59%, and Sp (CK-MB) = 90% for AMI [31].
RAPICHEK[b] (Handheld, disposable) Dainippon Pharmaceuticals Suita City, Osaka, Japan www.dainippon-pharm.co.jp	H-FABP	Sample: 150 µL WB Analysis time: 15 min Method: Chromatographic immunoassay	H-FABP panel test achieved 98.4% agreement with H-FABP mass concentration ELISA [22,32]. At 3 hours following onset of symptoms of AMI, RAPICHEK had Sn = 100%, Sp = 63%, PPV = 44%, and NPV = 100%. RAPICHEK versus TropT sensitivity were 100% versus 50%, respectively.
Stratus CS STAT (Transportable NPT) Dade Behring Deerfield, IL www.dadebehring.com	CK-MB Myoglobin cTnI D-dimer[a]	Sample: 2.7 mL heparainzed WB or plasma Analysis time: 14 min for first result, 4 min for each additional result Other analytes: β-hCG Method: Fluorescence-based immunoassay	Device correlated well with cTnI tests performed in a central laboratory; imprecision of troponin method has a CV of less than 10% at the 99th percentile of the reference population [33,34].
Triage Cardiac Panel (Portable) Biosite Diagnostics San Diego, CA www.biosite.com	CK-MB + myo + cTnI cTnI + CK-MB + myo + BNP (test clusters) D-dimer	Sample: 225 µL EDTA WB or plasma Analysis time: ~15 min Other analytes: acetaminophen, amphetamines, methamphetamines, cocaine, opiates, phencyclidine, tetrahydrocannabinol, barbiturates, benzodiazepines, propoxyphen, tricyclic antidepressants Method: Fluorescence-based immunoassay	Triage MeterPlus interprets Triage Cardiac Panels, includes built-in quality controls, and provides simultaneous analyses of multiple analytes. Study showed Triage Cardiac Panel comparable to established methods for detection of AMI [35]. Sn for cTnI, CK-MB, and Myo were 98%, 95%, and 81% respectively, and the Sp were 100%, 91%, and 92% respectively for AMI [35,36].
	TBA	Sample: fingerstick WB Analysis time: 2–5 min Method: under development	A faster quantitative fingerstick-based test strip using whole blood is being developed (Julie Doyle, M.D. Biosite Diagnostics, e-mail communication.).

Abbreviations: ACT, activated clotting time; ALT, alanine aminotransferase; β-hCG, β-human chorionic gonadotropin; BUN, blood urea nitrogen; ELISA, enzyme-linked immunoabsorbant assay; F, female; Hb, hemoglobin; Hct; hematocrit; HDL, high density lipoprotein; H-FABP, human-type fatty acid binding protein; M, male; MLC-1, myosin light chain-1; myo, myoglobin; NA, not available; NPT, near-patient testing; NPV, negative predictive value; PPV, positive predictive value; PT, prothombin time; QC, quality control; QUAL, qualitative; Sn, sensitivity; Sp, specificity; TBA, to be announced; TnI, troponin I; WB, whole blood; and WNV, West Nile Virus.

Notes: a) Under development, b) Not available in US, +) Indicates test cluster. Methods were provided by manufacturers or their web sites. Reference 20 cited for completeness. No current information available for the First Medical Alpha Dx system [37,38]. Chemometrics data given for emergency room or early diagnostic applications. See Jaffe chapter for general information of sensitivity, specificity, and predictive values.

Table 2
Clinical decision levels for cardiac biomarker POCT

Biomarker	Device(s)	Qualitative	Quantitative	Decision level
BNP	Triage Cardiac Panel		X	100 pg/mL
CK-MB	Cardiac STATus	X		5.0 ng/mL
	LifeSign MI	X		5.0 ng/mL
	Nexus Dx[a,b]		X	Under development
	One-Step Marker Test	X		5.0 ng/mL
	RAMP Reader		X	5.0 ng/mL
	Stratus CS STAT		X	3.5 ng/mL
	Triage Cardiac Panel		X	4.3 ng/mL
CRP	Cholestech LDX		X	Under development
	NycoCard CRP	X		Not available
cTnI	Cardiac STATus	X		0.5 ng/mL
	i-STAT 1 and PCA		X	0.1 ng/mL
	LifeSign MI	X		1.5 ng/mL
	One-Step Marker Test	X		0.5 ng/mL
	RAMP Reader		X	0.12 ng/mL
	Stratus CS STAT		X	0.06 ng/mL
	Triage Cardiac Panel		X	0.4 ng/mL
	Nexus Dx[a,b]		X	Under development
cTnT	Cardiac Reader		X	0.1 ng/mL
	TropT Sensitive	X		0.1 ng/mL
D-dimer	Cardiac Reader		X	0.5 µg/mL
	NycoCard D-dimer	X		Not available
	Triage Cardiac Panel		X	100 ng/mL
	Stratus CS STAT[a]		X	Under development
H-FABP	RAPICHECK		X	6.2 ng/mL
MLC-1	LifeSign MI[b]	X		Not available
Myoglobin	Cardiac Reader		X	76 ng/mL (M), 64 ng/mL (F)
	Cardiac STATus	X		80 ng/mL
	LifeSign MI	X		50 ng/mL
	Nexus Dx[a,b]		X	Under development
	One-Step Marker Test	X		50 ng/mL
	RAMP Reader		X	99.3 ng/mL
	Stratus CS STAT		X	98 ng/mL (M), 56 ng/mL (F)
	Triage Cardiac Panel		X	107 ng/mL
NT-proBNP	Cardiac Reader[a]		X	Under development
	LifeSign MI[b]	X		Not available
	Nexus Dx[a,b]		X	Under development

Abbreviations: CRP, C-reactive protein; cTnT, cardiac troponin T; F, female; H-FABP, human-type fatty acid binding protein; M, male; MI, myocardial infarction; MLC-1, myosin light chain-1; NT-proBNP, N-terminal proBNP; TnI, troponin I; TnT, troponin T.

Notes: a) Under development; b) Not available in United States.

Disclaimer: Tables 1 through 3 were compiled from reliable sources including company web sites and cited literature. However, during evaluation before implementation users should update and verify all data directly from manufacturers and product inserts. Users also should verify decision levels and reference methods, as well as FDA-approved clinical applications of each cardiac biomarker.

Qualitative versus quantitative testing: the American College of Cardiology/American Heart Association guidelines

Cardiac biomarkers linked with efficient triage and treatment strategies can facilitate resource use, risk stratification, therapeutic management, and clinical outcomes [59–64]. The American College of Cardiology/American Heart Association (ACC/AHA) 2002 guideline update [65] for patients who present with unstable angina (UA) and non–ST-segment elevation myocardial infarction (NSTEMI) states that "point-of-care assays at present are qualitative or, at best, semiquantitative. The evolution of technology

Table 3
Special applications of cardiac biomarker POCT

Special applications	Biomarker/concept	Device/index
ACS. Rapid test for ACS risk stratification utilizing cardiac myoglobin and CAIII for early specificity and sensitivity (Chris Wayne, Spectral Diagnostics, e-mail communication).	cMyo	Spectral Dx cMyo Test (under development)
CHF. Patients who died or were readmitted tend to have an increase in BNP concentration during their hospitalization (+ 239 ± 233 pg/mL). Patients who had successful treatment tend to have decreases in their BNP concentration during their hospitalization (−216 ± 69 pg/mL). The difference between these two groups were significant ($P < .05$). Therefore, POCT of BNP may be an effective way to improve in-hospital management of patients with decompensated CHF [45].	BNP	Triage BNP
Correctional facility. When the Cardiac STATus is combined with EKG results and medical history, a positive result leads to early diagnosis and subsequently faster, more effective treatment. A negative result can provide the confidence needed to safely treat the inmate on premises. In the end the correctional facility saved substantial funds (Chris Wayne, Spectral Diagnostics, e-mail communication).	Multivariate analysis	Cardiac STATus
Diabetes risk. Bhalla and colleagues [46] state BNP to be the most significant ($P < .001$) predictor of all-cause mortality in diabetic patients suspected of cardiac dysfunction.	BNP	Triage BNP
Diagnostic synthesis. "MMX" combines multiple biomarker test results in a continuous parameter that shows potential to discriminate patients with ACS from those without ACS (Julie Doyle, M.D., Boisite Diagnostics, e-mail communication). From ROCs, MMX AUC appears to outperform individual analyte (cTnI, CK-MB, myoglobin, or BNP) AUCs in ACS versus non-ACS and in other comparisons, such as MI versus UA or non-ACS, including for subsets of patients within 6 hours after the onset of chest pain. MMX algorithms have the potential to aid in the differential diagnosis of other conditions, such as stroke. Independent multimarker analysis also can be used for risk stratification [47,48].	Multimarker index	MMX (Anderberg J. and colleagues. AACC Oak Ridge Conference, 2005;63)
Early dysfunction. Mueller and colleagues [49] showed NT-proBNP comparable to BNP biomarkers for differential diagnosis in symptomatic and asymptomatic structural heart disease. However, results also suggested NT-proBNP was able to discern early cardiac dysfunction compared to BNP.	NT-proBNP	(Roche Elecsys) POCT under development
General practice environment. Dahler-Eriksen and colleagues [50] showed CRP testing in general practice identified significantly ($P = .002$) more new diseases (eg, infectious disease, inflammatory disease) compared to the control group. Additionally, cost-effectiveness analysis showed a reduction of $110,000 per year.	CRP	NycoCard Reader

Table 3 (*continued*)

Special applications	Biomarker/concept	Device/index
Home testing. Each year, more than a million persons in the United States have a heart attack, and about 50% of them die [51]. About 50% who die do so within 1 hour of the start of symptoms, such as pre-infarction angina. Home testing could improve outcomes.	Various cardiac biomarkers	Waived tests (to be developed)
Military. Cardiac troponin T can help exclude myocardial damage in patients who experience an elevated CK caused by skeletal muscle trauma [52].	cTnT	TropT Sensitive and Cardiac T
Military. The Cardiac STATus is available to every surface ship in the entire US Navy fleet (Chris Wayne, Spectral Diagnostics, e-mail communication).	Multimarker Analysis	Cardiac STATus
Mobile intensive care unit. When used within 2 to 12 hours from the onset of symptoms, the CK-MB/myoglobin multimarker test can prevent misdiagnosis of AMI or unnecessary hospitalization [53].	Multimarker Analysis	Cardiac STATus
Paramedic use. Use of the cTnI test helps Onslow County paramedics to quickly diagnose chest pain, and confidently rule-in or rule-out heart attacks while patients are in transit to the hospital. In certain cases, if the paramedic or ED physician confirms the patient is having a heart attack they can, following a protocol, implement therapy before they reach the hospital doors (Chris Wayne, Spectral Diagnostics, e-mail communication).	cTnI	Cardiac STATus
Potential new biomarker. For the diagnosis of AMI, quantitative ELISA-based measurement of H-FABP has been shown to be more sensitive than myoglobin or CK-MB, and more specific than myoglobin [22]. However, the ELISA process takes $\geq$ 90 minutes whereas the RAPICHEK takes 15 minutes. Additionally, the RAPICHEK test exhibited superior negative predictive values, which reached nearly 100% for patients in all time frames. Seino and colleagues [22] concluded that the H-FABP could be useful for emergencies.	H-FABP	RAPICHEK
Prehospital admission. Prehospital cTnT testing appears to be an objective marker for patients with poor outcomes [54].	cTnT	TropT Sensitive and Cardiac T
Renal dysfunction. McCullough and colleagues [55] showed myoglobin and CK-MB correlated with corrected creatinine clearance (r = −0.36, $P < 0.01$, and r = −0.10, $P = .01$, respectively), while cTnI did not (r = −0.10, $P = .12$). Multiple receiver operating characteristic curve testing showed cTnI to be the most consistent marker of myocardial injury over all strata of renal dysfunction including end-stage renal disease on dialysis [56]. Therefore, cTnI is applicable and superior to myoglobin or CK-MB in the evaluation of chest pain in patients with renal dysfunction [55].	cTnI	Triage Cardiac Panel
Renal failure. In patients with severe renal failure, cTnT could not be broken down and cleared by the kidneys, resulting in high serum cTnT levels [56].	cTnT	TropT Sensitive and Cardiac T

(*continued on next page*)

Table 3 (continued)

Special applications	Biomarker/concept	Device/index
Secondary referral. European Society of Cardiology recommendations include BNP testing to refer patients to secondary care.	BNP	BNP
Thrombosis. As a cardiac biomarker, Dempfle and colleagues [57] found the Roche Cardiac D Rapid Assay was also useful as a rule-out diagnostic tool for patients with suspected acute thrombosis [58]. The Roche Cardiac D Rapid Assay also can be used for diagnostic work-up for deep vein thrombosis [57].	D-dimer	Cardiac D

Abbreviations: AUC, area under curve; CAIII, cardiac anhydrase III; cMyo, cardiac myoglobin; CorrCrCl, corrected creatinine clearance; CRP, C-reactive protein; cTnT, cardiac troponin T; ELISA, enzyme-linked immunoabsorbant assay; F, female; H-FABP, human-type fatty acid binding protein; M, male; MI, myocardial infarction; MMX, multimarker index; NA, not available; NT-proBNP, N-terminal pro B-type natriuretic peptide; ROC, receiver operator curve; and UA, unstable angina.

that will provide quantitative assays of multiple markers that are simple to use will improve the diagnosis and management of patients with suspected acute coronary syndrome (ACS) in the ED". The 2004 ACC/AHA guidelines [66] for the management of patients with STEMI stated, "Although handheld bedside (point-of-care) assays may be used for a qualitative assessment of the presence of an elevated level of a serum cardiac biomarker, subsequent measurements of cardiac biomarker levels should be performed with a quantitative test…. in general, bedside assays are less sensitive and less precise than quantitative assays". Further, "A positive bedside test should be confirmed by a conventional quantitative test" [66]. These guidelines statements regarding qualitative assays allude to the various types of handheld formats and disposable test kits noted for convenience [67] and listed in Table 1. Qualitative versus quantitative assays are identified in Table 2. Much room for improvement exists in the detection of minor myocardial damage. The sensitivity and precision at the cutoff concentrations of qualitative and quantitative assays should be checked and deemed clinically appropriate before implementation [68] in chest pain centers.

Assay types, clinical applications, and testing sites create many alternatives, and the relevance of published studies will depend in part on the configuration and staffing of individual chest pain centers. Hamm and colleagues [69] found qualitative POC cardiac troponin T (cTnT) and cTnI tests to be sensitive and useful for ED triage. Schwartz and colleagues [70] documented diagnostically similar results from CK-MB and myoglobin qualitative testing in the ED and quantitative testing in the laboratory. Panteghini

and colleagues [25] studied the potential usefulness of rapid bedside qualitative myoglobin/CK-MB and cTnT tests in initiating revascularization therapy. James and colleagues [48] found rapid qualitative cTnI suboptimal for prediction of subsequent cardiac events at suspicion of unstable coronary syndromes. Hirschl and colleagues [71] found reliable clinical performance of qualitative cTnT testing, whether performed in laboratories or by nurses and physicians in critical care units. For "patients with suspicious AMI," Seino and colleagues [22] showed improved early sensitivity with a rapid whole-blood quantitative assay for heart-type fatty acid binding protein versus qualitative cTnT testing. Wu and colleagues [31] reported equivalent results for quantitative cardiac biomarker POCT and laboratory testing. Other studies [21,72] address quantitative bedside testing. Additionally, POCT encompasses near-patient testing (NPT), such as in ED satellite laboratories, where automated analyzers that provide quantitative testing (eg, Stratus CS STAT) often are placed.

In the ED, analytically sensitive quantitative cTn assays have blurred the distinction between patients who present with and without classically defined acute myocardial infarction (AMI) and have focused attention on the continuum of ACS from angina to transmural Q-wave myocardial infarction (MI) [73,74]. With first-draw specimens in the ED and *qualitative* POCT, Kratz and colleagues [75] showed that triple cardiac biomarkers (ie, a test cluster) may be needed to avoid weak positive predictive values for individual tests, and quantitative confirmation in the clinical laboratory yields additional improvement. In a five-hospital study of acute chest pain patients, Goldman and colleagues [18] reported equivalent results for quantitative POC cTnT and myoglobin testing in the ED versus testing in the clinical laboratory and stated that POC cTnT proved advantageous for rapid decision making. In the ED, optimal clinical sensitivity for ACS on first-draw specimens derives from myoglobin, a better adjunct test than CK-MB [76]. Although qualitative POC methods appear in routine and also several special settings (see Table 3), to expedite clinical assessment without missing cases of AMI, quantitative and highly sensitive POC assays are needed. POC assays also allow monitoring of release and clearance dynamics in the form of bedside changes (Δ, "delta values") [65]. A conservative approach, the evidence to date, and the guidelines above indicate a need for highly sensitive *and* quantitative cardiac biomarker POCT, and given a choice, chest pain centers should implement quantitative assays.

Ischemia markers: critical need

Any ischemia biomarker that works well clinically, that is, can detect ischemia in the absence of necrosis, would be an immediate success if used for POCT. Aggressive early triaging demands improved cardiac biomarkers for that purpose. A new biomarker, ischemia-modified albumin (IMA) (ACB, albumin Cobalt binding test; Ischemia Technologies, Denver, Colorado), has been approved and licensed by the Food and Drug Administration (FDA). Unfortunately, clinical data show that the current generation of the IMA assay lacks requisite specificity [77–87] like that possibly afforded, for example, by ultrahigh-sensitivity assays for troponins. In addition, IMA has not been implemented on any of the POC platforms listed in Table 1. Biomarkers of ischemia under evaluation include free fatty acid, glycogen phosphorylase isoenzyme BB, myeloperoxidase, nourin-1, pregnancy-associated plasma protein A, sphingosine-1-phosphate, soluble CD40L, and whole-blood choline. Future clinical studies of ischemia biomarkers should target low-risk patients in whom quick evaluation in the chest pain center can exclude AMI, and then attention can turn to the underlying cause of the chest pain.

Therapeutic turnaround time

Because it measures the *total* time from test ordering to treatment, TTAT (Fig. 1) represents an overall performance monitor (metric) useful for identifying the "bottleneck" route, that is, the critical path of acute cardiac care in chest pain centers and EDs. Expedited treatment influences patient survival, and TTAT can assess efficiency. If blood specimens are obtained first or before verbal orders are documented, as may occur in critical situations, TTAT starts with collection. In the algorithmic evaluation and treatment of chest pain using critical pathways and in concepts recommended by the ACC/AHA [65,66,88] (also ESC [89,90]), the AMI and the UA/NSTEMI pathways call for rapid cTn testing but not necessarily at the point of care. POCT, however, eliminates preanalytic delays. Caragher and colleagues [91] showed that POCT for myoglobin, CK-MB, and cTnI expedited diagnosis in the ED by decreasing the time to test results by 55% (39 versus 87 minutes) compared with the clinical laboratory. Hsu and colleagues [33] found a reduction from 65 to 26 minutes with POCT. McCord and colleagues [6] reported a median time from sampling to reporting of 24 minutes, and others [92,93] reported results availability in about 20 minutes. Stubbs and Collinson [94,95] showed that POCT of cardiac biomarkers decreased turnaround time by 52 minutes (central laboratory, 72; POCT, 20) and shortened hospital stay. Altinier and colleagues [96] reported a turnaround time of 82.5 minutes (50th percentile) versus 17 minutes with POCT, which facilitated faster discharge for some patients in the ED. In a study of five hospitals, Gaze and colleagues [97] documented that bedside cTnT testing in ED produced results in 12 to 22 minutes, a gain in time of 65 minutes (range 34 to 135 minutes) compared with central laboratory measurements. Thus, these studies have established POCT as fast and capable of producing clinical results in time spans comparable to the analysis times shown in Table 1.

Lee-Lewandrowski and colleagues [98] showed that when POC cardiac biomarkers were combined with other POC tests (ie, pregnancy testing and urine dipstick), the integration decreased test turnaround time by 87% and ED length of stay by 41.3 minutes. Performed at a time when Boston ambulance diversion was an issue, this study found that implementation of a POCT satellite laboratory in the ED decreased divert hours by 27%. POCT increased physician satisfaction [68]. Integration of testing plus synthesis of test results and other clinical evidence represents an essential pivot for knowledge optimization and decision making [3]. Collinson [94] suggested that POCT must be used if cardiac biomarker results are delayed more than 25% of the clinical decision time. In reality, POCT integrates decision making at the bedside. Widespread availability of POCT now makes fast TTAT an expectation in critical care management, the early recognition of life-threatening conditions, and the titration of commonly applied therapies [2,99–101]. Experience in United States legal deliberations has demonstrated that POCT may be deemed clinically necessary to achieve fast TTAT. Hence, well-conceived and mutually agreed upon goals for TTAT that are based on evidentiary needs [102] will improve cycles of individual patient care and overall performance in chest pain centers and emergency medicine.

Timeliness

Perception versus performance

Discordant viewpoints about how to measure the timeliness of diagnostic testing frustrate teamwork. Most clinicians measure response time as the interval starting with test ordering and ending with result reporting [103]. In contrast, laboratorians typically start the clock when they receive the sample in the laboratory and thereby discount preanalytic delays [103] that may degrade samples. Even for ED tests, such as potassium and hemoglobin, specimen transit times account for approximately one third of the total response time [104]. Active monitoring improves performance when the laboratory does not control the specimen handling process, but invariably, response time goals for EDs still are not met most of the time [105]. Significantly delayed outliers interrupt diagnostic-therapeutic processes. When finally reported, results from such delayed samples may no longer represent physiologically or medical relevant data, or they may sit in the laboratory information system unnoticed if the laboratory has not listed them as critical values. For enhanced clarity, communication, understanding, and teamwork, chest pain center physicians and laboratorians should agree on definitions of response time, jointly develop performance goals, and perpetually monitor key indicators.

In 2004, a College of American Pathologists (CAP) survey [106] of 159 hospital subscribers (mostly in the United States) to the Q-Probes program revealed critical deficiencies in the timeliness of cardiac biomarker services. Most (82%) laboratory participants deemed 1 hour or less a reasonable order-to-report response time for myocardial

injury markers (cTn or CK-MB), while most (75%) ED physicians wanted results within 45 minutes, in regards to patients presenting to the hospital ED with symptoms of AMI. Neither goal was met. Among the fastest performing 25% of laboratories, median order-to-report cTn and CK-MB response times equaled 50 and 48.3 minutes, respectively. On the average, 90% of results were reported in slightly more than 90 minutes measured from the time the tests were ordered. In about 50% of the hospitals, specimens were ordered by protocol before clinicians saw their patients. In 35.8% of participating hospitals, laboratory policies dictated that no results be reported until all results became available. In 10%, clinicians waited more than 2 hours for results. Shorter response times were associated with having specimens obtained by the laboratory rather than by nonlaboratory personnel and with performing marker assays in EDs or other peripheral laboratories compared with performing tests in central laboratories. For the CAP respondents, however, only 7.2% used an ED or other peripheral laboratory, and only 4.1% used POC instruments.

Evolution of guidelines and the standard of care for timeliness

The discipline inherent in applying practice guidelines can improve teamwork and outcomes [107–109]. In 1993 over one decade ago, the National Institutes of Health (NIH) published, "Emergency Department: Rapid Identification and Treatment of Patients with Acute Myocardial Infarction" [110], a product of the "60 Minutes to Treatment Working Group" of the National Heart Attack Alert Program Coordinating Committee, which had nearly forty member organizations at the time. The working group proposed a goal of 60 minutes for laboratory test results "…in patients with questionable symptoms and ECG findings…", and 30 minutes for algorithmic "door-to-drug" treatment of "patients with a clear diagnosis of AMI". The document stated, however, that "the value of rapidly available assays… [CK isoforms, troponin, myoglobin] is unknown at this [1993] time" [110].

Five years ago the ACC/AHA 2000 guidelines [88] for the management of patients with UA and NSTEMI recommended a target of 60 minutes with *30 minutes preferred* for completion of central laboratory test results, and stated further that, "Point-of-care systems, if implemented at the bedside, have the advantage of reducing delays due to transportation and processing in a central laboratory and can eliminate delays due to the lack of availability of central laboratory assays at all hours" [88]. The guidelines also stated of POCT that "The evolution of technology that will provide quantitative assays of multimarkers that are simple to use will improve the diagnosis and management of patients with suspected ACS in the ED" [88]. The 2002 update reiterated [65] that "When a central laboratory is used, results should be available within 60 minutes, preferably within 30 minutes".

The web-based draft of the National Academy of Clinical Biochemistry (NACB) guidelines [111] proposed that "The laboratory should perform cardiac marker testing with a turnaround time (TAT) of 1 hour, *optimally 30 minutes, or less.* The TAT is defined as the time from blood collection to the reporting of results." "Institutions that cannot consistently deliver cardiac marker TATs of approximately 1 hour should implement POC testing devices." The phrase, "...approximately 1 hour..." requires clarification to avoid misunderstandings. Nevertheless, over the past 12 years these NIH, ACC/AHA, and NACB guidelines have pointed consistently toward faster cardiac biomarker testing *within 30 minutes.* One must assess, therefore, whether POC technologies can meet or exceed expectations in these guidelines, positions tantamount to the standard of care. Additionally, the statistical distribution of performance times and outlier delays, and standards in critical care testing using WBA, must be considered to formulate cohesive rapid response criteria for chest pain centers. Lastly, the Society of Chest Pain Centers should consider adopting timeliness as a criterion for accreditation, as suggested in later discussion.

POCT has evolved substantially during the past decade, and so has the way it fits into clinical practice [112]. Now ubiquitous in the United States, POCT has established a new precedent for speed in *critical care testing.* Timeliness expectations for test results, such as electrolytes, blood gases, pH, and hematocrit or hemoglobin, in critical care medicine now have contracted to only 5 to 15 minutes, basically a little longer than WBA time [44,113]. This expectation for timeliness, a *de facto* legal requirement in the care of critically ill patients, prohibits diagnostic testing from prolonging TTAT and certainly from ever degrading efficiency in cases where AMI might be missed in an ED and patients

sent home prematurely. In chest pain centers, therefore, POCT should be approached not only from the perspective of cardiac biomarkers but also from the broader standpoint of garnering benefits that arise when integrating several test clusters. Delays could impede critical pathways, increase legal liability, aggravate risk exposure, and possibly also degrade medical and economic outcomes [3]. For some chest pain centers, fast TTAT and decision making will be achieved only by using POCT, in the form of bedside or near-patient testing.

The timeliness envelope (curve) in Fig. 2 traces progressive contraction of the time interval, test ordering → results receipt, the first of two intervals that make up TTAT (see Fig. 1), versus the year and conceptual evolution in POCT. To the right, standard-of-care milestones for cardiac biomarkers demarcate points that NIH and ACC/AHA published guidelines [88,110], practice standards, and chest pain centers have called for or actualized by virtue of published literature cited herein, faster response time. The performance (map) vector [2] consisting of POCT, focused multimarker innovations, faster immunotesting, and test cluster integration points to diagnostic-therapeutic (Dx-Rx) process optimization by which physicians in chest pain centers intuitively synthesize risk indices for individual patients. POCT provides not only immediate results but also acute awareness. The whole picture reflects a paradigm shift enabled by POCT and increasingly efficient solutions for the management of ACS patients. In the future, real-time in vivo and noninvasive function monitors, now embryonic or yet to be discovered, will supplant discrete in vitro diagnostic tests and lead to continuous knowledge optimization at the bedside, thus further improving the standard of care.

Cost-effectiveness, algorithmic strategies, and multimarkers

Cardiac biomarkers, especially cTn and myoglobin [114,115], play a pivotal role in cost-effectively triaging patients, assessing damage, gauging risk, determining prognosis, and economizing length of stay [116–121]. Decision analysis modeling showed that in patients who presented with acute undifferentiated chest pain, biochemical testing, observation for 2 to 6 hours, and then repeat testing, had a low incremental cost per quality adjusted life year, and that strategies

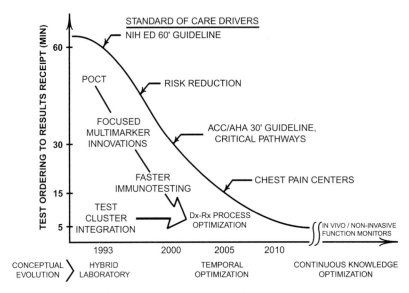

Fig. 2. The standard of care for timeliness of cardiac biomarker testing. Forceful clinical drivers mold the shape of the rapid response curve while the underlying performance vector enables it, aiming at optimization, first discrete, then in the future, continuous. Contemporary timeliness in critical care testing has set a continuum precedent for chest pain centers, which now can consider 15 minutes as reasonable criterion for accreditation. However, all cardiac biomarker results should be available within 30 minutes, the preference stated in ACC/AHA guidelines and the optimal stated in draft NACB guidelines.

requiring hospital admission had poor value [122]. Brogan and colleagues [26] recommended serial testing of CCU admissions to eliminate non-AMI causes and conserve resources. While serial testing of cardiac biomarkers, a hallmark for diagnosis of AMI, comes in at the low end of the cost spectrum of invasive procedures and hospitalization expenses [40], new POC multimarker approaches will redefine serial testing needs and temporal patterns. In the ED, cost and other issues, such as lack of connectivity or apparently modest value in STEMI, have slowed acceptance of POCT [123,124]. However, at a meeting in 2004, Kugelmass and colleagues [125] reported that in a broad group of four community-based hospitals, for 2248 consecutive admissions of patients who received a primary diagnosis of AMI, revascularization (PCI, CABG) rates increased significantly, and in-hospital mortality declined 24.7% (P = .049) following 1 year of implementation of POCT.

In the context of ACS and chest pain evaluation, chest pain centers can provide the dual efficiencies of expediting definitive treatment while managing patients with accelerated diagnostic-therapeutic protocols that proved cost-effective and beneficial to patient care [6–9,126,127].

Algorithmic strategies, however, using cardiac biomarkers need to be adapted to local settings [40]. The relative efficacy of diverse testing strategies reported in the literature remains uncertain, in part because sensitivity and specificity for AMI depend on: biomarkers selected, decision levels, timing of testing after symptom onset, natural discordance, unique settings, risk and age strata of patients [128], infarct size [129], and random stochastic events encountered commonly during emergencies. Nonetheless, Mant and colleagues [130] used Monte Carlo statistical simulation of management strategies for suspected ACS and found that POCT with cardiac troponins proved cost-effective.

In the CHECKMATE study, Newby and colleagues [131] showed that rapid quantitative multimarker (myoglobin, CK-MB, and cTnI) NPT identified positive patients earlier and provided better risk stratification for mortality than a local laboratory-based, single-marker approach. NPT was used to facilitate early detection. The study related marker status with 30-day death or infarction. All three markers discriminated 30-day death better than just CK-MB and cTnI, and the report identified the effect of NPT with multimarkers, despite lack of standardization and completion before guidelines suggested use of the 99th percentile of the normal interval and the 10% coefficient of variation precision level as the cutoff [132]. In 2001, McCord and colleagues [6] showed POC myoglobin and cTnI can help exclude AMI rapidly during the first 90 minutes after presentation to the ED. Using NPT in the CCU, Eggers and colleagues [133] showed that when a 10% coefficient of variation cutoff was used, POC multimarkers (cTnI + CK-MB + myoglobin) did not necessarily offer additional diagnostic value versus cTnI alone in the exclusion of MI. Thus, decision levels may affect the clinical efficiency of multivariate (multimarker) approaches, which need to be optimized mathematically and statistically.

Biomarkers of neurohormonal activation in heart failure include BNP and the N-terminal fragment of its prohormone (NT-proBNP), collectively called "BNP" here. In a recent University HealthSystem Consortium comprehensive review, Cummings and colleagues [134] cataloged the merits of BNP-facilitated decision making for early intervention, fewer echocardiograms, severity assessment, risk stratification, prognostic value, therapeutic monitoring, discharge decisions, postsurgical status, transplant rejection, sudden death, device alternatives, and so on. For example, a rapid bedside BNP assay recently was shown [135] cost-effective and efficient in accelerating hospital discharge for patients presenting to the ED with acute dyspnea. Outpatient reimbursement for BNP testing increased in 2003. BNP assays now reside, however, on several automated chemistry analyzers appropriate for main laboratories in hospitals where inpatient testing is covered under the capitated DRG reimbursement system. As noted earlier, the 2004 POCT survey [13] showed that institutions may move BNP to the main laboratory. Thus, the cost-effectiveness of future BNP testing depends on multiple dynamic factors that may change often. Chest pain centers are well advised to establish guidelines for BNP testing and its timeliness now and, with the aim of improving outcomes, reevaluate the guidelines periodically during the next 2 years.

BNP, other biomarkers, and POC test clusters (see Table 1) work synergistically. For example, although not POCT, Sabatine and colleagues [47] documented the value of including BNP and C-reactive protein (CRP) along with cTnI for risk stratification, "When patients were categorized on the basis of the number of elevated biomarkers at presentation, there was a near doubling of the mortality risk for each additional biomarker that was elevated ($P = .01$)". The investigators suggested using the number of elevated biomarkers at presentation to risk stratify patients for short- and long-term major cardiac events. Multimarker testing as historically configured [49,50] now embraces BNP, CRP, and other cardiac biomarkers to support patient evaluation and treatment. Speed, per se, can be achieved through efficient integration of all clinical pathology services, including the main laboratory (eg, using an automated transport system), NPT (eg, by placing a satellite laboratory in the emergency area), and bedside testing. The extent to which each of these modalities can be used conveniently for multimarker testing depends on individual health system facilities, organization, and priorities. However, to take advantage of multivariate analysis (eg, using cTnI, CK-MB, myoglobin, BNP, and CRP) and multimarker benefits—including improved triage, facilitated decision making, consistent ACS work-up of NSTEMI, enhanced communication, efficient cardiology consultation, shortened intervention wait times, scaling of treatment, decreased risk for inappropriate discharge, and reduced length of stay [47,133,136–140]—testing should be early, simultaneous, and quick, which can be accomplished conveniently with POCT.

Chest pain centers, risk management, and customer satisfaction

The largest dollar amount for liability recovery still involves chest pain with subsequent missed transmural MI [141]. Rather than treating patients in their offices, more physicians refer patients to EDs, and high-risk specialists progressively become unwilling to provide ED on-call coverage because of malpractice concerns and skyrocketing premiums [142]. Efficiency mandates that chest pain centers should use prompt rule-out schemes and that rapid cardiac biomarker testing should be performed (along with rapid EKG) to help physicians avoid missing patients who present with AMI, currently estimated to occur in 2% to 5% [109,143,144]. Chest pain centers that adopt a macroscopic viewpoint, aggressive leadership, and legal precautions generate excellent community relations and customer satisfaction [145]. Experience in legal case analysis has revealed patients were sent home before clinical laboratory results became available, only to discover too late an elevated cTnI or CK-MB. Also, physicians may order cardiac biomarker tests for which blood collection is delayed, and attend to other patients or leave the area, thereby inadvertently overlooking important results. POCT and "physician capture" [2] can help alleviate these types of errors and simultaneously provide other critical test results necessary for patient evaluation and triaging.

To reduce risk exposure each institution should identify bottlenecks in cardiac critical pathways and then determine specifically if cardiac biomarker POCT can accelerate evaluation and therapy. TTAT actually achieved not only should meet ACS/AHA guidelines but also should satisfy the current standard of care for rapid response testing of patients with life-threatening conditions. Table 1 includes tests (other than cardiac biomarkers) that are available on the same platforms. These other tests can help physicians synthesize critical care solutions [2,3]. For example, clinicians evaluating acutely ill patients who present with chest pain can order electrolyte measurements, such as potassium (K^+) and ionized calcium (Ca^{++}), and these analytes, already available on several POC platforms (possibly the same ones that perform cardiac biomarker testing), can be integrated increasingly as market demand and manufacturing efficiencies drive instrument consolidation in the cardiac biomarker field.

Summary: planning and implementing point-of-care testing

Table 4 presents 12 fundamental objectives and recommendations to consider when planning and implementing POCT in chest pain centers. If accurate, precise, safe, and cost-effective in the context of holistic cycles of patient care, no a priori reason exists to not use POCT. The discussion below highlights points from Table 4 and key considerations for chest pain centers.

Timeliness accreditation and the Society of Chest Pain Centers

For cardiac biomarkers, the evolution in clinical guidelines has shaped the standard-of-care envelope for timeliness (see Fig. 2). Response time is being decreased by minimizing the WBA time for on-site quantitative testing in vitro. Future ex vivo and in vivo techniques for assessing myocardial function can generate immediate real-time data. Needs assessment by leadership in individual chest pain centers will reveal how best to optimize

POCT, whether performed at the bedside or in near-patient satellite laboratories.

The 2004 United States survey of POCT [13] discussed earlier showed that some main laboratories may move tests, such as BNP, away from the point of care; however, timeliness must be preserved. The authors recommend, therefore, that the timeliness of cardiac biomarker testing and also the elimination of all delayed outlier results be adopted as criteria for accreditation by the Society of Chest Pain Centers. These criteria should be reassessed at least every 2 years as improved POC technologies for WBA grow progressively faster, more accurate, and better integrated.

Therapeutic turnaround time and risk reduction

POCT has set a general precedent for timeliness in the standard of care for critically ill patients. WBA facilitates that timeliness. TTAT (see Fig. 1) represents a common denominator for performance. Diagnostic testing must not compromise TTAT. Chest pain centers not using POCT or fast WBA of cardiac biomarkers eventually may have to prove, perhaps in a court of law if delayed test results lead to a missed diagnosis of AMI and adverse outcomes, that they consistently achieve requisite speed and TTAT without POCT.

Even if courier and pneumatic tube systems serve the ED, testing performed in a main laboratory may generate significantly and unpredictably delayed results that impair patient evaluation or treatment. Decision-makers must be cognizant of the medicolegal ramifications and reduce risk by optimizing performance, that is, by minimizing TTAT. TTAT represents an integrative performance indicator that can be applied to entire cycles of patient care. The time required to perform diagnostic testing should fit comfortably within the TTAT goals for different diagnoses in individual chest pain centers, so that testing does not delay the critical paths of care and increase risk exposure for patients.

User-friendly new cardiac biomarkers and instruments

In view of rapid growth, anticipate the appearance of several new cardiac biomarkers, some developed exclusively for POCT. For novel tests and new indices, chest pain centers should document clinical justification and assure cost-effectiveness. The benefits of on-site testing should outweigh the costs of innovating, implementing,

Table 4
Planning and implementing future POCT in chest pain centers

Objective	Recommendation
• Algorithmic integrative strategies	Embedding POCT within diagnostic-therapeutic algorithms, care paths, and critical pathways improves the overall efficiency and effectiveness of cardiac biomarker testing.
• Connectivity	CPCs should use primarily POC devices that provide connectivity to the electronic medical record and other computerized information systems.
• Critical limits and urgent notification	Urgent notification of critical results assures physician awareness and may help prevent premature discharge to home of patients with evidence of AMI.
• Error prevention and biohazard control	Security of instrument operation, validation of personnel skills, and certification of qualified operators who perform POCT help prevent errors, decrease risk, and contain biohazards.
• Home testing and early detection	Since up to 50% of AMI patients die before reaching the hospital, future home testing with automated communication of cardiac biomarker results may facilitate early life-saving detection and transport.
• Integration of critical care test clusters	POC technologies that combine simultaneous measurements of blood gasses, pH, electrolytes (eg, K^+ and Ca^{++}), metabolites (eg, glucose), and other essential critical care test clusters along with cardiac multimarkers will streamline holistic evaluation, diagnosis, and treatment of critically ill patients.
• Minimum analysis time and critical path	CPCs can provide cardiac biomarker test results as expeditiously as permitted by newer, smaller, and faster analytical methods, which soon may provide quantitative results on fingerstick whole-blood samples in 2 to 3 minutes, thereby facilitating the critical path of patient care.
• Multimarker synthesis and indices	Multimarker synthesis will facilitate differential diagnosis and risk profiling through evidence-based joint probabilities and mathematical heuristics using indices that help decipher myocardial ischemia, NSTEMI, STEMI, heart failure, and inflammation.
• POCT coordinator and hybrid staff	POCT should be managed by POC Coordinators who work collaboratively with nurses and physicians to enhance performance through education, quality control, compliance monitoring, and proficiency testing.
• Quantitative assay performance	Quantitative POC assays should achieve equivalent or better performance (detection threshold, accuracy, and 10% coefficient of variation for precision at the 99th percentile of normals) and clinical performance (sensitivity, specificity, and predictive values) versus main laboratory counterparts.
• Standardization, continuity, and consistency	Use of identical POC assays in the CPC and critical care areas (eg, CCU, ICU, and OR) promotes local consistency, while for clinical continuity dissimilar assays, if used, should be referenced to the same comparison method or better, standardized, and all methods should have compatible reference intervals, decision levels, and critical limits.
• Timeliness and accreditation	Expanding numbers of CPCs in the US will lead to higher expectations for fast cardiac biomarker results and codification of timeliness, potentially a Society of CPCs accreditation requirement, here suggested as the analysis time of 15 minutes for POCT, with all results received by the clinical team within the ACC/AHA guidelines preferred time of 30 minutes (order-to-receipt, 24 h/d, 7 d/wk).

Abbreviations: ACC, American College of Cardiology; AHA, American Heart Association; CCU, cardiac/coronary care unit; CPC, chest pain center; ICU, intensive care unit; NSTEMI, non-ST-elevation myocardial infarction; OR, operating room; STEMI, ST-elevation myocardial infarction; TTAT, therapeutic turnaround time.

and operating POCT or proprietary miltimarker indices. Economic analysis should assess the total benefits and costs of care episodes and determine the marginal effects of POCT alternatives. Analysis also should take into account hospital admissions that could have been prevented through timely cardiac biomarker POCT. Already valuable risk stratification will build as new POCT inventions and innovations appear, but lack of definitive biomarkers for myocardial ischemia represents an unmet need. Research should target discovery of highly sensitive and specific biochemical tests predictive for myocardial ischemia.

Because the 2004 POCT United States survey [13] showed hospitals evaluated but then rejected cardiac biomarker instrument platforms more frequently than other forms of POCT, user-friendly POC instrument designs also are needed badly. Solutions currently available will not satisfy the present or future needs of chest pain centers or busy EDs. Poorly integrated systems that lack connectivity to the electronic medical record threaten quality control monitoring and make the management tasks of the POC coordinator extremely difficult. Additionally, existing devices are poorly adapted for emergency field response and must be simplified substantially to garner waived status for home testing under federal regulations.

Algorithmic practice and quantitative testing

POCT can speed diagnostic synthesis in chest pain centers, and speed is essential in EDs overwhelmed with patients. For most cardiac biomarkers, accelerated algorithmic strategies will help position cardiac biomarkers temporally and optimally within the diagnostic decision tree and its treatment branches to take advantage of time-dependent kinetics, sensitivities, specificities, predictive values, and multivariate functions. The choice of test clusters, types of instruments, and sites, such as bedside or near-patient (eg, an ED satellite laboratory) and home or field (eg, ambulance, helicopter, ships, and airplanes), rests with collaborative care teams who must assure the continuity, efficiency, and efficacy of critical pathways in emergency situations.

Whether using cardiac biomarker POCT onsite or testing performed elsewhere, United States physicians (and physicians in United States jurisdictions abroad) must be aware of FDA-approved manufacturer claims to avoid clinical misuse of tests and unnecessary liability. Quantitative testing

is recommended by the ACC/AHA, ECS, and NACB guidelines discussed earlier, and also here. Qualitative testing remains beneficial in some cases to determine quickly whether a patient is "hot or not." Highly sensitive quantitative testing with well-defined detection limits [146], however, has several advantages and better fits the multidimensional, multimarker, and multivariate algorithmic practice of the future in chest pain centers.

Leadership vision and chest pain centers

With more than 150 sites in the United States in 2005, chest pain centers now can pool professional resources to: (a) consolidate care algorithms, (b) write guidelines for POCT, (c) systematize bedside and NPT, (d) consider adopting timeliness accreditation criteria, (e) form purchasing groups to obtain POC devices and reagents inexpensively, (f) facilitate rapid discovery of evidence to avoid missing patients with AMI, (g) monitor performance indicators, such as TTAT, regularly, and (h) provide outreach programs to extend cardiac biomarker testing to field and home sites to help reduce unacceptably high mortality rates there.

POCT should be approached from the standpoint of the laboratory-clinical-community interface and optimized by physicians, nurses, POC coordinators, and laboratorians working collaboratively [2,147]. Professional leadership groups, such as the Society of Chest Pain Centers, can help guide the current rapid growth of cardiac biomarker POCT to fulfill important practice goals, including accurate diagnosis of myocardial ischemia, improved triage, administration of proven treatment (eg, glycoprotein IIb/IIIa inhibitors), quantitative risk stratification, early invasive strategies, and improved economic and medical outcomes.

Acknowledgments

We thank Ms. Claudia Graham, University of California Artist, for drawing Fig. 1. We are indebted to Ms. Susan Farber of Enterprise Analysis Corporation for sharing the 2004 US POCT survey data on cardiac biomarkers. We thank colleagues in industry who responded when asked to review the data in Tables 1 through 3. Figures and tables were used permission and courtesy of Knowledge Optimization®, Davis, CA 95616.

References

[1] Kost GJ. Principles and practice of point-of-care testing. Philadelphia: Lippincott, Williams, and Wilkins; 2002.

[2] Kost GJ. The hybrid laboratory, therapeutic turn-around time, critical limits, performance maps, and Knowledge Optimization®. In: Kost GJ, editor. Principles and practice of point-of-care testing. Philadelphia: Lippincott, Williams, and Wilkins; 2002. p. 13–25.

[3] Kost GJ. Controlling economics, preventing errors, and optimizing outcomes in point-of-care testing. In: Kost GJ, editor. Principles and practice of point-of-care testing. Philadelphia: Lippincott, Williams, and Wilkins; 2002. p. 577–600.

[4] Bourke SE, Kirk JD, Kost GJ. Point-of-care testing in emergency medicine. In: Kost GJ, editor. Principles and practice of point-of-care testing. Philadelphia: Lippincott, Williams, and Wilkins; 2002. p. 99–118.

[5] Kost GJ, Bullock J, Despotis GJ. On-site and near-patient testing in the operating room. In: Kost GJ, editor. Principles and practice of point-of-care testing. Philadelphia: Lippincott, Williams, and Wilkins; 2002. p. 119–32.

[6] McCord J, Nowak RM, McCullogh PA, et al. Ninety-minute exclusion of acute myocardial infarction by use of quantitative point-of-care testing of myoglobin and troponin I. Circulation 2001;104: 1483–8.

[7] Ng SM, Krishnaswamy P, Morissey R, et al. Ninety-minute accelerated critical pathway for chest pain evaluation. Am J Cardiol 2001;88:611–7.

[8] Maisel AS. Point-of-care diagnosis and management of myocardial infarction and congestive heart failure. In: Kost GJ, editor. Principles and practice of point-of-care testing. Philadelphia: Lippincott, Williams, and Wilkins; 2002. p. 554–66.

[9] Hainut C, Gade W. The emerging roles of BNP and accelerated cardiac protocols in emergency laboratory medicine. Clin Lab Sci 2003;16:166–79.

[10] Amsterdam EA, Lewis WR, Kirk JD, et al. Acute ischemic syndromes. Chest pain center concept. Cardiol Clin 2002;20:117–36.

[11] Society of Chest Pain Centers. eNews Update. January 24, 2005. Available at: http://www.scpcp.org/accreditation/index.html.

[12] Kugelmass AD, Anderson AL, Brown PB, et al. Does having a chest pain center impact the treatment and survival of acute myocardial infarction patients [abstract no. 1932]? J Amer Heart Assoc (Suppl to Circulation) 2004;110(17):111–409.

[13] Farber S. US hospitals point-of-care survey. Cardiac makers section excerpt. January 24, 2005. Stanford (CT): Enterprise Analysis Corporation; 2004.

[14] Diller W. Hospitals' hang-ups with point-of-care testing. Around the Industry. Available at: http://www.windover.com; 2004. December: 2,8,9.

[15] Rosen S. Market outlook for IVDs. IVD Tech 2004;10(7):39–43. Available at: http://www.devicelink.com/ivdt/archive/04/06/001.html. Accessed December 28, 2004.

[16] Kost GJ. Goals, guidelines, and principles for point-of-care testing. In: Kost GJ, editor. Principles and practice of point-of-care testing. Philadelphia: Lippincott, Williams, and Wilkins; 2002. p. 3–12.

[17] Kost GJ. Preventing medical errors in point-of-care testing: security, validation, safeguards, and connectivity. Arch Pathol Lab Med 2001;125: 1307–15.

[18] Goldmann BU, Langenbrink L, Matschuck G, et al. Quantitative bedside testing of troponin T: is it equal to laboratory testing? The Cardiac Reader Troponin T (CARE T) study. Clin Lab 2004;50: 1–10.

[19] Agewall S. Evaluation of point-of-care test systems using the new definition of myocardial infarction. Clin Biochem 2003;36:27–30.

[20] Saadeddin S, Habbab M, Siddieg H, et al. Reliability of the rapid bedside whole-blood quantitative cardiac troponin T assay in the diagnosis of myocardial injury in patients with acute coronary syndrome. Med Sci Monit 2004;10:43–6.

[21] Yamamoto M, Komiyama N, Koizumi T, et al. Usefulness of rapid quantitative measurement of myoglobin and troponin T in early diagnosis of acute myocardial infarction. Circ J 2004;68: 639–44.

[22] Seino Y, Tomita Y, Takano T, et al. Office cardiologists cooperative study on whole blood rapid panel tests in patients with suspicious acute myocardial infarction. Comparison between heart-type fatty acid-binding protein and troponin T tests. Circ J 2004;68:144–8.

[23] Schwartz JG, Gage CL, Farley NJ, et al. Evaluation of the cardiac STATus CK-MB/myoglobin card test to diagnose acute myocardial infarctions in the ED. Am J Emerg Med 1997;15:303–7.

[24] Heeschen C, Goldmann BU, Moeller RH, et al. Analytical performance and clinical application of a new rapid bedside assay for the detection of serum troponin I. Clin Chem 1998;44:1925–30.

[25] Panteghini M, Cuccia C, Pagani F, et al. Comparison of the diagnostic performance of two rapid bedside biochemical assays in the early detection of acute myocardial infarction. Clin Cardiol 1998; 21:394–8.

[26] Brogan GX, Bock JL, McCuskey CF, et al. Evaluation of cardiac STATus CK-MB/myoglobin device for rapidly ruling out acute myocardial infarction. Clin Lab Med 1997;17:655–68.

[27] Shindelman J, Bellet N, Haley K, et al. Development of a high-sensitivity immunoassay for c-reactive protein on Cholestech LDX, a point-of-care analyzer. Point of Care: the Journal of Near-Patient Test and Technology 2004;3:191–4.

[28] Apple FS, Murakami MM, Christenson RH, et al. Analytical performance of i-STAT cardiac troponin I assay. Clin Chim Acta 2004;345:123–7.

[29] Drug Testing. Available at: http://www.drugtesting. com.au. Accessed January 7, 2005.

[30] Syn X Pharma. Available at: http://www.synxpharma. com/news_2004_1.html. Accessed January 7, 2005.

[31] Wu AHB, Smith A, Christenson RH, et al. Evaluation of a point-of-care assay for cardiac markers for patients suspected of acute myocardial infarction. Clin Chim Acta 2004;346:211–9.

[32] Wantanabe T, Ohkubo Y, Matsuoka H, et al. Development of a simple whole blood panel test for detection of human heart-type acid binding protein. Clin Biochem 2001;34:257–63.

[33] Hsu LF, Koh TH, Lim YL. Cardiac marker point-of-care testing: evaluation of rapid on-site biochemical marker analysis for diagnosis of acute myocardial infarction. Ann Acad Med Singapore 2000;29:421–7.

[34] Christenson RH, Cervelli DR, Bauer RS, et al. Cardiac troponin I method: performance characteristics including imprecision at low concentrations. Clin Biochem 2004;37:679–83.

[35] Apple FS, Christenson RH, Valdes R, et al. Simultaneous rapid measurement of whole blood myoglobin, creatine kinase MB, and cardiac troponin I by the Triage Cardiac Panel for detection of myocardial infarction. Clin Chem 1999;45:199–205.

[36] Clark TJ, McPherson PH, Buechler KF. Triage cardiac panel: cardiac markers for the triage system. Point of Care: the Journal of Near-Patient Test and Technology 2002;1:42–6.

[37] Apple FS, Anderson FP, Collinson P, et al. Clinical evaluation of the first medical whole blood, point-of-care testing device for detection of myocardial infarction. Clin Chem 2000;46:1604–9.

[38] Mulcahy K, Montalvo J, Tran L, Oltjenbruns X. The alpha dx point-of-need system: an evaluation with reference to the national association of clinical biochemistry recommendations for the use of cardiac markers in coronary artery disease. Point of Care: the Journal of Near-Patient Test and Technology 2002;1:58–61.

[39] Tang Z, Louie RF, Kost GJ. Principles and performance of point-of-care testing instruments. In: Kost GJ, editor. Principles and practice of point-of-care testing. Philadelphia: Lippincott, Williams, and Wilkins; 2002. p. 67–92.

[40] Cummings JP, Kost GJ, Matuszewski KA, et al. POC tests for cardiac injury markers: clinical improvement and effectiveness. Oak Brook (IL): University HealthSystem Consortium; 2000.

[41] Ammirati EB. Regulatory qualification of new point-of-care diagnostics. In: Kost GJ, editor. Principles and practice of point-of-care testing. Philadelphia: Lippincott, Williams, and Wilkins; 2002. p. 469–80.

[42] Poe SS, Case-Cromer DL. Nursing strategies for point-of-care testing. In: Kost GJ, editor. Principles and practice of point-of-care testing. Philadelphia: Lippincott, Williams, and Wilkins; 2002. p. 214–35.

[43] Anderson M. Assessing point-of-care testing programs. In: Kost GJ, editor. Principles and practice of point-of-care testing. Philadelphia: Lippincot, Williams, and Wilkins; 2002. p. 417–21.

[44] Kost GJ. New whole blood analyzers and their impact on cardiac and critical care. Crit Rev Clin Lab Sci 1993;30:153–202.

[45] Cheng V, Kazanagra R, Garcia A, et al. A rapid bedside test for B-type peptide predicts treatment outcomes in patients admitted for decompensated heart failure: a pilot study. J Am Coll Cardiol 2001;37:386–91.

[46] Bhalla MA, Chiang A, Epstheyn VA, et al. Prognostic role of b-type natriuretic peptide levels in patients with type 2 diabetes mellitus. J Am Coll Cardiol 2004;44:1047–52.

[47] Sabatine MS, Morrow DA, de Lemos JA, et al. Multimarker approach to risk stratification in non-ST elevation acute coronary syndromes. Simultaneous assessment of troponin I, C-reactive protein, and B-type natriuretic peptide. Circulation 2002;105:1760–3.

[48] James SK, Lindahl B, Armstrong P, et al. A rapid troponin I assay is not optimal for determination of troponin status and prediction of subsequent cardiac events at suspicion of unstable coronary syndromes. Int J Cardiol 2004;93:113–20.

[49] Mueller T, Gegenhuber A, Poelz W, et al. Head-to-head comparison of diagnostic utility of BNP and NT-proBNP in symptomatic and asymptomatic structural heart disease. Clin Chim Acta 2004; 341:41–8.

[50] Dahler-Eriksen BS, Lauritzen T, Lassen JF, et al. Near-patient test for c-reactive protein in general practice: assessment of clinical, organizational, and economic outcomes. Clin Chem 1999;45:478–85.

[51] http://www.nhlbi.nih.gov/health/dci/Diseases/Heart Attack/HeartAttack_WhatIs.html. Accessed February 13, 2005.

[52] Collinson PO, Chandler HA, Stubbs PJ, et al. Measurement of serum troponin T, creatine kinase MB isoenzyme, and total creatine kinase following arduous physical training. Ann Clin Biochem 1995; 32:450–3.

[53] Roth A, Malov N, Bloch Y, et al. Assessment of a creatine kinase-MB/myoglobin in the prehospital setting in patients presenting with acute nontraumatic chest pain: the "shahal" experience. Crit Care Med 1999;27:1085–9.

[54] Schuchert A, Hamm C, Scholz J, et al. Prehospital testing for troponin T in patients with suspected acute myocardial infarction. Am Heart J 1999; 138:45–8.

[55] McCullough PA, Nowak RM, Foreback C. Performance of multiple cardiac biomarkers measured in the emergency department in patients with chronic kidney disease and chest pain. Acad Emerg Med 2002;9:1389–96.

[56] Diris JH, Hackeng CM, Kooman JP, et al. Impaired renal clearance explains elevated troponin T fragments in hemodialysis patients. Circulation 2004;109:23–5.

[57] Dempfle C, Schraml M, Besenthal I, et al. Multicentre evaluation of a new point-of-care test for the quantitative determination of D-dimer. Clin Chim Acta 2001;307:211–8.

[58] Legnani C, Fariselli S, Cini M, et al. A new rapid bedside assay for quantitative testing of D-dimer (cardiac D-dimer) in the diagnostic work-up for deep vein thrombosis. Thromb Res 2003;111:149–53.

[59] Kost GJ, Omand K, Kirk JD. A strategy for the use of cardiac injury markers (troponin I and T, creatine kinase-MB mass and isoforms, and myoglobin) in the diagnosis of acute myocardial infarction. Arch Pathol Lab Med 1998;122:245–51.

[60] Hudson MP, Christenson RH, Newby LK, et al. Cardiac markers: point of care testing. Clin Chim Acta 1999;284:223–37.

[61] Ohman EM, Armstrong PW, White HD, et al. Risk stratification with a point-of-care cardiac troponin test in acute myocardial infarction. GUSTOIII. Am J Cardiol 1999;84:1281–6.

[62] Giannitsis E, Lehrke S, Wiegand UK, et al. Risk stratification in patients with inferior acute myocardial infarction treated by percutaneous coronary interventions: the role of admission troponin T. Circulation 2000;102:2038–44.

[63] Azzazy HM, Christenson RH. Cardiac markers of acute coronary syndromes: is there a case for point-of-care testing? Clin Biochem 2002;35:13–27.

[64] Lewandrowski K, Chen A, Januzzi J. Cardiac markers for myocardial infarction. A brief review. Am J Clin Pathol 2002;118:S93–9.

[65] Braunwald E, Antman EM, Beasley JW, et al. ACC/AHA guideline update for the management of patients with unstable angina and non-ST-segment elevation myocardial infarction—2002: summary article: a report of the American College of Cardiology/American Heart Association Task Force on Practice Guidelines (Committee on the Management of Patients with Unstable Angina). Circulation 2002;106:1893–900. Full text available at: www.acc.org. Accessed February 16, 2005.

[66] Antman EM, Anabe DT, Armstrong PW, et al. ACC/AHA guidelines for the management of patients with ST-elevation myocardial infarction—executive summary. J Amer Coll Cardiol 2004;44:671–719. Full text available at: www.aacc.org. Accessed January 22, 2005.

[67] Antman EM, Grudzien C, Sacks DB. Evaluation of a rapid bedside assay for detection of serum cardiac troponin T. JAMA 1995;273:1279–82.

[68] Lee-Lewandrowski E, Benzer T, Corboy D, et al. Cardiac marker testing as part of an emergency department point-of-care satellite laboratory in a large academic medical center: practical issues concerning implementation. Point of Care: the Journal of Near-Patient Testing and Technology 2002;1:145–54.

[69] Hamm CW, Goldmann BU, Heeschen C, et al. Emergency room triage of patients with acute chest pain by means of rapid testing for cardiac troponin T or troponin I. N Engl J Med 1997;337:1648–53.

[70] Schwartz JC, Gage CL, Farley NJ, et al. Evaluation of the Cardiac STATus CK-MB/myoglobin card test to diagnose acute myocardial infarctions in the ED. Am J Emer Med 1997;15:303–7.

[71] Hirschl MM, Herkner H, Laggner AN, et al. Analytical and clinical performance of an improved qualitative troponin T rapid test in laboratories and critical care units. Arch Pathol Lab Med 2000;124:583–7.

[72] Muller-Bardoff M, Rauscher T, Kampmann M, et al. Quantitative bedside assay for cardiac troponin T: a complementary method to centralized laboratory testing. Clin Chem 1999;45:1002–8.

[73] Plebani M, Zaninotto M. Cardiac markers: centralized or decentralized testing? Clin Chem Lab Med 1999;37:1113–7.

[74] Storrow AB, Gibler WB. The role of cardiac markers in the emergency department. Clin Chim Acta 1999;284:187–96.

[75] Kratz A, Januzzi JL, Lewandrowski KB, et al. Positive predictive value of a point-of-care testing strategy on first-draw specimens for the emergency department-based detection of acute coronary syndromes. Arch Pathol Lab Med 2002;126:1487–93.

[76] Melanson SF, Lee-Lewandrowski E, Januzzi JL, et al. Reevaluation of myoglobin for acute chest pain evaluation. Would false-positive results on "first-draw" specimens lead to increased hospital admissions? Am J Clin Pathol 2004;121:804–8.

[77] Apple FS, Quist HE, Otto AP, et al. Release characteristics of cardiac biomarkers and ischemia-modified albumin as measured by the albumin cobalt-binding test after a marathon race. Clin Chem 2002;48:1097–100.

[78] Quiles J, Roy D, Gaze D, et al. Relation of ischemia-modified albumin (IMA) levels following elective angioplasty for stable angina pectoris to duration of balloon-induced myocardial ischemia. Am J Cardiol 2003;92:322–4.

[79] Sinha MK, Gaze DC, Tippins JR, et al. Ischemia modified albumin is a sensitive marker of myocardial ischemia after percutaneous coronary intervention. Circulation 2003;107:2403–5.

[80] Wu AH. The ischemia-modified albumin biomarker for myocardial ischemia. Med Lab Obser 2003;35:36–40.

[81] Borderie D, YAllanore, Meune C, et al. High ischemia-modified albumin concentration reflects

oxidative stress but not myocardial ischemia in system sclerosis. Clin Chem 2004;50:2190–3.

[82] Garrido IP, Roy D, Calvino R, et al. Comparison of ischemia-modified albumin levels in patient undergoing percutaneous coronary intervention for unstable angina pectoris with versus without coronary collaterals. Am J Cardiol 2004;93:88–90.

[83] Roy D, Quiles J, Aldama G, et al. Ischemia modified albumin for the assessment of patients presenting to the emergency department with acute chest pain but normal or non-diagnostic 12-lead electrocardiograms and negative cardiac troponin T. Int J Cardiol 2004;97:297–301.

[84] Roy D, Quiles J, Sharma R, et al. Ischemia-modified albumin concentration in patients with peripheral vascular disease and exercise-induced skeletal muscle ischemia. Clin Chem 2004;50:1656–60.

[85] Roy D, Quiles J, Sinha M, et al. Effect of direct-current cardioversion on ischemia-modified albumin levels in patients with atrial defibrillation. Am J Cardiol 2004;93:366–8.

[86] Roy D, Quiles J, Sinha M, et al. Effect of radiofrequency catheter ablation on the biochemical marker ischemia modified albumin. Am J Cardiol 2004;94:234–6.

[87] Zapico-Muniz E, Santalo-Bel M, Merce-Muntanola J, et al. Ischemia-modified albumin during skeletal muscle ischemia. Clin Chem 2004;50:1063–5.

[88] Braunwald E, Antman EM, Beasley JW, et al. ACC/AHA guidelines for the management of patients with unstable angina and non-ST-segment elevation myocardial infarction: a report of the American College of Cardiology/American Heart Association Task Force on Practice Guidelines. J Am Coll Cardiol 2000;36:970–1062 and Circulation 2000;102:1193–209.

[89] Joint European Society of Cardiology/American College of Cardiology Committee. Myocardial infarction redefined—a consensus document of the joint European Society of Cardiology/American College of Cardiology Committee for the redefinition of myocardial infarction. J Am Coll Cardiol 2000;36:959–69.

[90] European Society of Cardiology Task Force for the Diagnosis and Treatment of Chronic Heart Failure. Guidelines for the diagnosis and treatment of chronic heart failure. Eur Heart J 2001;22:1527–60.

[91] Caragher TE, Fernandez BB, Jacobs FL, et al. Evaluation of quantitative cardiac biomarker point-of-care testing in the emergency department. J Emer Med 2002;22:1–7.

[92] Collinson PO, Gerhardt W, Katus HA, et al. Multicentre evaluation of an immunological rapid test for the detection of troponin T in whole blood samples. Eur J Clin Chem Clin Biochem 1996;34:591–8.

[93] Sylven C, Lindahl S, Hellkvist K, et al. Excellent reliability of nurse-based bedside diagnosis of acute myocardial infarction by rapid dry-strip creatine kinase MB, myoglobin, and troponin T. Am Heart J 1998;135:677–83.

[94] Collinson PO. The need for point of care testing: an evidence-based appraisal. Scand J Clin Lab Invest 1999;230(Suppl):67–73.

[95] Stubbs P, Collinson PO. Point-of-care testing: a cardiologist's view. Clin Chim Acta 2001;15:57–61.

[96] Altinier S, Zaninotto M, Mion M, et al. Point-of-care testing of cardiac markers: results from an experience in an emergency department. Clin Chim Acta 2001;311:67–72.

[97] Gaze D, Collinson PO, Haass M, et al. The use of a quantitative point-of-care system greatly reduces the turnaround time of cardiac marker determination. Point of Care: the Journal of Near-Patient Testing and Technology 2004;3:156–8.

[98] Lee-Lewandrowski E, Corboy D, Lewandrowski K, et al. Implementation of a point-of-care satellite laboratory in the emergency department of an academic medical center. Impact on test turnaround time and patient emergency department length of stay. Arch Pathol Lab Med 2003;127:456–60.

[99] Kilgore ML, Steindel SJ, Smith JA. Evaluating stat testing options in an academic health center: therapeutic turnaround time and staff satisfaction. Clin Chem 1998;44:1597–603.

[100] St-Louis P. Status of point-of-care testing: promise, realities, and possibilities. Clin Biochem 2000;33:427–40.

[101] Drenck N. Point of care testing in critical care medicine: the clinician's view. Clin Chim Acta 2001;307:3–7.

[102] Christenson RH, Collinson PO. Point-of-care testing for cardiac markers: an outcome-based appraisal. In: Price CP, St John A, Hicks JM, editors. Point-of-care testing. Washington DC: AACC Press; 2004. p. 375–94.

[103] Howanitz PJ, Cembrowski GS, Steindel SJ, et al. Physician goals and laboratory test turnaround times. A College of American Pathologists Q-Probes study of 2763 clinicians and 722 institutions. Arch Pathol Lab Med 1993;117:22–8.

[104] Howanitz PJ, Steindel SJ, Cembrowski GS, et al. Emergency department stat test turnaround times. A College of American Pathologists' Q-Probes study for potassium and hemoglobin. Arch Pathol Lab Med 1992;116:122–8.

[105] Steindel SJ, Howanitz PJ. Changes in emergency department turnaround time performance from 1990 to 1993. A comparison of two College of American Pathologists Q-Probes studies. Arch Pathol Lab Med 1997;121:1031–41.

[106] Novis DA, Jones BA, Dale JC, et al. Biochemical markers of myocardial injury test turnaround time: a College of American Pathologists Q-Probes study of 7020 troponin and 4368 creatine kinase-MB determinations in 159 institutions. Arch Pathol Lab Med 2004;128:158–64.

[107] Panteghini M, Apple FS, Christenson RH, et al. Use of biochemical markers in acute coronary syndromes. Clin Chem Lab Med 1999;37:687–93.

[108] Wu AHB, Apple FS, Gibler WB, et al. National Academy of Clinical Biochemistry standards for laboratory practice: recommendations for the use of cardiac markers in coronary diseases. Clin Chem 1999;45:1104–21.

[109] Kamineni R, Alpert JS. Acute coronary syndromes: initial evaluation and risk stratification. Prog Cardiovas Dis 2004;46:379–92.

[110] Lambrew CT, Smith MS, Annas GG, et al. National Heart Attack Alert Program Coordinating Committee 60 Minutes to Treatment Working Group. Emergency department: rapid identification and treatment of patients with acute myocardial infarction Bethesda (MD): National Institutes of Health; 1993. Ann Emerg Med 1994;23:311–29.

[111] Storrow AB. NACB recommendations—logistics (administrative, cost-effectiveness, point-of-care, what are the rules?) Laboratory Medicine Practice Guidelines (LMPG)—biomarkers of acute coronary syndrome and heart failure. Available at: http://www.nacb.org/lmpg/card_biomarkers_ LMPG_ draft_PDF.stm. Accessed September 23, 2005.

[112] Males RG, Stephenson J, Harris P. Cardiac markers and point-of-care testing: a perfect fit. Crit Care Nurs Q 2001;24:54–61.

[113] Henderson AR, Gerhardt W, Apple FS. The use of biochemical markers in ischemic heart disease: summary of the roundtable and extrapolations. Clin Chim Acta 1998;272:93–100.

[114] Kellett J, Hirschl MM, Derhaschnig U, et al. Bedside testing of cardiac troponin T and myoglobin for the detection of acute myocardial infarction in patients with a nondiagnostic electrocardiogram in the emergency department. Point of Care: the Journal of Near-Patient Testing and Technology 2004;3:159–61.

[115] Derhaschnig U, Hirschl MM, Collinson PO, et al. Diagnostic efficiency of a point-of-care system for quantitative determination of troponin T and myoglobin in the coronary care unit. Point of Care: the Journal of Near-Patient Testing and Technology 2004;3:162–4.

[116] Gomez MA, Anderson JL, Karagounis LA, et al. An emergency department-based protocol for rapidly ruling out myocardial ischemia reduces hospital time and expense: results of a randomized study (ROMIO). J Am Coll Cardiol 1996;28:25–33.

[117] Anderson FP, Fritz ML, Kontos MC, et al. Cost-effectiveness of cardiac troponin I in a systematic chest pain evaluation protocol: use of cardiac troponin I lowers length of stay for low-risk patients. Clin Lab Manage Rev 1998;12:63–9.

[118] Blomkalns AL, Gibler WB. Markers and the initial triage and treatment of patients with chest pain. Cardiovasc Toxicol 2001;1:111–5.

[119] Beyerle K. POC testing of cardiac markers enhances ED care. Nurs Manage 2002;33:37–9.

[120] Panteghini M. The measurement of cardiac markers: where should we focus? Am J Clin Pathol 2002;118:354–61.

[121] Panteghini M. Acute coronary syndrome: biochemical strategies in the troponin era. Chest 2002;122:1428–35.

[122] Goodacre S, Calvert N. Cost effectiveness of diagnostic strategies for patients with acute, undifferentiated chest pain. Emer Med J 2003;20:429–33.

[123] Gibler WB, Hoekstra JW, Weaver WD, et al. A randomized trial of the effects of early cardiac serum marker availability on reperfusion therapy in patients with acute myocardial infarction: the serial markers, acute myocardial infarction and rapid treatment trial (SMARTT). J Am Coll Cardiol 2000;36:1500–6.

[124] Fermann GJ, Suyama J. Point of care testing in the emergency department. J Emer Med 2002;22: 393–404.

[125] Kugelmass A, Anderson A, Katz M, et al. Point-of-care biomarkers: does it make a difference in acute myocardial infarction outcomes? Circulation 2004; 109:50 [abstract no. P248].

[126] Dadkhah S, Fisch C, Zonia C, et al. Accelerated coronary reperfusion through the use of rapid bedside cardiac markers. Case Reports. Angiology. J Vascular Dis 1999;50:55–62.

[127] Edmond JJ, French JK, Henny H, et al. Prospective evaluation of a chest pain pathway at Green Lane Hospital. N Z Med J 2002;115:U103.

[128] Polancyzk CA, Kuntz KM, Sacks DB, et al. Emergency department triage strategies for acute chest pain using creatine kinase-MB and troponin I assays: a cost-effectiveness analysis. Ann Intern Med 1999;131:909–18.

[129] de Winter RJ, Koster RW, Sturk A, et al. Value of myoglobin, troponin T, and CK-MB mass in ruling out an acute myocardial infarction in the emergency room. Circulation 1995;92:3401–7.

[130] Mant J, McManus RJ, Oakes RA, et al. Systematic review and modeling of the investigation of acute and chronic chest pain presenting in primary care. Health Tech Assess 2004;8:1–158.

[131] Newby LK, Storrow AB, Gibler WB, et al. Bedside multimarker testing for risk stratification in chest pain units. The chest pain evaluation by creatine kinase-MB, myoglobin, and troponin I (CHECK-MATE) study. Circulation 2001;103:1832–7.

[132] Apple FS, Jaffe AS. Bedside multimarker testing for risk stratification in chest pain units: the chest pain evaluation by creatine kinase-MB, myoglobin, and troponin I (CHECKMATE) study [Letter and Newby response]. Circulation 2001;104:E125.

[133] Eggers KM, Oldgren J, Nordenskjold A, et al. Diagnostic value of serial measurement of cardiac markers in patients with chest pain: limited value of adding myoglobin to troponin I for exclusion

of myocardial infarction. Am Heart J 2004;148: 574–81.

[134] Cummings JP, Kost GJ, Matuszewski KA, Ratko TA (contributing reviewers). UHC high-impact technology brief: B-type natriuretic peptide blood test. Oak Brook (IL): University HealthSystem Consortium; 2003.

[135] Mueller C, Scholer A, Laule-Kilian K, et al. Use of B-type natriuretic peptide in the evaluation and management of acute dyspnea. N Engl J Med 2004;350:647–54.

[136] Fonarow GC, Horwich TB. Combining natriuretic peptides and necrosis markers in determining prognosis in heart failure. Rev Cardiovasc Med 2003; (Suppl 4):S20–8.

[137] Gibler WB, Blomkalns AL, Collins SP. Evaluation of chest pain and heart failure in the emergency department: impact of multimarker strategies and B-type natriuretic peptide. Rev Cardiovasc Med 2003;4(Suppl 4):S47–55.

[138] de Lemos JA, Morrow DA. Combining natriuretic peptides and necrosis markers in the assessment of acute coronary syndromes. Rev Cardovasc Med 2003;4(Suppl 4):S37–46.

[139] James SK, Armstrong P, Barnathan E, et al. Troponin and C-reactive protein have different relations to subsequent mortality and myocardial infarction after acute coronary syndrome: a GUSTO-IV substudy. J Am Coll Cardiol 2003;41: 916–24.

[140] Blick KE. Economics of point-of-care (POC) testing for cardiac markers. In: the value of critical care and point of care testing: who benefits? Proceedings of the 20th International Symposium, Critical and Point of Care Testing Division, American Association for Clinical Chemistry. Wurzburg, Germany. June 9–12, 2004.

[141] Berenson RA, Kuo S, May JH. Medical malpractice liability crisis meets markets: stress in unexpected places. Issue Brief Cent Stud Health Syst Change 2003;68:1–7.

[142] Amon E, Winn HN. Review of professional medical liability insurance crisis: lessons learned from Missouri. Am J Obstet Gynecol 2004;190:1534–40.

[143] Pope HJ, Aufderheide TP, Ruthazer R, et al. Missed diagnosis of acute cardiac ischemia in the emergency department. N Engl J Med 2000;342:1163–70.

[144] Vukmir RB. Medical malpractice: managing the risk. Med Law 2004;23:495–513.

[145] Worthington K. Customer satisfaction in the emergency department. Emerg Med Clin North Am 2004;22:87–102.

[146] Clinical Laboratory and Standards Institute (CLSI). Protocols for Determination of Limits of Detection and Limits of Quantitation. NCCLS-IFCC (ISO) Joint Project. Wayne (PA): CLSI EP17-A; 2005.

[147] Kost GJ, Ehrmeyer SS, Chernow B, et al. The laboratory-clinical interface: point-of-care testing. Chest 1999;115:1140–54.

Markers of Cardiac Ischemia and Inflammation

Tracy Y. Wang, MD, MS[a], Wael A. AlJaroudi, MD, MS[b],
L. Kristin Newby, MD, MHS[c],*

[a]Division of Cardiology, Box 31246, Duke University Medical Center, Durham, NC 27710, USA
[b]Department of Medicine, Box 31184, Duke University Medical Center, Durham, NC 27710, USA
[c]Duke Clinical Research Institute, P.O. Box 17969, Durham, NC 27715-7969, USA

Coronary artery disease (CAD) is one of the leading causes of death in the United States. The challenge is not only to diagnose acute coronary syndromes (ACSs) in patients who present with the traditional combination of anginal pain and electrocardiography (ECG) changes but also to recognize disease in patients who have atypical symptoms and initially nondiagnostic ECGs. Advances in the understanding of the pathophysiology of cellular injury and in analytical technology have made possible the development of molecular markers that can be measured in serum or plasma. This development has already made a tremendous impact on our clinical assessment of myocardial injury. In September 2000, a committee comprising members representing the American College of Cardiology and the European Society of Cardiology redefined acute myocardial infarction (MI), including the manner in which biomarkers of myocardial necrosis, preferentially cardiac troponins, are used in addition to ischemic symptoms and ECG changes [1].

Because current biomarkers of myocardial necrosis only become positive in the setting of MI and disruption of cellular integrity, the diagnosis of MI can only be made in retrospect. Ideally, one would like to identify patients at risk for complications before myocardial necrosis

occurs. Insights into the pathophysiology of atherothrombosis have allowed development of novel markers to detect not only early ischemia without myocyte death, but also early indicators of coronary inflammation in patients with preclinical atherosclerosis.

Inflammation and atherothrombosis

There is extensive literature supporting the role of inflammation in CAD. Hemodynamic forces from hypertension and oxidative stressors, such as tobacco and hyperglycemia, result in vascular endothelial injury. The attachment of leukocytes, transformation of monocytes into macrophages, and subsequent uptake of cholesterol lipoproteins initiate the fatty streak. Cytokine release from the fatty streak recruits further inflammatory cells (macrophages, mast cells, activated T cells), with resulting uptake and oxidation of low-density lipoprotein (LDL). These cytokines also stimulate smooth muscle cell proliferation and development of a collagenous fibrous cap that covers this inflammatory mixture to form the mature atherosclerotic plaque [2].

Recent data show that the risk for an acute coronary event has less to do with the degree of angiographic luminal stenosis than with the underlying pathology of the atherosclerotic plaque that makes it susceptible to rupture [3]. Activated T cells within the atheromatous core secrete interferon gamma that decreases smooth muscle cell production of collagen [4]. Inflammatory cytokine-activated macrophages secrete matrix metalloproteinases that degrade the extracellular matrix, further weakening the fibrous cap and making it prone to rupture [5,6]. Disruption of

Dr. Newby has received consulting honoraria from Ischemia Diagnostics, Inc. and Ortho-Clinical Diagnostics and research grant support from Roche Diagnostics Corporation.

* Corresponding author.

E-mail address: newby001@mc.duke.edu (L.K. Newby).

the cap exposes the atheronecrotic core to blood, after which further inflammatory reactions lead to platelet activation, coagulation cascade, further vasomotor dysfunction [7,8], and ultimately luminal occlusion.

Thus, all stages of atherothrombosis implicate inflammation as a key pathogenic mechanism. Several clinical studies have therefore targeted inflammatory factors as potential markers for cardiovascular risk assessment.

Markers of inflammation

Several inflammatory factors involved in the cascade described earlier have been studied in clinical trials in the last decade. These include the proinflammatory cytokines interleukin (IL)-1, IL-6, tumor necrosis factor α), catalysts of the inflammatory reaction (CD40 ligand), cellular adhesion molecules (intercellular cell adhesion molecule [ICAM]-1, vascular cell adhesion molecule [VCAM]-1, selectins), and acute phase reactants (fibrinogen, white blood count, C-reactive protein [CRP], serum amyloid A).

C-reactive protein

CRP is the best studied of the inflammatory markers in cardiovascular disease. It is an acute-phase protein that has been shown to be a marker of systemic inflammation, elevated in response to acute injury, infection, and other inflammatory stimuli [9]. Hepatic production is directly related to IL-6 stimulation and, unlike other acute phase reactants, its levels remain stable over long periods of time in the absence of new stimuli [10]. Traditional CRP assays with limits of quantification of 3 to 8 mg/L lack adequate sensitivity to detect levels required for atherosclerotic risk prediction. The development of a standardized high-sensitivity CRP (hsCRP) assay has improved precision at low concentrations of CRP that permits its use in cardiovascular risk assessment.

In several studies of patients who have ACS (Chimeric c7E3 AntiPlatelet Therapy in Unstable angina REfactory to standard treatment, Thrombolysis In Myocardial Infarction [TIMI]-11a, and FRagmin during InStability in Coronary artery disease [FRISC] trials), elevated hsCRP at hospital admission independently predicted increased mortality [11–13]. In a Global Use of Strategies to open Occluded arteries IV substudy, hsCRP elevation during the acute stage of unstable CAD was associated with an increased 30-day mortality

independent of troponin levels; there was no association with recurrent MI [14]. However, in stable post-MI patients, elevated hsCRP predicted a significantly higher risk for recurrent nonfatal MI or fatal coronary events (75% higher in the highest versus lowest quintile of hsCRP), suggesting that it is not merely a marker for the extent of myocardial damage [15].

In the European Concerted Action on Thrombosis and Disabilities Angina Pectoris Study, 2121 patients admitted with angina were followed over a 2-year period. A plasma concentration of CRP greater than 3.6 mg/L at study entry was associated with a 45% increase in the relative risk for nonfatal MI or sudden cardiac death (95% confidence interval [CI], 1.15–1.83) [16]. However, the usefulness of measuring hsCRP in patients who have ACS is limited because there is already sufficient evidence warranting maximal lipid-lowering, antiplatelet, and other cardioprotective drug therapies in these patients, so that measurement of hsCRP does not provide incremental information.

The setting in which hsCRP may be most useful is primary prevention. A population-based cross-sectional study in Great Britain showed that the prevalence of CAD increased 1.5 fold (95% CI, 1.25–1.92) for each doubling of hsCRP among men aged 50 to 69 years [17]. In the Multiple Risk Factor Intervention Trial cohort of middle-aged men who had traditional high cardiovascular risk factors, CRP was elevated more in smokers versus nonsmokers. Over 17 years of follow-up, an elevated baseline CRP was associated with a 2.8-fold increased risk for coronary heart disease mortality (95% CI, 1.4–5.4) [18].

Several prospective studies of hsCRP in apparently healthy individuals have also shown that elevated baseline levels of hsCRP are correlated with higher risk for future cardiovascular morbidity and mortality after adjustment for potential confounders. The Physicians Health Study, a prospective, nested case-control study of men who did not have prior history of CAD and had low rates of cigarette use, showed that men in the highest quartile of hsCRP (≥2.1 mg/L) had a significant 2.9-fold increase in risk for MI that was independent of smoking status, lipid levels, and other traditional risk factors for CAD [19]. This finding was confirmed in the Monitoring Trends and Determinants of Cardiovascular Disease (MONICA)–Augsburg prospective study in Europe that followed 936 healthy, middle-aged men over 8 years and noted a 19% increase in risk for future coronary event for each standard deviation increase in baseline hsCRP after adjustment for multiple risk factors [20].

This relationship also bears out in women. In a prospective nested case-control study involving postmenopausal women enrolled in the Women's Health Study, Ridker and colleagues [21] showed hsCRP to be the most powerful predictor of cardiovascular risk compared with other inflammatory markers, baseline lipid levels, and homocysteine. Women in the highest quartile had a relative risk of 4.4 (95% CI, 2.2–8.9, $P < .001$) compared with those in the lowest quartile. Addition of hsCRP to cholesterol measurement increased the area under the receiver operating characteristic (ROC) curve from 0.59 to 0.66 ($P < .001$). Furthermore, in women who had LDL levels less than 130 mg/dL (the target level recommended for primary prevention by the National Cholesterol Education Program), those who had elevated baseline CRP were still at increased risk for future events with a 3.1 relative risk in the highest quartile compared with the lowest (95% CI, 1.7–11.3, $P = .002$) after adjustment for traditional risk factors and high-density lipoprotein (HDL) cholesterol levels.

Prospective data show that hsCRP levels minimally correlate with lipid levels and are a stronger predictor of risk than LDL cholesterol (area under the ROC curve 0.64 versus 0.60) [22]. Therefore, the role of CRP is adjunctive to lipid screening and the additive predictive value of hsCRP to the Framingham 10-year risk score, LDL, total, and HDL cholesterol measurements has been demonstrated in several studies [23,24]. However, there is not yet a consensus that the degree of hsCRP elevation correlates with atherosclerotic burden.

Tataru and colleagues [25] showed that in survivors of MI, there was a significant association of hsCRP level with angiographically detected degree of coronary artery stenosis. In addition, patients who had coronary disease who had sonographically detectable peripheral arterial disease had even higher levels of hsCRP compared with those who had CAD alone. In a small Denmark study of 269 patients referred for elective coronary angiography, hsCRP levels were significantly higher in patients who had coronary stenoses than those who did not, but no difference in hsCRP levels were found comparing groups with single, 2-, or 3-vessel disease [26]. In a nested case-control substudy of the Prospective Army Coronary Calcium trial that looked at healthy men between the age of 40 and 45 years who did not have coronary disease, the prevalence of coronary artery calcium as assessed by electron-beam CT was similar across all hsCRP quartiles [27]. Therefore, although hsCRP has good risk assessment value, there is no definitive evidence supporting its role in selecting patients for coronary angiography.

The role of hsCRP in predicting CAD has been established. What remains uncertain at this time is whether CRP should be a target of therapy or used to guide therapy. In vitro and in vivo studies show that hsCRP contributes to plaque development by increasing monocyte adherence, inducing expression of cell surface adhesion molecules [28], and increasing LDL scavenger cell uptake of cholesterol [29]. Furthermore, high CRP is associated with decreased nitric oxide availability impacting vasomotor activity [30] and increased monocyte production of tissue factor [31]. CRP is also shown to activate complement and neutrophils [32] and decrease fibrinolytic capacity [33], thereby contributing to plaque instability and thrombus formation.

In the Physicians Health Study, use of aspirin was associated with a statistically significant, 55.7% risk reduction for first MI among men who had hsCRP levels in the highest quartile compared with a nonsignificant 13.9% reduction in those who had hsCRP levels in the lowest quartile [19]. No follow-up levels were drawn to deduce whether aspirin directly lowered hsCRP levels.

The anti-inflammatory effects of statins are still unclear; experimental evidence posits statin-mediated reduction in macrophage activation, antiproliferative effects on smooth muscle cells, improvements in endothelial function and vasomotion, and antithrombotic effects [34,35]. At 5-year follow-up of stable post-MI patients randomized in the Cholesterol and Recurrent Events trial, mean hsCRP levels decreased by 37.8% in those randomized to pravastatin therapy, whereas levels increased in the placebo patients [36]. This reduction in hsCRP was independent of the magnitude of changes in lipid levels. Furthermore, patients randomized to pravastatin therapy had a twofold reduction in risk for recurrent MI or fatal coronary event in the elevated hsCRP group compared with the group that did not have elevated hsCRP, even though baseline lipid levels were identical in both groups [15].

More recently, PRavastatin Or atorVastatin Evaluation and Infection Therapy (PROVE-IT) trial demonstrated that intensive statin therapy that lowered hsCRP levels to a mean of less than 2 mg/L resulted in a decreased risk for recurrent MI or death from coronary causes, irrespective of the degree of LDL lowering [37]. In the PRavastatin Inflammation CRP Evaluation (PRINCE) study, pravastatin was shown to also reduce hsCRP levels in patients who did not have prior history of cardiovascular disease [38]. There is not yet evidence linking hsCRP reduction to a reduction in cardiovascular events in the primary prevention setting.

The Centers for Disease Control and Prevention/American Heart Association consensus statement advocates use of hsCRP for risk assessment in patients who are at intermediate risk for cardiovascular events (10% to 20% 10-year risk of coronary event) [39]. However, there is no prospective randomized clinical trial yet examining the benefits or harm of screening with hsCRP. Presently the guidelines rate a hsCRP level less than 1 mg/L as normal, 1 to 3 mg/L intermediate, and more than 3 mg/L as high. A level greater than 10 mg/L indicates a noncardiovascular source of inflammation and should prompt a search for a source of infection or other inflammation. For patients who have ACS, hsCRP may provide some prognostic information, and a cutoff level of more than 10 mg/L is most predictive of risk for adverse outcomes.

Interleukin-6

IL-6 is an inflammatory cytokine that induces hepatic synthesis of all the acute phase proteins and is the primary determinant of CRP levels. The presence of IL-6–expressing macrophages in coronary atherosclerotic plaques [40] suggests that increased IL-6 levels are not just a marker of inflammation but also play a direct role in increasing plaque vulnerability to fissuring and thrombosis. In addition to its proinflammatory effects, it also has procoagulant effects by modulating fibrinogen synthesis, enhancing platelet adhesion, and impairing endothelial vasodilation. High IL-6 levels in healthy men correlated with increased risk for future MI independently of hsCRP [41]. In patients who had ACS, IL-6 elevation (>5 ng/mL) was associated with 3.5-fold higher 1-year mortality than levels less than 5 ng/mL, independent of troponin and hsCRP [42]. Furthermore, in this study it appeared that patients who had inflammation as determined by IL-6 levels greater than 5 ng/mL had a greater response to an invasive versus conservative strategy than patients who had IL-6 levels less than 5 ng/mL.

Lipoprotein-associated phospholipase A2

Lipoprotein-associated phospholipase A2 (Lp-PLA_2), previously described as platelet-activating factor acetylhydrolase, is a novel marker whose role in atherosclerosis has been heavily debated. Initially considered atheroprotective because of its ability to degrade platelet-activating factor, this enzyme has since been discovered to cleave oxidized phosphatidylcholine into lysophosphatidylcholine and oxidized free fatty acids which promote the inflammatory process of atherosclerosis. Lp-PLA_2 is produced by macrophages and T lymphocytes and can be detected in human atherosclerotic lesions [43]. In humans, Lp-PLA_2 is predominantly bound to LDL cholesterol particles and is activated once LDL particles undergo oxidative damage [44].

The West of Scotland Coronary Prevention Study first demonstrated that baseline Lp-PLA_2 elevation in hyperlipidemic men predicted risk for coronary events independently of other inflammatory markers, such as CRP and fibrinogen. There was a 60% statistically significant increase in risk between the highest and lowest quintile of Lp-PLA_2 [45]. However, in a lower risk population of women (in a nested case-control analysis of the Women's Health Study), the predictive ability of Lp-PLA_2 was not statistically significant after adjustment for traditional risk factors [46].

The Atherosclerosis Risk in Communities study enrolled men and women who had a wide range of LDL levels and found that in patients who had LDL levels below 130 mg/dL, Lp-PLA_2 was significantly and independently associated with CAD [47]. This finding suggests a role for Lp-PLA_2, similar to CRP, in identifying high-risk patients who may benefit from drug therapy and are not targeted for statin use under the current Adult Treatment Panel (ATP) III guidelines. In the most recent study by Brilakis and colleagues [48], Lp-PLA_2 levels correlated with extent of angiographic CAD; however, this was not independently predictive after adjusting for CRP, lipid status, and other traditional risk factors. Inhibition of Lp-PLA_2 in animal models has been shown to be effective in reversing atherosclerosis in animal models [49], and phase II trials of SB-480848, a specific Lp-PLA_2 inhibitor, as a potential treatment of atherosclerosis are currently underway.

CD40 ligand

CD40 ligand (CD40L) is a transmembrane protein expressed on CD4+ T cells, macrophages, and activated platelets. Its interaction with the CD40 receptor on endothelial cells, smooth muscle cells, and phagocytes has been shown to stimulate expression of proinflammatory cytokines, cellular adhesion molecules, matrix metalloproteinases, and procoagulant tissue factor [50]. Furthermore, CD40 ligand has a KGD sequence that is a known binding motif for platelet integrin αIIβ3. T cells expressing CD40L are found in atherosclerotic plaques [51], and disruption of the CD40-CD40L interaction in vitro diminishes atheroma formation and promotes stabilization of the established plaque [52].

Biologically active soluble CD40L (sCD40L) released from stimulated lymphocytes can be measured in plasma. Healthy women who have high levels of sCD40L have been shown to be at increased risk for cardiovascular events [53]. In patients who have ACS, sCD40L elevation (>5 μg/L) correlated with increased 6-month mortality (18.6% versus 7.1%, $P < .001$) [54]. Treatment of these patients with abciximab before coronary angioplasty reduced risk for death or nonfatal MI (hazard ratio 0.12; 95% CI, 0.08–0.49; $P < .001$). However, patients who had lower levels of sCD40L did not experience the same treatment benefit. Among troponin-negative patients, those who had elevated sCD40L had an increased risk for cardiac events (13.6%) similar to that of patients who were troponin-positive (14%). Treatment of these patients with abciximab also reduced risk for cardiac events (5.5% versus 13.6%, $P = .03$).

Selectins

Selectins (P-selectin, E-selectin) and cellular adhesion molecules (VCAM-1, ICAM-1) mediate the initial leukocyte rolling along the endothelium and attachment/subintimal transmigration, respectively, that are the initial steps of atherosclerosis. Immunohistochemical studies have demonstrated expression of these molecules, stimulated by oxidized LDL, in the endothelium overlying the atherosclerotic plaque. Circulating levels of VCAM-1, ICAM-1, and P- and E-selectin have been detected in plasma and are thought to arise from proteolytic cleavage from endothelial cells, particularly during inflammatory conditions [55]. In a nested case-control analysis of the Physicians Health Study, risk for future MI was 60% higher in patients who had soluble ICAM-1 elevation, and this increased risk was independent of smoking status or lipid levels [56]. Elevated baseline soluble

P-selectin levels in healthy women in the Women's Health Study were also associated with increased cardiovascular risk [57]. The levels of ICAM-1 and E-selectin, but not VCAM-1, have been shown to correlate with atherosclerotic burden as measured by carotid ultrasound, suggesting the usefulness of circulating adhesion molecules as indicators of subclinical disease [58]. Despite these intriguing data, the challenges of sample handling (samples are unstable unless frozen) currently limit the clinical usefulness of these markers.

Serum amyloid A

Like CRP, serum amyloid A (SAA) is an acute-phase protein that is synthesized in the liver in response to stress, injury, or inflammation. During the acute phase, SAA becomes the predominant apolipoprotein on HDL cholesterol, thus altering HDL-mediated cholesterol delivery to cells [59]. In the Women's Ischemia Syndrome Evaluation study of women referred for coronary angiography for suspected myocardial ischemia, SAA level correlated with 3-year risk for cardiovascular events and with angiographic severity of CAD [60].

Interleukin-10

IL-10 is a cytokine whose function is to limit the inflammatory reaction once the pathogen is eliminated. Its effects on macrophages include down-regulation of proinflammatory cytokine production and adhesion molecule expression. It also inhibits synthesis of matrix metalloproteinases implicated in plaque destabilization [61]. Overexpression of human IL-10 compensates for the rapid atherosclerosis of LDL-receptor knockout mice [62]. A small study in the United Kingdom showed higher IL-10 levels in patients who had stable versus unstable coronary syndrome [63].

Markers of ischemia

Commonly used biomarkers such as creatine kinase (CK), CK-MB, and troponin are not detected in blood until several hours after symptom onset, and their presence is almost always correlated with myocardial necrosis. The challenge is to identify patients who develop symptoms of ischemia, such as plaque rupture with partial occlusion of the vessel lumen, before myocyte death. In this early stage of ACS, traditional biomarkers are not yet detectable in blood. Recent efforts have focused on identifying new markers of ischemia. The main difficulty is the lack of a gold standard to diagnose myocardial ischemia, and many studies rely on clinical diagnosis with inconsistent objective data end points.

Ischemia modified albumin

Human serum albumin is a complex protein with an N-terminus capable of binding metals such as cobalt. During ischemic events, free radicals are released, resulting in acetylation of the N-terminus and alteration of the cobalt binding site. Therefore, ischemia-modified albumin (IMA) is unable to bind cobalt, and the free metal can be detected using a specific assay. The higher the amount of free cobalt detected, the greater the degree of ischemia [64]. The advantage of this test is that IMA becomes positive within a few minutes of the ischemic event. A positive test despite negative troponin places the patient at high risk for a cardiac event [65]. It has a sensitivity of 83%, specificity of 69%, negative predictive value (NPV) of 96%, and a positive predictive value (PPV) of 33%. Sensitivity increases to 92% when combined with positive ECG findings, and 95% when combined with positive troponin and ECG. Conversely, a combination of negative IMA, negative troponin, and negative ECG has 99% NPV of a cardiac event [66]. Rapid hepatic clearance (6 hours) allows specificity for an acute event, but the main disadvantage is that IMA is not specific for cardiac ischemia; any ischemia can result in a positive test [67]. It can also be elevated in patients who have cancer, acute infections, cirrhosis, and end-stage renal disease.

The Food and Drug Administration recently approved the Albumin-Cobalt Binding Test, which measures ischemia-modified albumin, for use in evaluating patients who have suspected myocardial ischemia. In its labeling, this test is intended to be used in conjunction with troponin testing and ECG evaluation to facilitate risk stratification of patients who have chest pain or other symptoms of suspected ischemic origin. Based on its sensitivity and specificity profile and excellent NPV, a negative ischemia-modified albumin level in conjunction with a negative troponin and nondiagnostic ECG can rule out ACS in low-risk patients. Thus, it is ideal for use in chest pain units. The results of an ongoing prospective study are expected to provide more information on the prognostic value of a positive IMA result.

Unbound free fatty acid

Unbound free fatty acid (u-FFA) is a new marker recently found to be elevated in patients who have ACS before more traditional biomarkers become positive. It is thought to be released as a marker of ischemia and plaque instability, with greater than 90% sensitivity [68]. In patients undergoing PCI, the elevation of u-FFA correlated with ST-segment changes and PCI-induced transient ischemic changes [69]. The clinical applicability of this test still needs to be determined and validated in a larger population.

B-type (brain) natriuretic peptide

B-type natriuretic peptide (BNP) is a peptide hormone released from cardiac ventricles in response to myocardial stretch or increased wall tension. Its actions include vasodilation, natriuresis, and inhibition of the renin-angiotensin aldosterone and sympathetic nervous systems [70]. BNP is produced as a prohormone, pro-BNP, which is enzymatically cleaved into BNP and N-terminal pro-BNP (NT-pro-BNP). Initially identified as highly sensitive diagnostic markers for congestive heart failure, BNP and NT-pro-BNP levels are highly correlated, although NT-pro-BNP may be slightly more sensitive for ventricular dysfunction. BNP and NT-pro-BNP have been found to predict increased mortality independently of left ventricular function when elevated in patients who have acute MI and unstable angina [71–73]. In patients who have unstable angina or non–ST-elevation MI, a BNP greater than 80 pg/mL was associated with angiographically tighter culprit lesions or left anterior descending coronary artery involvement, implicating more severe ischemia as a cause of increased mortality [74]. However, the role of BNP levels in terms of therapy decisions in ACS is still unclear. In the Treat Angina with Aggrastat and Determine Cost of Therapy with Invasive or Conservative Strategy (TACTICS-TIMI 18) population, an elevated baseline BNP did not predict significant benefit from an early invasive management strategy [75]. However, in the FRISC II study, baseline NT-pro-BNP in concert with IL-6 elevation were useful for identifying patients who derive survival benefit from an early invasive strategy [76].

Recent data have shown that BNP is elevated in the setting of myocardial ischemia even in the absence of necrosis. Plasma NT-pro-BNP levels are higher in patients who have unstable angina compared with age-matched controls who have stable angina or no coronary disease [77]. Patients who have stable CAD and BNP elevation are more likely to have inducible ischemia on exercise treadmill testing [78]. BNP increases transiently after exercise in patients who have stable CAD and is correlated with size of ischemic territory as assessed by single-photon emission computed tomography [79]. In patients undergoing PCI, plasma BNP levels increase immediately after balloon inflation [80] and remain elevated 24 hours postintervention independent of intracardiac filling pressures [81].

Experimental studies confirm that acute cardiac hypoxia induces BNP expression in the ventricular myocardium [82] and BNP is released in the setting of coronary artery occlusion [83]. In the rat heart model, the degree of BNP elevation correlates with duration of ischemia (induced up to 20 minutes by reversible ligation of the left main coronary artery). Exogenous infusion of BNP limits infarct size in a dose-dependent manner, suggesting that BNP is released in response to ischemia such that its vasodilatory effect attenuates ischemic injury. These basic and clinical data suggest that plasma measurement of BNP and NT-pro-BNP can be useful in detecting myocardial ischemia. However, this finding still needs to be validated in larger studies.

Markers of plaque instability or rupture

Recognition of the role of plaque rupture in the pathogenesis of cardiac ischemia has led to investigation of serum markers for plaque instability. These markers include whole blood choline levels, pregnancy-associated plasma protein-A (PAPP-A), and malondialdehyde-modified LDL.

Whole blood choline

Choline is thought to be released from leukocytes and platelets in response to activation of phospholipase D during plaque rupture. In patients presenting with symptoms of ACS and negative troponin levels on admission, an elevated choline level predicts higher risk for cardiac death, nonfatal cardiac arrest, life-threatening arrhythmias, heart failure, and future angioplasty within 30 days [84]. Furthermore, in the absence of MI, choline detects patients who have high-risk unstable angina (prolonged chest pain, ischemia-related pulmonary edema, rest pain with dynamic ECG changes, or hypotension) with a sensitivity and

specificity of 86%. Unlike troponin, choline is not a marker of myocardial cell necrosis. Its use as an early biomarker of MI is limited, with a sensitivity of 41%, specificity of 79%, PPV of 51%, and NPV of 71%. The weak association of choline with ST-elevation MI has been attributed to the possibility a different mechanism of plaque rupture, whereby rapid red thrombus formation leaves limited time for the injured endothelium and collagen tissue to activate phospholipase D [85]. Intermittent formation of nonoccluding white thrombi in the setting of unstable angina leads to phospholipase D activation in platelets and choline release. Therefore, choline may provide early detection of patients who have high-risk unstable angina, indicating subendocardial rather than transmural injury.

Pregnancy-associated plasma protein-A

Another emerging marker of plaque instability is PAPP-A, a zinc-binding matrix metalloproteinase that activates insulin-like growth factor I (IGF-I), a mediator of atherosclerosis. IGF-I induces migration of vascular smooth muscle cells, monocyte chemotaxis, and release of cytokines. Histologically, PAPP-A is abundantly expressed in ruptured or eroded plaques but not in stable plaques, suggesting a potential enzymatic role in extracellular matrix degradation and fibrous cap weakening that contributes to plaque rupture [86]. Circulating levels of PAPP-A were significantly higher in patients who had unstable angina or MI compared with patients who did not have an ACS; the areas under the receiver operating curve were 0.94 and 0.88, respectively, at the threshold level of 10 mIU/L. The sensitivity and specificity were 89.2% and 81.3%, respectively. PAPP-A levels did not correlate with markers of cardiac necrosis such as troponin and CK-MB, suggesting its role as a marker of early ischemia but not infarction [86]. In troponin-negative patients presenting with ACS, those who had elevated PAPP-A levels had a 4.6-fold higher risk for cardiovascular morbidity at 6 months compared with those who had low PAPP-A levels [87].

Malondialdehyde-modified low-density lipoprotein

During ischemic injury of the endothelium, a cascade of platelet adhesion and activation involving the prostaglandin pathway results in the release of aldehydes that bind to the apo-B100 moiety of LDL, forming malondialdehyde (MDA)-modified LDL [88]. Plasma levels of

MDA-modified LDL become elevated in patients who have ACS within the first 6 hours of symptom onset. In patients presenting with ACS, the sensitivity of admission MDA-modified LDL was 95% compared with 38% for troponin I in the diagnosis of unstable angina [89], and the specificity was 95%. The use of troponin I and MDA-modified LDL in combination achieved a sensitivity of 98%. MDA-modified LDL levels were threefold higher in patients who had unstable angina compared with those who had stable CAD. In acute MI, MDA-modified LDL is 95% sensitive when used alone, troponin I is 90% when used alone, and the combination had a sensitivity approaching 100% [89]. This evidence suggests that MDA-modified LDL, reflecting endothelial injury and plaque rupture, is useful in discriminating unstable from stable angina, in contradistinction to troponin, which helps to discriminate between unstable angina and myocardial infarction.

Summary

Recent advances have identified many promising new molecular markers of ischemia and inflammation. Their clinical usefulness requires satisfaction of the following criteria: they must (1) be easily available, simple, and standardized assay, (2) have trial-based evidence of association with clinical end points, (3) be generalizable to various population groups, and (4) demonstrate adequate sensitivity and specificity.

There is a growing recognition of the role of hsCRP in further risk assessment, particularly in patients at intermediate cardiovascular risk and for risk stratification in patients who have ACS. However, it has limited diagnostic usefulness in chest pain patients. Ischemia-modified albumin is now available clinically to rule out acute coronary ischemia in conjunction with standard troponin and ECG evaluation, and whole blood choline and MDA-modified LDL are two markers of plaque instability that have been shown in small trials to diagnose unstable angina with good sensitivity and specificity. However, larger clinical trials will be needed to validate their clinical value.

As understanding of the pathophysiology of atherothrombosis evolves, the number of candidate markers meriting clinical consideration will increase exponentially. The hope is that these markers will permit earlier detection of disease, allowing time for interventions to circumvent myocardial damage and other complications. The challenge for clinicians will be to integrate marker testing into practice without overwhelming, or substituting for, clinical judgment and rational decision making.

References

[1] Alpert JS, Thygesen K, Antman E, et al. Myocardial infarction redefined—a consensus document of the Joint European Society of Cardiology/American College of Cardiology Committee for the redefinition of myocardial infarction. J Am Coll Cardiol 2000;36:959–69.

[2] Mantovani A, Bussolino F, Dejana E. Cytokine regulation of endothelial cell function. FASEB J 1992;6:2591–9.

[3] Libby P. Molecular bases of the acute coronary syndromes. Circulation 1995;91:2844–50.

[4] Amento EP, Ehsani N, Palmer H, et al. Cytokines and growth factors positive and negatively regular interstitial collagen gene expression in human vascular smooth muscle cells. Arterioscler Thromb Vasc Biol 1991;11:1223–30.

[5] Galis ZS, Muszynski M, Sukhova GK, et al. Cytokine stimulated human vascular smooth muscle cells synthesize a complement of enzymes required for extracellular matrix digestion. Circ Res 1994;75:181–9.

[6] Galis ZS, Sukhova GK, Lark MW, et al. Increase expression of matrix metalloproteinases and matrix degrading activity in vulnerable regions of human atherosclerotic plaques. J Clin Invest 1994;94:2493–503.

[7] Moreno PR, Bernardi VH, Lopez-Cuellar J, et al. Macrophages, smooth muscle cells, and tissue factor in unstable angina: Implications for cell-mediated thrombogenicity in acute coronary syndromes. Circulation 1996;94:3090–7.

[8] Neri Serneri G, Abbate R, Gori A, et al. Transient intermittent lymphocyte activation is responsible for the instability of angina. Circulation 1992;86:790–7.

[9] Deodhar SD. C-reactive protein: the best laboratory indicator available for monitoring disease activity. Cleve Clin J Med 1989;56:126–30.

[10] Macy E, Hayes T, Tracy R. Variability in the measurement of C-reactive protein in healthy subjects: Implications for reference interval and epidemiologic applications. Clin Chem 1997;43:52–8.

[11] Heeschen C, Hamm CW, Bruemmer J, et al. Predictive value of C-reactive protein and troponin T in patients with unstable angina: a comparative analysis. CAPTURE Investigators. Chimeric c7E3 Anti-Platelet Therapy in Unstable angina REfractory to standard treatment trial. J Am Coll Cardiol 2000;35:1535–42.

[12] Morrow DA, Rifai N, Antman EM, et al. C-reactive protein is a potent predictor of mortality

independently of and in combination with troponin T in acute coronary syndromes: a TIMI 11a substudy. J Am Coll Cardiol 1998;31:1460.

[13] Lindahl B, Toss H, Siegbahn A, et al. Markers of myocardial damage and inflammation in relation to long-term mortality in unstable coronary artery disease. FRISC Study Group. Fragmin during Instability in Coronary Artery Disease. N Engl J Med 2000;343:1139–47.

[14] James S, Armstrong P, Barnathan E, et al. Troponin and C-reactive protein have different relations to subsequent mortality and myocardial infarction after acute coronary syndrome: a GUSTO-IV study. J Am Coll Cardiol 2003;41:916–24.

[15] Ridker P, Rifai N, Pfeffer M, et al. Inflammation, pravastatin, and the risk of coronary events after myocardial infarction in patients with average cholesterol levels. Circulation 1998;98:839–44.

[16] Haverkate F, Thompson SG, Pyke SD, et al. Production of C-reactive protein and risk of coronary events in stable and unstable angina. European Concerted Action on Thrombosis and Disabilities Angina Pectoris Study Group. Lancet 1997;349: 462–6.

[17] Mendall MA, Patel P, Ballam L, et al. C-reactive protein and its relation to cardiovascular risk factors: a population base cross sectional study. BMJ 1996;3–12:1061–5.

[18] Kuller LH, Tracy RP, Shaten J, et al. Relation of C-reactive protein and coronary heart disease in the MRFIT nested case control study. Multiple Risk Factor Intervention Trial. Am J Epidemiol 1996; 144:537–47.

[19] Ridker PM, Cushman M, Stampfer MJ, et al. Inflammation, aspirin and the risk of cardiovascular disease in apparently healthy men. N Engl J Med 1997;336:973–9.

[20] Koenig W, Sund M, Frohlich M, et al. C-reactive protein, a sensitive marker of inflammation, predicts future risk of coronary heart disease in initially healthy middle aged men. Circulation 1999;99: 237–42.

[21] Ridker P, Hennekens CH, Buring JE, et al. C-reactive protein and other markers of inflammation in the prediction of cardiovascular disease in women. N Engl J Med 2000;342:836–43.

[22] Ridker P, Rifai N, Rose L, et al. Comparison of C-reactive protein and low-density lipoprotein cholesterol levels in the prediction of first cardiovascular events. N Engl J Med 2002;347: 1557–65.

[23] Ridker P, Glynn R, Hennekens C. C-reactive protein adds to the predictive value of total and HDL cholesterol in determining risk of first myocardial infarction. Circulation 1998;97:2007–11.

[24] Ridker PM. High sensitivity C-reactive protein: potential adjunct for global risk assessment in the primary prevention of cardiovascular disease. Circulation 2001;103:1813–8.

[25] Tataru MC, Heinrich J, Junker R, et al. C-reactive protein and the severity of atherosclerosis in myocardial infarction patients with stable angina pectoris. Eur Heart J 2000;21:1000–8.

[26] Masden T, Skou HA, Hansen VE, et al. C-reactive protein, dietary n-3 fatty acids, and the extent of coronary artery disease. Am J Cardiol 2001;88:1139–42.

[27] Hunt ME, O'Malley PG, Vernalis MN, et al. C-reactive protein is not associated with the presence or extent of calcified subclinical atherosclerosis. Am Heart J 2001;141:206–10.

[28] Pasceri V, Willerson J, Yeh E. Direct pro-inflammatory effect of C-reactive protein on human endothelial cells. Circulation 2000;102:2165–8.

[29] Zwaka T, Homback V, Torzewski J. C-reactive protein-mediated low density lipoprotein uptake by macrophages: implications for atherosclerosis. Circulation 2001;103:1194–7.

[30] Venugopal S, Devaraj S, Yuhanna I, et al. Demonstration that C-reactive protein decreases ENOS expression and bioactivity in human aortic endothelial cells. Circulation 2002;106:1439–41.

[31] Cermak J, Key NS, Bach RR, et al. C-reactive protein induces human peripheral blood monocytes to synthesize tissue factor. Blood 1993;82:513–20.

[32] Wolbink GJ, Brouwer MC, Buysmann S, et al. CRP-mediated activation of complement in-vivo: assessment by measuring circulating complement-C-reactive protein complexes. J Immunol 1996;157: 473–9.

[33] Deveraj S, Xu D, Jialal I. C-reactive protein increases plasminogen activator inhibitor-1 expression and activity in human aortic endothelial cells: implications for the metabolic syndrome and atherothrombosis. Circulation 2003;107:398–404.

[34] Vaughan CJ, Murphy MB, Buckley BM. Statins do more than just lower cholesterol. Lancet 1996;348: 1079–82.

[35] Rosenson RS, Tangney CC. Antiatherothrombotic properties of statins: Implications for cardiovascular event reduction. JAMA 1998;279:1643–50.

[36] Ridker P, Rifai N, Pfeffer M, et al. Long term effects of pravastatin on plasma concentration of C-reactive protein. Circulation 1999;100:230–5.

[37] Ridker PM, Cannon CP, Morrow D, et al. C-reactive protein levels and outcomes after statin therapy. N Engl J Med 2005;352:20–8.

[38] Albert MA, Danielson E, Rifai N, et al. Effect of statin therapy on C-reactive protein levels: the pravastatin inflammation/CRP evaluation (PRINCE): a randomized trial and cohort study. JAMA 2001; 286:64–70.

[39] Pearson TA, Mensah GA, Alexander RW, et al. Markers of inflammation and cardiovascular disease – application to clinical and public health practice: a statement for healthcare professionals for the Center for Disease Control and Prevention and the American Heart Association. Circulation 2003;107: 499–511.

[40] Scheiffer B, Scheiffer E, Hilfker-Kleiner D, et al. Expression of angiotensin II and interleukin-6 in human coronary atherosclerotic plaques: potential implications for inflammation and plaque instability. Circulation 2000;101:1372–8.

[41] Ridker P, Rifai N, Stampfer MJ, et al. Plasma concentration of interleukin-6 and the risk of future myocardial infarction among apparently healthy men. Circulation 2000;101:1767–72.

[42] Lindmark E, Diderholm E, Wallentin L, et al. Relationship between interleukin-6 and mortality in patients with unstable coronary artery disease. JAMA 2001;286:2107–13.

[43] Hakkinen T, Luoma JS, Hiltunen MO, et al. Lipoprotein-associated phospholipase A2, platelet activating factor acetylhydrolase, is expressed by macrophages in human and rabbit atherosclerotic lesions. Arterioscler Thromb Vasc Biol 1999;19: 2909–17.

[44] Caslake MJ, Packard CJ, Suckling KE, et al. Lipoprotein-associated phospholipase A2, platelet activating factor acetylhydrolase: a potential new risk factor for coronary artery disease. Atherosclerosis 2000;50:413–9.

[45] Packard CJ, O'Reilly DS, Caslake MJ, et al. Lipoprotein-associated phospholipase A2, as an independent predictor of coronary heart disease. N Engl J Med 2000;343:1148–55.

[46] Blake GJ, Dada N, Fox JC, et al. A prospective evaluation of lipoprotein-associated phospholipase A2 levels and the risk of future cardiovascular events in women. J Am Coll Cardiol 2001;38:1302–6.

[47] Ballantyne CM, Hoogeveen RC, Bang H, et al. Lipoprotein-associated phospholipase A2, high sensitivity C-reactive protein, and risk for incident coronary heart disease in middle aged men and women in the Atherosclerosis Risk in Communities (ARIC) study. Circulation 2004;109:837–42.

[48] Brilakis ES, McConnell JP, Lennon RJ, et al. Association of lipoprotein-associated phospholipase A2 levels with coronary artery disease risk factors, angiographic coronary artery disease, and major adverse events at follow-up. Eur Heart J 2005;26: 137–44.

[49] Leach CA, Hickey DM, Ife RJ, et al. Lipoprotein-associated PLA2 inhibition–a novel, non-lipid lowering strategy for atherosclerosis therapy. Farmaco 2001;56:45–50.

[50] Henn V, Slupsky JR, Grafe M, et al. CD40 ligand on activated platelets triggers an inflammatory reaction of endothelial cells. Nature 1998;351:591–4.

[51] Mach F, Schonbeck U, Sukhova GK, et al. Functional CD40 ligand is expressed on human vascular endothelial cells, smooth muscle cells, and macrophages: implications for CD40–CD40 ligand signaling in atherosclerosis. Proc Natl Acad Sci U S A 1997;94:1931–6.

[52] Schonbeck U, Sukhova GK, Shimizu K, et al. Inhibition of CD40 signaling limits evolution of established atherosclerosis in mice. Proc Natl Acad Sci U S A 2000;97:7456–63.

[53] Schonbeck U, Varo N, Libby P, et al. Soluble CD40L and cardiovascular risk in women. Circulation 2001;103:2266–8.

[54] Heeschen C, Dimmeler S, Hamm C, et al. Soluble CD-40 ligand in acute coronary syndromes. N Engl J Med 2003;348:1104–11.

[55] Gearing AJ, Newman W. Circulating adhesion molecules in disease. Immunol Today 1993;14:506–12.

[56] Ridker P, Hennekens CH, Roitman-Johnson B, et al. Plasma concentration of soluble intracellular adhesion molecule 1 and risks of future myocardial infarction in apparently healthy men. Lancet 1998; 351:88–92.

[57] Ridker P, Buring JE, Rifai N. Soluble P-selectin and the risk of future cardiovascular events. Circulation 2001;103:491–5.

[58] Hwang SJ, Ballantyne CM, Sharrett R, et al. Circulating adhesion molecules VCAM-1, ICAM-1, and E-selectin in carotid atherosclerosis and incident coronary heart disease cases: the Atherosclerosis Risk in Communities Study. Circulation 1997;96: 4219–25.

[59] Artl A, Marsche G, Lestavel S, et al. Role of serum amyloid A during metabolism of acute phase HDL by macrophages. Arterioscler Thromb Vasc Biol 2000;20:763–72.

[60] Johnson BD, Kip KE, Marroquin OC, et al. Serum amyloid A as a predictor of coronary artery disease and cardiovascular outcome in women. Circulation 2004;109:726–32.

[61] Girndt M, Kohler H. Interleukin-10 (IL-10): an update on its relevance for cardiovascular risk. Nephrol Dial Transplant 2003;18:1976–9.

[62] Von der Thusen JH, Kuiper J, Fekkes ML, et al. Attenuation of atherogenesis by systemic and local adenovirus-mediated gene transfer of interleukin-10 in LDLr–/– mice. FASEB J 2001;15:2730–2.

[63] Smith DA, Irving SD, Sheldon J, et al. Serum levels of the anti-inflammatory cytokine interleukin-10 are decreased in patients with unstable angina. Circulation 2001;104:746–9.

[64] Bar-Or D, Lau E, Winkler JV. A novel assay for cobalt-albumin binding and its potential as a marker for myocardial ischemia: A preliminary report. J Emerg Med 2000;19:311–5.

[65] Pollack CV, Sieck S. Use of ischemia-modified albumin in emergency department risk stratification of chest pain is both clinically effective and cost effective. Ann Emerg Med 2003;(Suppl 42):S37.

[66] Christenson RH, Duh SH, Sanhai WR, et al. Characteristics of an albumin cobalt binding test for assessment of acute coronary syndrome patients: A multicenter study. Clin Chem 2001;47:464–70.

[67] Kontos MC, Schorer S, Kirk JD. Ischemia modified albumin, a new biomarker of myocardial ischemia, for the emergency diagnosis of acute coronary syndrome. J Am Coll Cardiol 2003;41:340A.

[68] Panteghini M. Role and importance of biochemical markers in clinical cardiology. Eur Heart J 2004; 25:1187–96.

[69] Kleinfeld AM, Prothro D, Brown DL, et al. Increases in serum unbound free fatty acid levels following coronary angioplasty. Am J Cardiol 1996;78: 1350–4.

[70] Stein BC, Levin RI. Natriuretic peptides: physiology, therapeutic potential and risk stratification in ischemic heart disease. Am Heart J 1998;135:914–23.

[71] Omland T, Aakvaag A, Bonarjee VV, et al. Plasma brain natriuretic peptide as an indicator of left ventricular systolic function and long term survival after acute myocardial infarction. Comparison with plasma atrial natriuretic peptide and N-terminal proatrial natriuretic peptide. Circulation 1996;93: 1963–9.

[72] de Lamos JA, Morrow DA, Bentley JH, et al. The prognostic value of B-type natriuretic peptide in acute coronary syndromes. N Engl J Med 2001; 345:1014–21.

[73] James SK, Lindahl B, Seigbahn A, et al. N-terminal pro-brain natriuretic peptide and other risk markers for the separate prediction of mortality and subsequent myocardial infarction in patients with unstable coronary artery disease. Circulation 2003;108: 275–81.

[74] Sadanandan S, Cannon CP, Chekuri K, et al. Association of elevated B-type natriuretic peptide levels with angiographic findings among patients with unstable angina and non-ST-segment elevation myocardial infarction. J Am Coll Cardiol 2004;44:564–8.

[75] Morrow DA, de Lemos JA, Sabatine MS, et al. Evaluation of B-type natriuretic peptide for risk assessment in unstable angina/non ST-elevation myocardial infarction: B-type natriuretic peptide and prognosis in TACTICS-TIMI 18. J Am Coll Cardiol 2003;41:1264–72.

[76] Jernberg T, Lindahl B, Siegbahn A, et al. N terminal pro-brain natriuretic peptide in relation to inflammation, myocardial necrosis and the effect of invasive strategy in unstable coronary syndrome. J Am Coll Cardiol 2003;42:1909.

[77] Talwar S, Squire IB, Downie PF, et al. Plasma N terminal pro-brain natriuretic peptide and cardiotrophin 1 are raised in unstable angina. Heart 2000;84:421–4.

[78] Bibbins-Domingo K, Ansari M, Schiller NB, et al. B-type natriuretic peptide and ischemia in patients with stable coronary disease. Circulation 2003;108: 2987–92.

[79] Marumoto K, Hamada M, Hiwada K. Increased secretion of atrial and brain natriuretic peptides during acute myocardial ischemia induced by dynamic exercise in patients with angina pectoris. Clin Sci 1995;88:551–6.

[80] Kyriakides ZA, Markianos M, Michalis L, et al. Brain natriuretic peptide increases acutely and much more prominently than atrial natriuretic peptide during coronary angioplasty. Clin Cardiol 2000;23:285.

[81] Tateishi J, Masutani M, Ohyanagi M, et al. Transient increase in plasma brain (B-type) natriuretic peptide after percutaneous transluminal coronary angioplasty. Clin Cardiol 2000;23:776–80.

[82] Goetze JP, Gore A, Moller CH, et al. Acute myocardial hypoxia increases BNP gene expression. FASEB J 2004;18:1928–30.

[83] D'Souza SP, Yellon DM, Martin C, et al. B-type natriuretic peptide limits infarct size in rat isolated hearts via KATP channel opening. Am J Physiol Heart Circ Physiol 2003;284:H1592–600.

[84] Danne O, Mockel M, Lueders C, et al. Prognostic implications of elevated whole blood choline levels in acute coronary syndromes. Am J Cardiol 2003; 91:1060–7.

[85] Mizuno K, Satomura K, Miyamoto A, et al. Angioscopic evaluation of coronary artery thrombi in acute coronary syndromes. N Engl J Med 1992; 326:287–91.

[86] Bayes-Genis A, Conover CA, Overgaard MT, et al. Pregnancy-associated plasma protein A as a marker of acute coronary syndromes. N Engl J Med 2001; 345:1022–9.

[87] Lund J, Qin QP, Ilva T, et al. Circulating pregnancy-associated plasma protein A predicts outcome in patients with acute coronary syndrome but no troponin I elevation. Circulation 2003; 108:1924–6.

[88] Lynch SM, Morrow JD, Roberts LJ, et al. Formation of non-cyclooxygenase-derived prostanoids in plasma of low density lipoprotein exposed to oxidative stress in vitro. J Clin Invest 1994;93: 998–1004.

[89] Holvoet P, Collen D, van de Werf F. Malondialdehyde-modified LDL as a marker of acute coronary syndromes. JAMA 1999;281:1719–21.

ELSEVIER
SAUNDERS

CARDIOLOGY
CLINICS

Cardiol Clin 23 (2005) 503–516

Exercise Testing in Chest Pain Units: Rationale, Implementation, and Results

Ezra A. Amsterdam, MD, FACC[a,*], J. Douglas Kirk, MD, FACEP[b],
Deborah B. Diercks, MD[b], William R. Lewis, MD, FACC[a],
Samuel D. Turnipseed, MD[b]

[a]*Department of Internal Medicine, University of California School of Medicine (Davis) and Medical Center,
4860 Y Street, Suite 2820, Sacramento, CA 95817, USA*
[b]*Department of Emergency Medicine, University of California School of Medicine (Davis) and Medical Center,
4150 V Street, PSSB Suite 2100, Sacramento, CA 95817, USA*

Although new diagnostic approaches have enhanced the evaluation of patients presenting to the emergency department (ED) with chest pain, this syndrome remains a major clinical challenge [1]. This symptom accounts for more than 8 million ED visits per year in this country, accounting for more than 2 million hospital admissions at a cost of $8 billion for presumed acute coronary syndrome (ACS) [2]. However, a coronary event is actually confirmed in only a minority of these patients [3]. This population poses a dilemma to the clinician of inadvertent discharge of those with a life-threatening condition versus unnecessary admission for a benign process with its associated expense and the potential risks of further tests. A low threshold for admission of these patients was advocated early in the coronary care unit (CCU) era by the admonition that "patients should be admitted to the CCU solely on suspicion of having a myocardial infarction" [4]. This approach has persisted because of the focus on patient welfare as well as the litigation potential of missed ACS [5]. Inadvertent discharge of patients with ACS persists at a rate of 4% to 5% and the mortality and morbidity of this group are substantial [6]. However, a consequence of the low threshold for admission has been large numbers of unnecessary hospitalizations, suboptimal patient management, and inefficient resource use. This problem is reflected by the recent demonstration that an appreciable number of patients with coronary artery disease (CAD) who present with acute chest pain respond to proton pump inhibitors, reflecting the gastrointestinal cause of their symptoms [7].

The development of chest pain units (CPUs) is a response to the need for a strategy to effect accurate, safe, and cost-effective management of patients presenting with possible ACS. Although their initial purpose was to facilitate rapid coronary reperfusion therapy, these units have evolved into centers for management of the lower risk population that composes the majority of patients presenting with chest pain. The latter include those without initial, objective evidence of myocardial ischemia/infarction in whom accelerated risk stratification can identify those requiring admission and those who can be safely discharged with outpatient follow-up [8–15]. A basic element of this accelerated diagnostic protocol (ADP) is stress testing after a negative initial assessment for myocardial infarction (MI) or unstable angina. The primary method of testing has been treadmill exercise electrocardiography (ECG) in the context of the ADP. Fundamental to this approach is the identification of patients with low clinical risk on presentation to the ED.

Indicators of low clinical risk

There is abundant evidence that low risk in patients presenting with chest pain can be

---

* Corresponding author.
E-mail address: eaamsterdam@ucdavis.edu
(E.A. Amsterdam).

recognized on presentation and that this group neither requires nor benefits from traditional intensive care or extended observation in a monitoring unit. Lee and colleagues [16] reported that in patients admitted to rule out a coronary event, those with < 5% probability of acute MI could be identified by type of chest pain, past history, and initial ECG. Extension of this approach to over 4600 such patients demonstrated that the initial clinical assessment could distinguish those with < 1% probability of major complications [17]. The prognostic utility of the initial ECG alone in patients admitted to rule out MI was demonstrated by Brush and colleagues [18] in their report that a negative ECG on admission was associated with a 0.6% rate of serious complications during hospitalization compared with a 14% incidence in those with an abnormal ECG [18]. An earlier study indicated that a normal ECG in patients admitted for preinfarction angina predicted benign early and late outcomes in contrast to ECG evidence of ischemia, which correlated with markedly increased cardiac morbidity and mortality [19]. These findings were confirmed by Schroeder and colleagues [20] in their report that in patients in whom MI was ruled out, ECG evidence of ischemia was associated with a 1-year mortality similar to that of post-MI patients. An important concept to emerge from these studies is that although the cause of chest pain is frequently elusive, basic clinical tools provide powerful estimates of cardiac risk.

Recognition of low clinical risk stimulated alternative approaches to conventional coronary care, such as reduced time in the CCU [21,22], direct admission to a step-down unit [23], and observation in a short stay unit [24]. Recent innovations in the management of low-risk patients include guidelines, critical pathways, new serum markers of cardiac injury, novel ECG monitoring systems, early noninvasive cardiac imaging, early treadmill exercise testing, coronary calcium screening in the ED, noninvasive coronary angiography by CT and conventional coronary angiography [8–15,21].

Chest pain units

Although risk is low in patients selected for admission to a CPU, it is not negligible. Contemporary CPUs (also known as chest pain observation units, chest pain emergency units, and chest pain evaluation units) provide an integrated approach to the patient with chest pain that affords: (1) early identification of clinical risk and (2) further risk stratification of low-risk patients to identify those who require admission and those who can be discharged [8–15,21]. CPUs vary in form and may either occupy a designated structural area or function as virtual units comprising primarily personnel and process. Close coordination between ED physicians and cardiologists is an essential element for successful functioning of the unit. The strategy is based on a protocol-driven process that uses current standards of care for efficient and timely treatment in conformity with the guidelines of the American College of Cardiology (ACC) and American Heart Association (AHA) [25] as depicted in Fig. 1.

Accelerated diagnostic protocols

ADPs have been increasingly used in low-risk patients, usually culminating in one of the methods of cardiac stress evaluation, depending on the results of the clinical assessment. This process usually entails 6 to12 hours of clinical observation, serial 12-lead ECGs, continuous ECG monitoring, and measurement of serial serum markers of cardiac injury [11,13,15,21,25]. Positive findings indicate ACS (usually non-ST elevation ACS, rarely ST elevation ACS) and mandate admission for further management. Negative findings are consistent with absence of MI and no evidence of ischemia at rest. In these cases, the evaluation proceeds to a stress test to determine if the patient has inducible ischemia. Those with a positive test are admitted and those with a negative result are discharged to outpatient follow-up. Multiple methods are currently available to detect stress-induced ischemia, the most widely available and readily applicable of which is treadmill exercise testing. The utility of ADPs has been well demonstrated with this method, as indicated by its safety and the very low clinical risk in patients designated as appropriate for early discharge.

Development and evolution of early exercise testng

Initial recommendations

Incorporation of treadmill exercise testing into current ADPs is a recent development based on ample data that has overcome initial concern regarding the possible hazards of this technique in potentially unstable patients. This early,

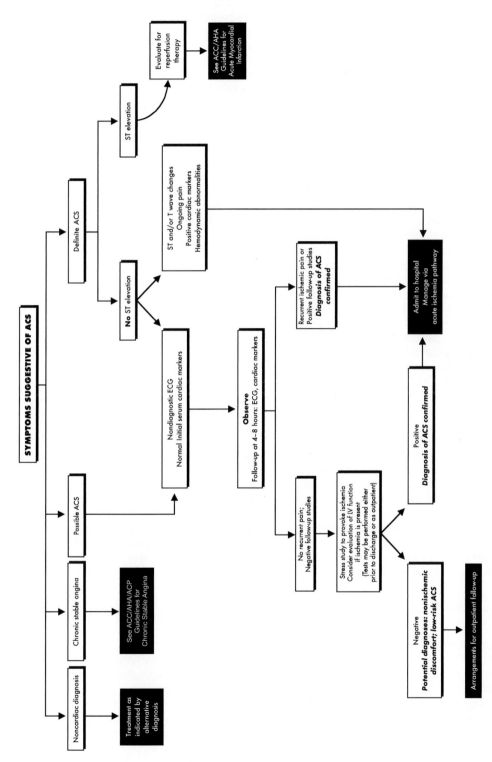

Fig. 1. Management of patients presenting with symptoms suggestive of an acute coronary syndrome (ACS). ACC, American College of Cardiology; AHA, American Heart Association. (*Adapted from* Braunwald E, Antman E, Beasley JW, et al. ACC/AHA guidelines for the management of patients with unstable angina and non-ST elevation myocardial infarction. http://www.acc.org/clincal/guidelines/unstable/unstable.pdf.)

cautionary approach and its evolution into current concepts is reflected in the progressive alteration of recommendations by expert panels that have considered exercise testing in patients presenting with possible ACS. Such caution is reflected in the Clinical Practice Guideline on Unstable Angina published in 1994 [26]. Noting that "In many cases, noninvasive stress testing provides a useful supplement to clinically based risk assessment," this guideline recommended that "unless cardiac catheterization is indicated, stress testing should be should be performed in patients hospitalized with unstable angina who have been free of angina and congestive heart failure for a *minimum of 48 hours.*" The strength of the evidence for this recommendation was rated "B" (B = evidence from well conducted clinical studies but no randomized clinical trials). The report of the American College of Emergency Physicians in 1995 emphasized the efficacy of CPUs in reducing both missed ACS and unnecessary hospitalizations [27]. However, its only reference to stress testing as part of the patient evaluation was that "Many patients, upon discharge from the CPU, are scheduled for a form of testing that is reliable for identifying ischemic heart disease." A year later, the Working Group Report of the National Heart Attack Alert Program published an extensive evaluation of technologies to detect ischemia in the ED [10]. This body concluded that "the expedited ECG exercise test may offer the benefit of an expedited workup and may reduce hospital admissions for chest pain. However, ECG exercise stress testing in the ED cannot be recommended in the absence of additional data demonstrating safety and effectiveness." The quality of the evidence at the time of publication was rated "C," indicating its basis in limited studies, and the test was viewed as modestly accurate with little or unknown clinical impact.

Current guidelines

Subsequent clinical studies demonstrating the safety and efficacy of exercise testing in ADPs have provided firm support for this approach. The 31st Bethesda Conference on Emergency Cardiac Care held in 1999 noted that "ADPs, including exercise testing as a key element, have been associated with reduced hospital stay and lower costs" [11]. The absence of adverse effects and the accurate identification of low post-discharge prognostic risk were also recognized. A subsequent Science Advisory of the AHA concluded that

contemporary studies "confirmed the safety of symptom-limited treadmill exercise ECG testing after 8 to 12 hours of evaluation in patients who have been identified as being at low to intermediate risk by a clinical algorithm that uses serum markers of myocardial necrosis and resting ECGs" [28]. This strategy is incorporated in the 2002 guidelines of the ACC/AHA for management of patients with non-ST elevation ACS in which it is recommended that exercise testing can be performed in stable, low risk patients if "a follow-up 12-lead ECG and cardiac marker measurements after 6 to 8 hours of observation are normal" [25]. Recent exercise testing guidelines are in accord with these recommendations [29,30]. These updated guidelines reflect evolution from earlier versions that advised exercise testing only after patients had been symptom-free for a "minimum of 48 hours" [31]. Thus, during the course of less than a decade, recommendations for exercise testing in low-risk patients progressed from admonitions for a pretest 48-hour period of clinical stability to expert consensus supporting its application after a much briefer interval.

Initial studies of early exercise testing

All studies of early exercise testing in patients presenting with chest pain have required that patients are clinically stable with no ECG evidence of ischemia/injury. The criteria for a positive test for myocardial ischemia are the standard indicators: ≥ 1.0 mm horizontal or downsloping ST segment shift. Other exercise-induced alterations that indicate an abnormal test and the need for further evaluation include angina, arrhythmias, and fall in blood pressure. Although the first two studies of this method included only small numbers of patients, they demonstrated the safety of exercise testing in low-risk patients in the ED setting, and the utility of this method was confirmed in multiple subsequent investigations (Table 1). There have been no reports of adverse events in any study of early exercise testing of low-risk patients.

Tsakonis and colleagues [32] evaluated 28 patients "several hours" after hospital arrival with treadmill ECG using a symptom-limited modified Bruce protocol (see Table 1). These patients had unexplained chest pain consistent with—but not diagnostic of—angina and normal baseline ECGs. The exercise test was negative in 23 patients and positive in 5. The latter group was admitted and the former was discharged. The

Table 1
Studies of exercise electrocardiography (ECG) testing in chest pain centers[a]

Author	Number of patients	Percent positive tests[b]	Percent negative predictive value[c]	Percent positive predictive value[c]	Adverse exercise test events
Tsakonis et al [32]	28	17.8	100		0
Kerns et al [33]	32	0	100		0
Lewis and Amsterdam [34]	93	13.0	100	46	0
Gibler et al [35]	782	1.2	99	44	0
Gomez et al [37]	100	7	100	0	0
Zalenski et al [39]	224	8	98	16	0
Polanczyk et al [40]	276	24	98	15	0
Kirk et al [44]	212	12.5	100	57	0
Amsterdam et al [45]	1000[d]	13	88.7	33	0

[a] Includes studies in which results of exercise ECG tests could be distinguished from those of other forms of stress testing.
[b] Positive exercise ECG.
[c] Based on clinical follow-up or further cardiac evaluation.
[d] Includes a small number of patients in Kirk and colleagues [44].

investigators reported no cardiac morbidity or mortality at 6 months in the patients with negative exercise tests. These findings were confirmed in the subsequent report of Kerns and colleagues [33] who performed exercise testing in 32 ED patients with atypical chest pain, normal ECGs, and cardiac risk factor stratification (see Table 1). Compared with similar patients admitted for evaluation of atypical chest pain, those with negative results during ED exercise testing had shorter length of stay (5.5 hours versus 2 days) and lower costs ($467 versus $2340). All patients in the accelerated protocol had negative exercise tests and no evidence of CAD at 6 months follow-up. In addition to their small numbers, limitations of these two studies include the very low risk of the patients (none had been designated for admission), the lack of any positive tests in Kerns' patients, and no further evaluation for CAD in Tskanosis's patients with positive tests.

The first study of exercise testing in patients with the clinical profile of those currently included in CPU ADPs was published from the authors' institution in 1994. In this investigational protocol, selected patients presenting with chest pain who were designated for admission by ED physicians to rule out ACS underwent immediate treadmill testing (see Table 1) [34] . The study group comprised 93 patients in whom ED symptom-limited exercise testing was performed by a cardiologist using a modified Bruce protocol without prior measurement of any markers. The test was performed within a median time of less

than 1 hour from the decision to admit and in less than 24 hours in all patients. Positive tests occurred in 13% of patients, negative in 64%, and nondiagnostic (no ischemia but peak heart rate < 85% of age-predicted maximum) in 13%. Ischemic ECG changes occurred at a significantly lower percentage of age-predicted maximal heart rate (70%) in patients with true-positive tests compared with those with false-positives (>90%) (Fig. 2). No complications were associated with exercise testing. Coronary angiography revealed significant CAD in 6 of the 13 patients with positive tests, 5 of whom had multivessel involvement. A majority (54%) of the 81 patients with negative or nondiagnostic results was discharged immediately after the exercise test. At 6 months follow-up, there were no coronary events in patients with negative or nondiagnostic exercise tests. Several unique aspects of this study demonstrated the utility of early exercise testing in low-risk patients and provided the basis for the authors' current approach of "immediate" exercise testing in low-risk patients without excluding MI by a traditional series of negative cardiac serum markers. In contrast to the preceding studies, it included only patients who were assigned to admission for a traditional rule out MI protocol. In these patients, exercise testing was performed before the latter process, there were no adverse effects of testing, true and false positive tests were related to the heart rate at ST-segment depression, the majority of patients were discharged immediately after a negative or nondiagnostic test, and there were

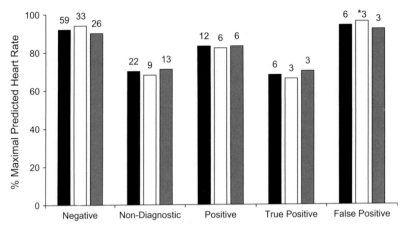

Fig. 2. Treadmill exercise results. Percent maximal predicted heart rate attained versus exercise electrocardiographic result for all patients (*solid bars*), men (*open bars*), women (*shaded bars*). Numbers above bars represent number of patients. *Percent maximal predicted heart rate for patients with true-positive tests versus false-positive tests, $P < .01$.

no coronary events during the posthospital course. One patient with a positive test was found to have non-ST elevation MI by subsequent serial serum enzymes. Coronary angiography revealed right coronary artery disease, coronary angioplasty was performed, and the clinical course was uncomplicated.

Exercise testing in chest pain units

Gibler and associates [34] demonstrated the utility of early exercise testing in 782 patients in whom low risk was by an ADP (see Table 1) [35]. Their protocol included serial ECGs and serum CK-MB, 9 hours of continuous ST-segment monitoring, and a resting echocardiogram followed by symptom-limited exercise testing in those with negative findings. There were no adverse effects and no mortality at 30-day follow-up in the patients with negative tests. The negative predictive value of the exercise test was 99%. Although the positive predictive value was less than 50%, only 9 of 782 patients ($<2\%$) had positive exercise tests, which was lower than in the authors' initial investigation [34].

Emerging from these studies [32–35] is recognition of the safety and excellent predictive value of negative exercise tests in patients identified as low risk (see Table 1). Further, a large majority of patients selected for exercise testing by an ADP had negative findings and, although the positive predictive value was modest, positive tests were infrequent and resulted in the need for further

evaluation in only small numbers of patients (see Table 1). The utility of this strategy was confirmed in its ability to safely and efficiently reduce unnecessary admissions in low-risk patients. Indeed, the relative frequency of patients with true- and false-positive exercise tests in this setting is actually similar to that seen in asymptomatic individuals [36], confirming the value of clinical indicators in identifying the probability of disease in patients presenting to the ED with chest pain [12,16,17,21,34,35].

The Rapid Rule-Out of Myocardial Ischemia Observation (ROMIO) study of Gomez and coworkers [37] was the first prospective, controlled investigation of ADP-exercise testing (see Table 1). It evaluated 100 patients with chest pain, half of whom were randomly assigned to admission for regular care and half to a chest pain center protocol consisting of a 12-hour observation period with standard ECGs, continuous ST-segment monitoring, and serial CK-MBs. Observation and monitoring were negative in 44 patients in the accelerated protocol in whom symptom-limited exercise testing was performed without adverse effects, demonstrating normal tests in 93% and positive results in 7%. The latter were all false-positives based on coronary angiography. All patients with negative tests were discharged after the exercise evaluation, and there were no coronary events at 30-day follow-up. However, compared with regular care, the observation protocol was associated with substantial reductions in length of stay (11.0 versus 22.8 hours) and total cost ($624 per patient at 30 days). This was the first study to document the anticipated cost savings by an observation unit protocol.

By the latter part of the last decade, the efficacy of ADP-exercise test protocols was evident for low-risk patients. However, although the potential for cost savings was suggested, this advantage had not been firmly established. Additionally, there was also the possibility, as suggested by Roberts and co-workers [38], that this strategy could actually lead to higher costs by capturing very low-risk patients who would previously have been discharged directly from the ED. These investigators addressed this issue in a prospective, randomized trial in which the primary outcomes were length of stay and total cost [38]. The study group comprised 165 low-risk chest pain patients enrolled in a 12-hour ADP followed by an exercise test in appropriate subjects. There were no deaths or serious complications associated with the ADP, which also resulted in fewer indeterminate evaluations than standard care (16% versus 54%, $P <$ .001). Length of stay and cost were significantly less for ADP patients than those receiving standard care (33 versus 45 hours, $P <$ .01; and $1528 versus $2095, $P <$ .001) (Table 2). Extrapolation of this cost benefit by the authors indicated a potential annual national saving of over $238 million.

In a prospective, cross-sectional study, Zalenski and colleagues [39] evaluated 317 patients by a 12-hour ADP followed by exercise testing (see Table 1). A unique aspect of this trial was admission of all patients to obtain a diagnosis to which the ADP evaluation could be compared. Exercise testing was performed in 224 patients with negative observation data and was negative in 66%, positive in 8%, and inconclusive in 26% because of failure of patients to reach 85% of age-predicted maximal heart rate. There were no adverse effects of exercise testing. There were no follow-up data in this study, in which the accuracy of the ADP-exercise strategy was based on diagnoses obtained during admission. In combination with the

Table 2
Primary outcomes

Outcome	ADP (n = 82)	Control (n = 83)	P
Hospitalized, %	45.1	100	<.001
Total cost, mean	1528	2095	<.001
LOS, mean, h	33.1	44.8	<.01

Abbreviations: ADP, accelerated diagnostic protocol; CI, confidence interval; LOS, length of stay.

CK-MB data and serial ECGs, the exercise test had a high sensitivity (90%) and excellent negative predictive value (98%); as in prior studies, specificity and positive predictive value were low (51% and 16%, respectively). Cost analysis demonstrated a savings of $567 per patient managed by the ADP-exercise test strategy.

The report of Polanczyk and colleagues [40] evaluated the prognostic significance of the exercise test performed within 48 hours of presentation in 276 low-risk patients admitted for chest pain (see Table 1). Twenty-six percent of these patients had a prior history of CAD. The test was performed within 12 hours in 7% of patients, at 12 to 24 hours in 45%, and after 24 hours in 48%. The Bruce treadmill protocol was used in 84% of the patients, and the modified version was used in 12%. A negative test was defined by achievement of at least 3 METs (one stage of the Bruce protocol) without evidence of ischemia. Positive tests were "those in which the results were interpreted as highly predictive of significant coronary disease or strongly positive" and "inconclusive tests were those consistent with but not diagnostic of ischemia" or without evidence of ischemia at a peak work of < 3 METs. There were no adverse effects of exercise testing. The test was negative in 71% of patients, positive in 24%, and inconclusive in 5%. Outcome data were available at 6 months for 92% of the study group. Events during the follow-up period were defined as cardiac death, MI, or myocardial revascularization. During this interval, there was no mortality and the event rate in the negative exercise test cohort was 2% compared with 15% in those with positive or equivocal tests. In the negative test group, compared with those with positive/equivocal tests, there were also fewer repeat ED visits (17% versus 21%, $P <$ .05) and fewer readmissions (12% versus 17%, $P <$ .01). The negative predictive value of the exercise test was 98%; sensitivity and specificity were 73% and 74%, respectively. In addition to the documented prognostic utility of the exercise test, this study afforded other noteworthy features. The investigators demonstrated the safety of the early exercise test in patients with a history of CAD and their definition of test results yielded a low rate of inconclusive diagnoses, increasing the clinical utility of the test in clinical decision-making.

Mandatory stress testing in a chest pain center was evaluated by Mikhail and co-workers [41] for its safety, utility, and cost-effectiveness. After negative findings for myocardial ischemia/infarction, a total of 424 patients underwent cardiac stress evaluation, which included 247 exercise treadmill tests. The remainder of the tests included stress imaging studies; no data are given on the results of the separate test modalities. The tests were negative in 392 (92.6%) patients, and average stay in the CPU was 12.8 hours. At 5 months follow-up, there was no mortality or MI in any of the patients discharged after a negative evaluation. A final diagnosis of ischemic heart disease was made in 44 patients admitted from the chest pain center, 24 (55%) of whom were identified only on stress testing with which there were no adverse effects. Evaluation in the CPU with mandatory stress testing was associated with a cost-per-case saving of 62% for each patient who would otherwise have been admitted to the inpatient service.

The largest and most recent prospective, randomized trial comparing management by an ADP-stress test with regular inpatient care is that of Farkouh and co-investigators [42]. They studied 424 patients with a diagnosis of unstable angina based on symptoms and considered to be at intermediate risk. Patients with ECG evidence of ischemia were excluded. The observation protocol, which included ECGs, ST-segment monitoring, and serial serum creatine kinase–MB measurements, differed from prior studies in its duration of only 6 hours. Patients with negative ADP findings who were sufficiently ambulatory underwent exercise testing while pharmacologic stress imaging was performed in the others. No adverse events occurred with the stress tests but the proportion of patients receiving the various tests is not specified. Patients with negative tests were discharged and those with positive or equivocal results were admitted. Forty-six percent of patients in the ADP-stress test group had a negative overall evaluation and were directly discharged after a median stay of 9.2 hours. At 6 months, there was no significant difference in cardiac events in the ADP-stress test group versus the regular care patients (6.6% versus 8.5%, respectively). Events were broadly defined (primary: death, MI, heart failure, stroke, cardiac arrest; secondary: any revisit to the ED or hospitalization for cardiac diagnosis or care). There were no primary events in the ADP-stress patients with negative evaluations and early discharge. The investigators emphasized that this group represented 46% of patients who ordinarily would have been admitted but in whom the accelerated protocol avoided admission. Finally, the use of cardiac procedures and hospitalization for cardiac care during the follow-up period was significantly higher in the hospital admission patients ($P = .003$), amounting to an estimated 61% increase in costs.

The impact of CPUs compared with regular hospital care was analyzed by Graff and colleagues [27] in the report of the Chest Pain Evaluation Registry (CHEPER) Study. Results were assessed in terms of the proportion of patients undergoing a complete "rule out MI" investigation, the number of missed MIs, and costs. Outcomes in over 23,000 patients managed in eight chest pain observation units were compared with results in over 12,000 patients in five studies from hospitals without these units. Although data on exercise testing were not provided in the report, the investigators note that all CPUs complied with standards of the American College of Emergency Physicians [8,43] and the Clinical Practice Guidelines for Management of Unstable Angina [26], which include recommendations on exercise testing in their management algorithms. CPUs were associated with an increase in evaluations to rule out MI (67% versus 57%, $P < .001$), a lower rate of missed MIs (0.4% versus 4.5%, $P < .001$) and a lower admission rate (47% versus 57%, $P < .001$). The latter effect equated to a potential for 2314 admissions avoided and more than $4 million saved.

The foregoing studies of the last decade reflect the parallel and interdependent development of chest pain centers, ADPs, and early exercise testing in low-risk patients presenting to the ED with chest pain. Integration of these methods into a protocol-driven process has firmly established the contemporary chest pain center and its capacity for safe, accurate, and rapid patient management. After a negative observation period of 12 hours or less to exclude MI and ischemia at rest, exercise testing has been feasible to detect or exclude inducible ischemia. The negative predictive accuracy of this strategy is very high ($\sim 98\%$) and the low positive predictive accuracy is not problematic because the frequency of positive exercise tests is low, resulting in a small number of patients requiring admission for further inpatient evaluation. Additionally, the exercise test avoids inappropriate discharge of patients not identified by the observation process. Estimates of cost-effectiveness indicate the potential for substantial savings by chest pain centers through reduction of unnecessary admissions and decrease of inadvertent discharges of ACS patients. The chest pain center is a relatively recent development, and investigation is ongoing to determine optimal implementation of this concept, which will vary with the resources of individual institutions and the expertise and experience of the responsible physicians. In this regard, as previously noted [12–15,34], the authors have used a unique approach to the management of low-risk patients at their institution.

Immediate exercise testing

The authors' evaluation of low-risk patients in the University of California (Davis) CPU differs from that of the previous studies in that they apply exercise testing "immediately" after identification of low-risk patients on presentation. Serial cardiac injury markers are not obtained in this selected group, as described in their first study 10 years ago [34]. Since then, more than 3000 patients have been assessed by this strategy with no adverse effects. The current approach embodies several modifications based on their continuing experience, as documented in their second study (see Table 1) [44]. In this investigation of 212 patients, those with a history of CAD were not excluded, exercise testing was performed by internists trained in this technique, who serve as attending physicians on the CPU, and cardiac injury markers were not obtained before testing. Strict selection criteria for exercise testing included, as before, absence of hemodynamic dysfunction or cardiac arrhythmias, normal or near-normal ECGs, and no evidence of a noncardiac cause of chest pain on screening examination (Box 1). Symptom-limited treadmill exercise was performed by a modified Bruce protocol with the following endpoints: ischemic ST-segment shift (1.00 mm horizontal or downsloping depression 60 to 80 msec after the J point), symptoms, or arrhythmias, any of which is an indication for immediate termination of the test (Box 2). Negative exercise tests were obtained in 59% of patients, positive in 13%, and nondiagnostic in 28% (negative exercise ECG but failure to reach ≥ 85% of age-predicted maximum heart rate). Patients with positive tests were admitted and all patients with negative exercise tests and 93% with nondiagnostic results were discharged directly from the ED. In the latter group, the decision to discharge was based on achievement of adequate functional capacity (eg, ≥ 2 stages of the Bruce protocol or ≥ 75% of maximum predicted heart rate). Further evaluation

demonstrated CAD in 57% of those with a positive test and 30-day follow-up revealed no mortality or morbidity in the negative or nondiagnostic groups. This study demonstrated the safety of proceeding to exercise testing in carefully selected patients on the basis of the initial presentation without serial ECGs or cardiac injury markers. However, its limited numbers required a larger patient population for confirmation of the feasibility of this strategy.

In the largest single center study of exercise testing in low-risk patients, the authors reported results in 1000 patients (see Table 1) [45]. This study incorporated their current approach, which includes confirmation of a single negative cardiac

---

Box 1. Selection criteria for immediate exercise test

Chest pain suspicious for myocardial ischemia
Able to exercise
ECG normal, minor ST-T changes, or no change from previous abnormal ECG
Hemodynamically stable, no arrhythmia
A single negative serum marker is measured in selected patients

---

Box 2. Immediate exercise test procedure and end-points

Modified Bruce treadmill protocol[a]
Symptom-limited
Other end-points
    Ischemia (≥1.0 mm ST segment shift for 80 msec after the J point)
    ↓ Blood pressure (≥10 mm Hg systolic)
    Significant arrhythmia (sustained supraventricular tachyarrhythmia; high-grade ventricular ectopy [≥2 consecutive beats, sustained bigeminy])
Positive result: ≥ 1.0 mm horizontal ST segment shift
Nondiagnostic result: < 85% maximum predicted heart rate with no ST shift

[a] Includes two initial 3-minute states (1.7 mph, 0% grade and 1.7 mph, 5% grade) before the standard Bruce protocol.

injury marker before exercise testing. Almost two-thirds of the patients had negative immediate exercise tests, approximately 13% were positive and less than 25% were nondiagnostic (Fig. 3). There was no mortality during the 30-day follow-up interval. The negative predictive value for a cardiac event was 99.7% at 30 days. In the nondiagnostic group, all events were accounted for by revascularization in 32% of the 79 patients who had further evaluation. The positive predictive value of the exercise test was 33% for a cardiac event (four non-Q MIs detected after admission, 12 myocardial revascularizations) or a confirmatory imaging test for CAD (two patients). These results extended the authors' previous findings to a large, heterogeneous population in that testing was uncomplicated, the bulk of patients had negative tests and could be released directly from the ED, negative predictive value was excellent, and the low positive predictive value involved a relatively small group with positive exercise tests. The safety and accuracy of this method has been confirmed in patients with known CAD by a specific study of immediate exercise testing of 100 consecutive patients with this disease [46]. Although exercise testing is considered to have limited value in women, the authors' experience has confirmed the reliability of a negative immediate exercise test in this group. The negative predictive value of the test was 99% in 661 women with a mean age of 54 years studied in the CPU [47].

Comparison of exercise testing and myocardial scintigraphy

The utility of myocardial scintigraphy has been well established in patients presenting with chest pain [48]. However, the cost and logistics of this

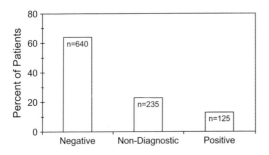

Fig. 3. Proportion of 1000 patients with negative, positive, and nondiagnostic immediate exercise tests. Numbers in bars indicate number of patients.

method are prohibitive for many institutions. In this regard, the authors have shown that > 70% of low-risk patients presenting with chest pain qualify for immediate exercise testing and that more complex and expensive stress imaging techniques can be appropriately reserved for the remainder of patients [49]. Moreover, a comparative study of 239 low risk patients by Senaratne and colleagues [50] revealed that early treadmill testing was as informative and more cost-effective than scintigraphy in identifying low-risk patients who did not require hospitalization. In this study, in which the follow-up period was 20 months, exercise testing was applicable in all but 9.6% of patients. These investigators report that, compared with scintigraphy as the initial cardiac study, exercise testing yielded a savings of more than $86,000 in this group of patients. In contrast to our strategy in which noncardiologists assess patients and perform immediate exercise testing, with cardiology consultation available as required, Senaratne and colleagues [50] emphasize the essential role of cardiologists in these processes. In this regard, the expertise of the authors' noncardiology CPU physicians in performing exercise testing has been confirmed by their accuracy in test interpretation and the complete absence of complications [51]. Analysis of 645 immediate exercise ECGs revealed a concordance of greater than 98% between the interpretations of these physicians and the authors' staff cardiologists.

Immediate exercise testing in special groups

The authors have recently explored a number of other issues presented by early exercise testing in patients presenting with chest pain. The use of beta-blockers or rate-limiting calcium channel-blockers often precludes diagnostic exercise testing because of attenuation of exertional heart rate by these agents. These drugs are associated with reduction of peak exercise heart rate and rate-pressure product, resulting in an increased frequency of nondiagnostic tests compared with patients not receiving these agents [52]. However, a majority (>60%) of patients taking these medications did have a diagnostic test. Therefore, it is our experience that use of these drugs should not preclude early exercise testing.

Recent trials of non-STE ACS have demonstrated the prognostic importance of multiple clinical factors in patients presenting with this diagnosis, including elevated cardiac injury markers, ST-segment deviation, age ≥ 65 years,

≥ three coronary risk factors, known CAD, ≥ two anginal episodes in the previous 24 hours and aspirin use in the previous 7 days. These factors comprise the TIMI risk score for prediction of fatal and nonfatal coronary events, which increase directly with the number of these risk factors [53]. However, in patients presenting to their CPU, the authors have found that, with the exception of elevated cardiac injury markers and ST-segment deviation, both of which preclude exercise testing, the test can be safely performed for reliable risk stratification regardless of the presence of the other TIMI risk factors [54]. Because it has recently been reported that augmenting the standard exercise ECG with additional leads enhances its sensitivity for detecting ischemia [55], the authors evaluated this innovation in their CPU patients. In this setting, the addition of four leads (two posterior and two right-sided) to the standard 12-lead ECG enhanced the sensitivity of the test minimally without altering specificity [56]: sensitivity rose only minimally from 7.6% to 8.0% based on detection of two patients who were positive only in the additional leads compared with 37 patients with positive findings in the standard exercise ECG. These additional leads were also not useful in detecting ischemia or injury in the resting ECG in patients admitted to the CPU [57]. In a study of 2021 patients referred for elective outpatient treadmill testing, the authors also found that the 16-lead exercise ECG did not afford increased sensitivity in this setting [58], thereby failing to confirm the prior study of Michaelides and colleagues [55].

A notable aspect of the authors' CPU experience has been the high recidivism rate of patients discharged from the unit with a negative evaluation. During a 7.5-year period, 13% of 1960 patients had ≥ two or more negative immediate exercise tests and accounted for 26% of the CPU visits [59]. Further, of the latter group, almost 10% had ≥ four negative exercise tests during this period. The multi-exercise test patients were relatively young (mean age 52 years) and most of them were women. Beyond the traditional differential diagnosis of multiple somatic causes of chest pain [60], common and underdiagnosed conditions responsible for this symptom include anxiety syndromes and somatoform disorders [11,60–62].

Further issues

Several aspects of the authors' application of immediate exercise testing in CPU patients warrant comment. As previously noted, patients in whom this method is used are carefully screened to confirm their low-risk status, as outlined in Box 1. The test is terminated at the initial appearance of any abnormality (see Box 2). Although noncardiologists perform the clinical assessment and exercise tests in CPU patients, these specially trained physicians have ready availability of consultation by staff cardiologists. In regard to the relatively large proportion (>20%) of patients with nondiagnostic tests (negative but peak heart rate < 85% of predicted maximum), the authors have found that those with negative tests at ≥ 80% of maximum predicted heart rate had uneventful outcomes on follow-up [45]. Therefore, use of this lower heart rate for a diagnostic test for the purpose of risk stratification appears prudent and would reduce the nondiagnostic group by 25% [45]. Although follow-up is only 30 days, the purpose of this approach is to determine short-term risk. This strategy is predicated on timely follow-up and further outpatient evaluation. Finally, although clinical assessment is basically reliable in identifying low-risk patients, it is imperfect and can result in inadvertent exercise testing in patients with ACS. This possibility is minimized by physician expertise and experience together with continued caution in the selection of patients for testing and in the indications for test termination.

A recurrent question concerns the necessity of performing exercise testing before discharge after a negative ADP rather than a short time after discharge. The former approach provides the most efficient completion of the evaluation and obviates concern regarding lack of return of patients for the outpatient test, which would contribute to the hazard of incomplete assessment and missed ACS [6]. However, where testing is not feasible and the system and patient characteristics are conducive to early return for testing (within 48 hours), it is reasonable to consider this approach. The authors have discharged selected very low-risk patients from their CPU without a predischarge exercise test. They have specifically studied this approach in a group of very low-risk women presenting to the ED with chest pain who were les than 50 years old, nondiabetic, and nonsmokers [63]. Of the entire group of 346 women, 175 were discharged from the CPU without exercise testing. At 30 days follow-up, none of these patients had confirmatory evidence of CAD or ACS. The results suggest that the risk of ACS is very minimal in women with low-risk profiles who present with chest pain and that stress testing in the CPU may not be necessary to determine disposition in these patients. These findings have implications for optimal use of limited resources.

Summary

CPUs are now established centers for assessment of low-risk patients presenting to the ED with symptoms suggestive of ACS. ADPs, of which treadmill testing is a key component, have been developed within these units for efficient evaluation of these patients. Studies of the last decade have established the utility of early exercise testing, which has been safe, accurate, and cost-effective in this setting. Specific diagnostic protocols vary, but most require 6 to12 hours of observation by serial ECGs and cardiac injury markers to exclude infarction and high-risk unstable angina before proceeding to exercise testing. However, in the CPU at UC Davis Medical Center, the approach includes "immediate" treadmill testing without a traditional process to rule out MI. Extensive experience has validated this approach in a large, heterogeneous population. The optimal strategy for evaluating low-risk patients presenting to the ED with chest pain will continue to evolve based on current research and the development of new methods.

References

[1] Gibler WB, Cannon CP, Blomkains AL, et al. Practical implementation of the guidelines for unstable angina/non-st-segment elevation myocardial infarction in the emergency department. Ann Emerg Med 2005;46:185–97.

[2] Pozen MW, D'Agostino RB, Selker HP, et al. Predictive instrument to improve coronary-care-unit admission practices in acute ischemic heart disease: a prospective multicenter clinical trial. N Engl J Med 1984;310:1273–8.

[3] Karlson BW, Herlitz J, Wiklund O, et al. Early prediction of acute myocardial infarction from clinical history, examination and electrocardiogram in the emergency room. Am J Cardiol 1991;68:171–5.

[4] Lown B, Vassaux C, Hood WB, et al. Unresolved problems in coronary care. Am J Cardiol 1967;20: 494–508.

[5] Karcz A, Holbrook J, Burke MC, et al. Massachusetts emergency medicine closed malpractice claims: 1988–1990. Ann Emerg Med 1993;22:553–9.

[6] Pope JH, Aufderheide TP, Ruthazer R, et al. Missed diagnoses of acute cardiac ischemia in the emergency department. N Engl J Med 2000;342: 1163–70.

[7] Liuzzo JP, Ambrose JA, Diggs P. Proton pump inhibitors for patients with coronary artery disease with reduced chest pain, emergency department visits, and hospitalizations. Clin Cardiol 2005;28: 369–74.

[8] Graff L, Joseph T, Andelman R, et al. American College of Emergency Physicians Information Paper: chest pain units in emergency departments—a report from the short-term observation services section. Am J Cardiol 1995;76(14):1036–9.

[9] Jesse RL, Kontos MC, Roberts CS. Evaluation of chest pain in the emergency department. Curr Prob Cardiol 1997;22:151–236.

[10] Selker HP, Zalenski RJ, Antman EM, et al. An evaluation of technologies for identifying acute cardiac ischemia in the emergency department. Executive summary of a National Heart Attack Alert Program Working Group report. Ann Emerg Med 1997;29: 1–87.

[11] Hutter AM, Amsterdam EA, Jaffe AS. Task force 2: acute coronary syndromes: section 2B-chest discomfort evaluation in the hospital, 31st Bethesda Conference. J Am Coll Cardiol 2000;35:853–62.

[12] Lewis WR, Amsterdam EA. Chest pain emergency units. Curr Opin Cardiol 1999;14:321–8.

[13] Kirk JD, Diercks DB, Turnipseed SD, Amsterdam EA. Evaluation of chest pain suspicious for acute coronary syndrome: use of an accelerated diagnostic protocol in a chest pain evaluation unit. Am J Cardiol 2000;85(5A):40B–8B.

[14] Lewis WL, Amsterdam EA. Observation units, clinical decision units and chest pain centers. In: Becker RC, Alpert JS, editors. Cardiovascular medicine: practice and management. London: Arnold; 2001. p. 85–103.

[15] Amsterdam EA, Lewis WR, Kirk JD, et al. Acute ischemic syndromes: chest pain center concept. Cardiol Clin 2002;20:117–36.

[16] Lee TH, Cook EF, Weisberg M, et al. Acute chest pain in the emergency room: identification and examination of low-risk patients. Arch Intern Med 1985;145:65–9.

[17] Goldman L, Cook F, Johnson PA, et al. Prediction of the need for intensive care in patients who come to emergency departments with acute chest pain. N Engl J Med 1996;334:1498–504.

[18] Brush JE Jr, Brand DA, Acampora D, et al. Use of the initial electrocardiogram to predict in-hospital complications of acute myocardial infarction. N Engl J Med 1980;312:1137–41.

[19] Gazes PC, Mobley EM Jr, Faris HM, et al. Preinfarctional (unstable) angina, a prospective study—a ten year follow-up. Prognostic significance of electrocardiographic changes. Circulation 1973;48: 331–7.

[20] Schroeder J, Lamb IH, Hu M. Do patients in whom myocardial infarction has been ruled out have a better prognosis after hospitalization than those surviving infarction? N Engl J Med 1980;303:1–5.

[21] Lee TH, Goldman L. Evaluation of the patient with acute chest pain. N Engl J Med 2000;342: 1187–95.

[22] Mulley AG, Thibault GE, Hughes RA, et al. The course of patients with suspected myocardial infarction: the identification of low-risk patients for early transfer from intensive care. N Engl J Med 1980; 302:943–8.

[23] Fineberg HV, Scadden D, Goldman L. Care of patients with a low probability of acute myocardial infarction: cost effectiveness of alternatives to coronary-care-unit admission. N Engl JM Med 1984; 310:1301–7.

[24] Gaspoz JM, Lee TH, Weinstein MC, et al. Cost-effectiveness of a new short-stay unit to "rule out" acute myocardial infarction in low risk patients. J Am Coll Cardiol 1994;24:1249.

[25] Braunwald E, Antman EM, Beasley JW, et al. ACC/AHA 2002 guideline update for the management of patients with unstable angina and non-ST-segment elevation myocardial infarction. http://www.acc. org/clincal/guidelines/unstable/unstable.pdf.

[26] Braunwald E, Mark DB, Jones RH, et al. Unstable angina: diagnosis and management. Agency for Health Care Policy and Research Publication No. 94–06062, Rockville, MD. 1994.

[27] Graff LG, Dallara J, Ross MA, et al. Impact on the care of the emergency department chest pain patient from the chest pain evaluation registry (CHEPER) study. Am J Cardiol 1997;80:563–8.

[28] Stein RA, Chaitman BR, Balady GJ, et al. Safety and utility of exercise testing in emergency room chest pain centers. An advisory from the Committee on Exercise, Rehabilitation, and Prevention, Council on Clinical Cardiology, American Heart Association. Circulation 2000;102:1463–7.

[29] Fletcher GF, Balady GJ, Amsterdam EA, et al. Exercise standards for testing and training. A statement for healthcare professionals from the American Heart Association. Circulation 2001; 104:1694–740.

[30] Gibbons RJ, Balady GJ, Bricker JT, et al. ACC/AHA 2002 guideline update for exercise testing: summary article. A report of the American College of Cardiology/American Heart Association task force on practice guidelines (committee to update the 1997 exercise testing guidelines). J Am Coll Cardiol 2002;40:1531–40.

[31] Gibbons RJ, Balady GJ, Beasley JW, et al. ACC/AHA guidelines for exercise testing. A report of the American College of Cardiology/American Heart Association task force on practice guidelines (committee on exercise testing). J Am Coll Cardiol 1997;30:260–315.

[32] Tsakonis JS, Shesser R, Rosenthal R, et al. Safety of immediate treadmill testing in selected emergency department patients with chest pain: a preliminary report. Am J Emerg Med 1991;9:557–9.

[33] Kerns JR, Shaub TF, Fontanarosa PB. Emergency cardiac stress testing in the evaluation of emergency department patients with atypical chest pain. Ann Emerg Med 1993;22:794–8.

[34] Lewis WL, Amsterdam EA. Utility and safety of immediate exercise testing of low-risk patients admitted to the hospital for suspected acute myocardial infarction. Am J Cardiol 1994;74:987–90.

[35] Gibler WB, Runyon JP, Levy RC, et al. A rapid diagnostic and treatment center for patients with chest pain in the emergency department. Ann Emerg Med 1995;25:1–8.

[36] Laslett LJ, Amsterdam EA. Management of the asymptomatic patient with an abnormal exercise ECG. JAMA 1984;252:1744–6.

[37] Gomez MA, Anderson JL, Labros AK, et al. An emergency department-based protocol for rapidly ruling out myocardial ischemia reduces hospital time and expense: results of randomized study (ROMIO). J Am Coll Cardiol 1996;28:25–33.

[38] Roberts RR, Zalenski RJ, Mensah EK. Costs of an emergency department-based accelerated diagnostic protocol vs hospitalization in patients with chest pain. JAMA 1997;278:1670–6.

[39] Zalenski RJ, McCarren M, Roberts R, et al. An evaluation of a chest pain diagnostic protocol to exclude acute cardiac ischemia in the emergency department. Arch Int Med 1997;157:1085–91.

[40] Polanczyk CA, Johnson PA, Hartley LH, et al. Clinical correlates and prognostic significance of early negative exercise tolerance test in patients with acute chest pain seen in the hospital emergency department. Am J Cardiol 1998;81:288–92.

[41] Mikhail MG, Smith FA, Gray M, et al. Cost-effectiveness of mandatory stress testing in chest pain center patients. Ann Emerg Med 1997;29:88–98.

[42] Farkouh MI, Smars PA, Reeder GS, et al. A clinical trial of a chest-pain observation unit for patients with unstable angina. N Engl J Med 1998;339:1882–8.

[43] Brillman J, Mathers-Dunbar L, Graff L, et al. Short term observation services section of the American College of Emergency Physicians. Management of observation units. Ann Emerg Med 1995;25:923–30.

[44] Kirk JD, Turnipseed S, Lewis WR, Amsterdam EA. Evaluation of chest pain in low-risk patients presenting to the emergency department: the role of immediate exercise testing. Ann Emerg Med 1998;32:1–7.

[45] Amsterdam EA, Kirk JD, Diercks DB, et al. Immediate exercise testing to evaluate low-risk patients presenting to the emergency department with chest pain. J Am Coll Cardiol 2002;40:251–6.

[46] Lewis WL, Amsterdam EA, Turnipseed S, Kirk JD. Immediate exercise testing of low risk patients with known coronary artery disease presenting to the emergency department with chest pain. J Am Coll Cardiol 1999;33:1843–7.

[47] Diercks DB, Kirk JD, Turnipseed S, Amsterdam EA. Exercise treadmill testing in women evaluated

in a chest pain unit [abstract]. Acad Emerg Med 2001;8:565.

[48] Kontos MC, Jesse RL, Schmidt KL, et al. Value of acute rest sestamibi perfusion imaging for evaluation of patients admitted to the emergency department with chest pain. J Am Coll Cardiol 1997;30:976–82.

[49] Amsterdam EA, Kirk JD, Diercks DB, et al. Assessment of low risk patients presenting to the emergency department with chest pain: immediate treadmill test or cardiac stress imaging [abstract]? J Am Coll Cardiol 2001;37:149A.

[50] Senaratne MJ, Carter D, Irwin M. Adequacy of an exercise test in excluding angina on patients presenting to the emergency department with chest pain. Ann Noninvas Electrocardiol 1999;4: 408–15.

[51] Kirk JD, Turnipseed S, Diercks DB, et al. Interpretation of immediate exercise treadmill test: interreader reliability between cardiologist and noncardiologist in a chest pain evaluation unit. Ann Emerg Med 2000;36:10–4.

[52] Diercks DB, Kirk JD, Turnipseed S, Amsterdam EA. Utility of immediate exercise treadmill testing in patients taking beta blockers or calcium channel blockers. Am J Cardiol 2002;90:882–5.

[53] Antman EM, Cohn M, Bernin PJLM, et al. The TIMI risk score for unstable angina/non–ST elevation MI. JAMA 2000;284:835–42.

[54] Amsterdam EA, Diercks DB, Kirk JD, et al. Multiple clinical risk factors do not preclude immediate exercise testing in a chest pain evaluation unit. J Am Coll Cardiol 2003;41:349A.

[55] Michaelides AN, Psomdaki ZD, Dilaveris PE, et al. Improved detection of coronary artery disease by exercise electrocardiography with the use of right precordial leads. N Engl J Med 1999;340:340–5.

[56] Diercks DB, Kirk JD, Turnipseed S, Amsterdam EA. Use of additional electrocardiographic leads in low-risk patients undergoing exercise treadmill testing [abstract]. Acad Emerg Med 2001;8:564.

[57] Ganim RP, Lewis WR, Diercks DB, et al. Right precordial and posterior electrocardiographic leads do not increase detection of ischemia in low-risk patients presenting with chest pain. Cardiology 2004;102:100–3.

[58] Sabapathy R, Bloom HL, Lewis WR, Amsterdam EA. Right precordial and posterior chest leads do not increase detection of positive response in electrocardiogram during exercise treadmill testing. Am J Cardiol 2003;91:75–7.

[59] Amsterdam EA, Kirk JD, Diercks DB, et al. Coronary artery disease in patients with multiple emergency department visits and negative immediate exercise tests for chest pain: an important minority in a total cohort of over 3,000 low risk patients presenting with chest pain [abstract]. J Am Coll Cardiol 2004;43:225A.

[60] Lewis WR, Amsterdam EA. Chest pain. In: Gershwin ME, Hamilton ME, editors. The pain management handbook: a concise guide to diagnosis and treatment. Totowa, NJ: Humana Press; 1998. p. 79–115.

[61] Carter C, Maddock R, Amsterdam EA, et al. Panic disorder and chest pain in the coronary care unit. Psychosomatics 1992;33:302–9.

[62] Thurston RC, Keefe FJ, Bradley L, et al. Chest pain in the absence of coronary artery disease: a biopsychosocial perspective. Pain 2001;93:95–100.

[63] Amsterdam EA, Diercks D, Kirk JD, et al. Evaluation of low risk women presenting to the emergency department with chest pain: is early stress testing necessary for risk stratification? Circulation, in press.

ELSEVIER
SAUNDERS

CARDIOLOGY
CLINICS

Cardiol Clin 23 (2005) 517–530

Imaging in the Evaluation of the Patient with Suspected Acute Coronary Syndrome

Michael C. Kontos, MD[a,b,*], James L. Tatum, MD[a]

[a]*Virginia Commonwealth University, VCU Medical Center, Room 7–074 North Hospital, 1300 E Marshall Street, PO Box 980051, Richmond, VA 23298–0051, USA*
[b]*Room 7-074, Heart Station, North Hospital, P.O. Box 980051, Medical College of Virginia, 12th and Marshall Streets, Richmond, VA 23298-0051, USA*

Over the last decade, major advances have been made in the treatment of acute coronary syndromes (ACSs). However, effective implementation of these treatments requires timely and accurate identification of the high-risk patient among all those presenting to the emergency department (ED) with symptoms suggestive of ACS. In the patient population presenting with a diagnostic ECG or those who have typical chest pain and a history of coronary disease, the initial triage and treatment strategies are straight-forward and guideline driven. However, for most patients the diagnosis is not clear-cut and further evaluation is required. The population of patients considered low risk after the initial evaluation accounts for nearly two thirds of ED chest pain patients [1,2], representing as many as 4 million patients a year in the United States. An additional consideration is that the opportunity for improving outcomes is time-dependent, so that early identification of the patient who has true ACS is essential. This necessity further increases the need for rapid triage tools, especially in the current setting of ED and hospital overcrowding that has become the norm in large urban centers.

In an effort to better identify patients who do not have myocardial ischemia, ED physicians have increasingly relied on technological advances, such as new bedside biomarkers and advanced imaging techniques. As these tools have become more available in the ED, triage decisions can be made with more rapid and comprehensive information. Advantages of rapid, accurate diagnosis are obvious and include early initiation of appropriate therapy for those who have myocardial infarction (MI) or unstable angina; reduction in the inadvertent discharge of patients who have ongoing ischemia; and shortened length of stay and reduced admissions for patients who have noncardiac chest pain.

Before implementing a new diagnostic tool or test, several questions require an affirmative answer, including whether it is accurate (ie, sensitive and specific), if it adds incremental diagnostic information to that which is already available, and if it is cost-effective. Over the last 15 years, numerous studies examining the usefulness of acute ED myocardial perfusion imaging (MPI) have confirmed that the answer to these questions is "yes."

Acute myocardial perfusion imaging

Knowledge of the ischemic cascade presupposes that "in vivo" noninvasive imaging of myocardial perfusion should provide an optimal technique for not only detecting (diagnosis) but also grading (risk stratification) ACS. This presumption is confirmed by studies dating back over 3 decades. Wackers and colleagues [3] and others used planar myocardial perfusion imaging with thallium in the 1970s to demonstrate that acute imaging had significant incremental diagnostic power in patients who had non–ST-elevation ACS [4]. However, the intrinsic characteristics of thallium as a radiotracer and the inherent

---

* Corresponding author.
E-mail address: mckontos@vcu.edu (M.C. Kontos).

limitations of planar imaging prevented wide-spread adoption of the technique in the clinical management of ACS. Although some of the issues related to the radionuclide could be mitigated by performing imaging immediately in the ED [5,6], the limitations of planar imaging required improvements in technology to overcome the low sensitivity for detecting small areas of ischemia and for detecting ischemia in the posterior distribution. The development of single-photon emission computed tomography (SPECT) in combination with the superior image quality provided by technetium-labeled myocardial perfusion agents led to observational studies followed by clinical trials demonstrating the usefulness of acute ED MPI. Technetium 99m (Tc-99m) sestamibi and tetrofosmin are taken up by the myocardium in proportion to blood flow, similar to thallium, but do not undergo significant redistribution [7]. Therefore, patients can be injected while experiencing symptoms and imaged up to several hours later, making it possible to perform high-quality SPECT imaging outside of the ED setting in the absence of dedicated equipment.

The favorable energy and dosimetry of Tc-99m also allow gated acquisition and reconstruction of dynamic functional images, thereby providing simultaneous assessment of regional and global ventricular function that can be correlated with perfusion defects [8]. In the setting of acute infarction or ischemia, wall motion is typically abnormal; in contrast, an apparent perfusion defect in the presence of normal wall motion and thickening on gated SPECT usually indicates an artifact such as tissue attenuation. The ability to perform simultaneous wall motion and perfusion significantly improves specificity [9,10] and is particularly valuable in the acute setting where serial images are not available.

In the presence of significant ischemia, the concomitant presence of a wall motion abnormality in conjunction with perfusion defects on acute imaging not only adds specificity but is a additional prognostic indicator. Recent data indicate this is true. A recent multicenter study by Kaul and colleagues [11] found that perfusion plus regional function provided substantially greater diagnostic and prognostic value for predicting outcomes in 163 patients who had possible ACS. In our study of 2286 consecutive patients who were admitted for exclusion of ischemia following acute rest MPI, we found that among the patients who had Troponin-I (TnI) elevations (4.0% versus 3.5%), creatine kinase-myocardial band (CK-MB) MI (1.7% versus 1.5%), or who underwent revascularization (5.6% versus 5.1%), there was no difference in the proportion of patients who had perfusion defects but had normal wall motion in that area and those who had normal perfusion and function. In contrast, those who had perfusion defects associated with abnormal wall motion were significantly more likely to have TnI elevations (15%), CK-MB MI (10%), and undergo revascularization (16%).

Diagnostic value

Sensitivity: acute myocardial infarction

Several studies to assess the diagnostic accuracy of acute ED MPI have found a high sensitivity for identifying patients who have MI (Table 1) [3,12–18]. However, because acute MPI is performed predominantly in low-risk patients, the absolute numbers of patients who have MI in any individual study is small, resulting in an imprecise measurement of sensitivity. In a study that included 141 patients who had CK-MB MI, we found that sensitivity was 89% (95%

Table 1
Diagnostic accuracy of rest myocardial perfusion imaging in patients who have acute chest pain syndrome and normal or nonischemic rest electrocardiograms

	Year	N	Tracer	Sensitivity	Specificity	NPV	End point
Wackers et al [3]	1979	203	Tl-201	100%	72%	100%	AMI
Varetto et al [12]	1993	64	Tc-mibi	100%	92%	100%	CAD
Hilton et al [13]	1994	102	Tc-mibi	94%	83%	99%	CAD/AMI
Tatum et al [14]	1997	438	Tc-mibi	100%	78%	100%	AMI
Kontos et al [15]	1997	532	Tc-mibi	93%	71%	99%	AMI
Heller et al [16]	1998	357	Tc-tetro	90%	60%	99%	AMI
Kontos et al [17]	1999	620	Tc-mibi	92%	67%	99%	AMI
Udelson et al [18]	2002	1215	Tc-mibi	96%	NR	99%	AMI

Abbreviations: AMI, acute myocardial infarction; CAD, angiographic coronary artery disease; NPV, negative predictive value; NR, not reported; Tc-mibi, Tc-99m-sestamibi; Tc-tetro, Tc-99m-tetrofosmin; Tl-201, thallium 201.

confidence interval, 83%–94%), similar to prior reported studies. As would be expected, patients who had negative MPI had small MIs as estimated by peak creatine kinase (CK) values, with an average CK of 313 ± 227 U/L, compared with 590 ± 620 U/L ($P < .001$) in those who had positive MPI [19].

Another confounding issue with these studies is that most used elevations in either CK or CK-MB as the diagnostic standard for MI. However, because of its high sensitivity and specificity for detecting myocardial necrosis [20,21], current guidelines recommend that cardiac troponin be the diagnostic standard for MI [22]. Because approximately 3% to 4% of the left ventricle must be ischemic to allow detection by MPI [23], the number of patients who have troponin elevations and negative MPI would be expected to be higher than the previous standard. This assumption has been supported by several small studies that reported that, although the sensitivity of MPI was high, it was significantly lower than that of TnI or Troponin-T [17,24]. In a larger study, we analyzed outcomes in 319 patients who were initially considered low risk for MI and underwent acute rest MPI as part of standard chest pain evaluation protocol and were subsequently found to have elevated TnI values [25], thus meeting the ACC/ESC definition for MI [22]. Seventy-seven patients had negative MPI, giving a sensitivity of only 76%; much lower than when CK or CK-MB was used as the diagnostic standard for MI. However, among the 77 patients who had negative MPI, more than half (n = 47, 61%) had a peak CK-MB of more than 8 ng/mL and therefore would not previously have been diagnosed with MI (Fig. 1). Patients who had negative MPI had significantly lower peak CK-MB values (15 ± 25 ng/mL versus 45 ± 78 ng/mL, $P < .001$), had higher ejection fractions (56% ± 15% versus 47% ± 13%, $P < .01$), and were more likely to have nonsignificant disease (60% versus 85%, $P < .001$) than those who had positive MPI. These findings demonstrate that acute MPI continues to provide additional risk/prognostic information even with the introduction of a newer generation of biomarkers.

Acute coronary syndrome without myocardial infarction

In the past 15 years, a large body of evidence has demonstrated that acute MPI using Tc-99m myocardial perfusion agents can accurately identify patients who have unstable angina. In one of the first studies, Bilodeau and colleagues [9] imaged 45 patients who did not have a previous history of MI and had been admitted for unstable angina. The presence of a perfusion defect had a sensitivity of 96% and specificity of 79% for predicting angiographic coronary disease in patients injected during an episode of pain, compared with a sensitivity of only 65% for the ECG. Although specificity of acute MPI appears low when MI is used as the end point, an important advantage is to remember that the entire continuum of ACS remains a diagnostic dilemma. Using revascularization or significant disease as a surrogate for unstable angina, abnormal images are found in a high proportion, and overall specificity and predictive value are increased. For example, we found that in 532 patients admitted after acute rest MPI in the ED, acute MI as assessed by CK-MB elevations was present in only 15% of patients who had positive MPI (Fig. 2) [15]. However, most patients who have positive MPI had an end point consistent with ACS, including acute infarction, subsequent revascularization, or significant coronary disease (>70% stenosis) on coronary angiography.

Negative predictive value and prognosis

A high negative predictive value is critical for the value of acute MPI to serve as a risk stratification tool. The ability to exclude significant ischemia in more than 99% of patients allows effective identification of those who can be placed in lower-intensity settings other than the coronary care unit (CCU) or can be discharged home (see Table 1). The predictive value of a negative acute MPI also extends beyond the immediate setting in identifying patients at low risk for short- and long-term cardiac complications. For example, Hilton and colleagues [26] found that patients who had normal perfusion imaging had an excellent prognosis, with no late events at 90-day follow-up. Similarly, we reported that patients who had negative acute MPI had a cardiac event rate of only 3% during the subsequent year [14]. In our experience over the last 9 years, low-risk patients discharged from the ED after undergoing acute ED rest MPI (n = 10,775) demonstrated a 30-day cardiac mortality of only 0.08%, with only nine cardiac deaths during the follow-up period.

An important prognostic parameter provided by acute MPI is that it not only identifies patients

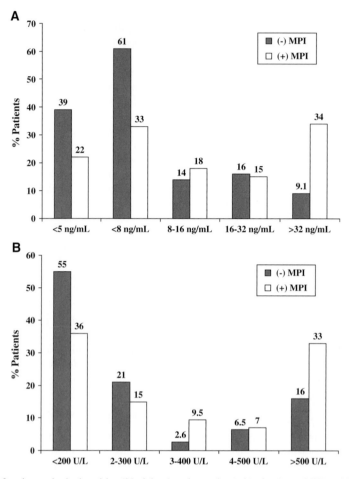

Fig. 1. Proportion of patients who had positive (*black bars*) and negative (*white bars*) rest MPI and levels of (*A*) CK-MB and (*B*) CK elevations. Of 104 patients who had creatine kinase myocardial band (CK-MB) level <8 ng/mL, 61% had negative images, whereas of 192 patients who had CK-MB ≥8 ng/mL, only 27% had negative images (sensitivity 83%). (*Modified from* Kontos MC, Fratkin MJ, Jesse RL, et al. Sensitivity of acute rest myocardial perfusion imaging for identifying patients with myocardial infarction based on a troponin definition. J Nucl Cardiol 2004;11:12–9; with permission.)

who have ACS but also provides a validated measurement of the ischemic risk area. The size of a perfusion defect is of significant clinical importance, as patients who have larger defects have a worse long-term prognosis [27,28]. The most important determinant of infarct size is the ischemic risk zone or the amount of myocardium in jeopardy [29]. MPI is the only technique among those commonly available that can determine the ischemic risk zone [30,31]. In studies in which post-MI patients had MPI before discharge, defect size correlated well with other outcome predictors, including left ventricular ejection fraction [32,33], regional wall motion index [32], end-systolic volume [33], and peak CK levels [34].

Even in the absence of ischemic ECG changes, the ischemic risk area can be large. We found that the ischemic risk area ranged from 0% to 62% of the left ventricle, with a mean risk area of 18% ± 11%. Even patients who had normal ECGs at the time of presentation had risk areas similar to those of patients who had abnormal but non-ischemic ECGs (16% ± 12% versus 19% ± 12%, $P = .25$) (Fig. 3) [35]. One explanation for this finding is that MI in these patients is often caused by occlusion of the left circumflex coronary artery, and the myocardial territory supplied by it is "silent" on a surface ECG [36]. In a small study that included patients who had ST-segment depression, Christian and colleagues [37] performed

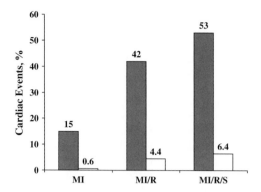

Fig. 2. Outcomes associated with results of acute rest MPI. Patients who had positive rest MPI (*dark bars*) had significantly (*P* < .0001) more MI; MI or revascularization (MI/R); and MI, revascularization, or significant coronary artery disease (>70% stenosis) (MI/R) or significant disease than patients who had negative rest myocardial perfusion imaging (*white bars*). (*Modified from* Kontos MC, Jesse RL, Schmidt KL, et al. Value of acute rest sestamibi perfusion imaging for evaluation of patients admitted to the emergency department with chest pain. J Am Coll Cardiol 1997;30:976–82; with permission.)

early MPI in 14 patients who did not have ST-segment elevation and later underwent coronary angiography. The culprit vessel was the circumflex coronary artery in six (43%) patients. In another study of 79 patients presenting with a nonischemic ECG and acute MI, we found that the left circumflex coronary artery was the infarct-related artery in 42% of the cases [35].

In patients who have left circumflex occlusions, the absence of ischemic ECG changes does not

predict small MIs [36]. O'Keefe and colleagues [38] reported that the risk area was not significantly different in patients who had left circumflex occlusion associated with ST-segment elevation, left circumflex occlusion without ST-elevation, and right coronary artery occlusion. Consistent with these results, we found that the ischemic area at risk was similar in patients in whom the infarct-related artery was the left circumflex (18% ± 10%, median 19%), the right coronary (18% ± 13%, median 17%), or the left anterior descending artery (18% ± 10%, median 19%) [35].

Incremental diagnostic value

Although a new test may offer high diagnostic accuracy, it may have limited value unless it provides significant incremental value over the current standard of care. Because the existing standard usually includes testing that is readily available and less expensive, the barrier to inclusion of techniques such as acute MPI is that they must demonstrate a clear benefit.

Studies performed in lower-risk patients have demonstrated that acute ED MPI does offer incremental value. In one of the first studies, Hilton and colleagues [13] used Tc-99m sestamibi SPECT imaging to study 102 patients presenting to the ED with typical angina and either a normal or nondiagnostic ECG. Seventy patients had a normal perfusion scan, only one of whom had a cardiac event. In comparison, 2 of the 15 (13%) patients who had equivocal scans and 12 of the 17 (71%) patients who had perfusion defects had cardiac events. When equivocal scans were classified as

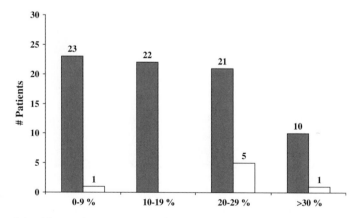

Fig. 3. Distribution of the risk area sizes as a percent of the left ventricle. Dark bars represents patients who had ECG evidence of prior infarction. (*Modified from* Kontos MC, Kurdziel KA, Ornato JP, et al. A nonischemic electrocardiogram does not always predict a small myocardial infarction: Results with acute myocardial perfusion imaging. Am Heart J 2001;141:360–66; with permission.)

abnormal, the sensitivity and specificity of an abnormal study for predicting adverse cardiac events were 94% and 83%, respectively.

Similarly, we found that abnormal MPI was the most important independent predictor of MI or revascularization in 532 patients who underwent acute ED MPI [15]. Finally, Heller and colleagues [16] found that that abnormal SPECT was the most important multivariate predictor of MI in 357 patients who underwent acute MPI. In addition, acute MPI added significant incremental diagnostic value after consideration of demographic, clinical, and ECG variables (Fig. 4).

In an interesting intent-to-treat survey study, Knott and colleagues [39] performed acute MPI on 120 patients in the ED. The requesting physician completed a questionnaire before imaging, asking what the proposed management would be had the test not been available. They found a 34% reduction in overall hospital admissions and a 59% reduction in planned CCU admissions. Overall, CCU admissions were not reduced because 17 patients initially considered low risk were admitted to the CCU after MPI was found to be abnormal.

Data from several observational studies were confirmed in the Emergency Room Assessment of Sestamibi for Evaluating Chest Pain (ERASE) study, a large prospective randomized controlled study. This study demonstrated that acute MPI was effective when compared with standard management of low-risk chest pain patients [18]. In this study, 2475 patients were randomized to routine care or ED MPI, in which patients were injected with sestamibi in the ED and subsequently underwent acute imaging, with the results called back to the ED physician [18]. All patients, whether admitted or discharged, underwent marker analysis and diagnostic evaluation. There was no difference in the percentage of patients who had ACS and either MI (97% versus 96%) or unstable angina (83% versus 81%) who were admitted, with one patient who had MI from each group discharged from the ED. However, there was a significantly lower admission rate and a higher rate of direct discharge from the ED in the ED MPI arm compared with the standardized care arm.

Other issues

Radiopharmaceutical

Although most studies were performed with sestamibi, comparable results have been obtained with tetrofosmin. In a multicenter study, Heller and colleagues [16] found a sensitivity of 90% in 357 patients who underwent acute MPI. Negative predictive value (NPV) was equally high at 99%, with only two patients who had small non–Q-wave MIs having negative acute MPI. In our study in which 319 patients had TnI elevations, sensitivity of those who had acute MPI with sestamibi (75%) and tetrofosmin (80%) were similar, as was the proportion who had CK-MB MI (84% versus 87%) [16].

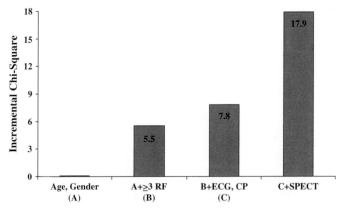

Fig. 4. Incremental prognostic value of rest tetrofosmin SPECT imaging over clinical variables. Model A: clinical variables; Model B: A plus three or more risk factors (RF); Model C: B plus admission ECG and chest pain (CP) at the time of tetrofosmin injection. (*Modified from* Heller GV, Stowers SA, Hendel RC, et al. Clinical value of acute rest technetium-99m tetrofosmin tomographic myocardial perfusion imaging in patients with acute chest pain and nondiagnostic electrocardiograms. J Am Coll Cardiol 1998;31:1011–17; with permission.)

Comparison with troponin

Although markers of necrosis, such as troponin, are considered the gold standard for identifying MI, rest MPI does have some important advantages over using markers alone. First, myocardial markers are by definition abnormal only in patients who have necrosis, and therefore are negative in patients who have ischemia alone. Also, given the time required for imaging and processing, acute MPI results can be available within 1 to 2 hours after injection. In contrast, markers of necrosis are not detectable in the blood until several hours after the damage has occurred. To achieve a high sensitivity, sampling must be performed over an 8- to 9-hour period [40]. Thus, the sensitivity of MPI is significantly higher than that of the initial troponin (Fig. 5).

A second advantage of acute MPI is that it can identify risk area, and therefore better quantitate overall cardiac risk. For example, two patients who have similar low-peak TnI values—one secondary to occlusion of a small branch vessel and the other resulting from a brief occlusion of the proximal portion of a major vessel—have markedly different areas at risk and the potential for markedly different outcomes, which can be readily determined using MPI.

Acute MPI has some limitations when used to assess patients who have chest pain. Acute MI, acute ischemia, and prior MI all cause perfusion defects, and differentiation is not possible based on the images alone. However, patients who have prior MI are at higher risk for acute events and are usually not candidates for primary triage to a subsequent outpatient evaluation. Sensitivity for identifying necrosis is imperfect for MPI, as at least 3% to 5% of the left ventricle must be ischemic for a defect to be detected. However, the many patients who have negative rest MPI despite marker elevations have nonsignificant disease on coronary angiography [25], and therefore are at low risk for short-term adverse outcomes, although aggressive risk factor modification would still be indicated. Therefore, rather than being seen as competitive diagnostic tools for evaluating patients presenting to the ED with chest pain, markers and MPI should be considered complementary.

Timing of tracer injection

Although it appears that sensitivity of acute MPI decreases as the symptom-free interval increases, the reduction is highly variable. In the case of thallium, Wackers and colleagues [3] performed thallium-201 scintigraphy in 98 patients admitted with chest pain who had MI excluded. When imaged within 6 hours of the last anginal symptoms, 57% of the patients had abnormal studies; however, when imaged after 12 hours, only 8% had abnormal studies. Similar results have been reported by Van der Wieken and colleagues [4].

Studies using technetium agents also demonstrate higher sensitivity when injection is

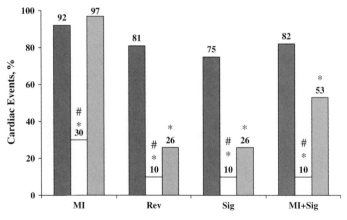

Fig. 5. Sensitivity of MPI (*dark bars*), the initial troponin I (*open bars*), and troponin I (*light bars*) for identifying end points. Asterisk denotes $P < .001$ compared with perfusion imaging; # denotes $P < .001$ compared with serial troponin. Rev, revascularization; Sig, significant disease (>70% stenosis). (*Data from* Kontos MC, Jesse RL, Anderson FP, et al. Comparison of myocardial perfusion imaging and cardiac troponin I in patients admitted to the emergency department with chest pain. Circulation 1999;99:2073–8.)

performed during or soon after pain. Bilodeau and colleagues [9] found that the sensitivity of MPI for detection of coronary artery disease was 96% in 45 patients injected with tracer during chest pain. When the same patients were reinjected later while pain-free, the sensitivity had decreased to 65%. However, in both cases the sensitivity was significantly higher than that of the initial ECG. In contrast, we found that when patients were injected within 6 hours of symptoms, sensitivity was similar for identifying patients who had MI, revascularization, or significant coronary disease between those who were injected with and without symptoms [15]. Others have also reported high sensitivity despite the absence of symptoms during injection [12].

One explanation relates to the difference in the underlying mechanisms causing perfusion defects in patients who have ACS as compared with those undergoing stress testing. Rather than causing true ischemia, stress perfusion defects result from flow heterogeneity between areas supplied by coronary arteries with and without significant stenoses. The perfusion tracer is injected at the time of maximal flow imbalance, with a rapid return of coronary flow to baseline once the patient stops exercising. In contrast, in patients who have ACS, perfusion defects result from the combination of intermittent thrombotic occlusion and vasoconstriction in the setting of complex coronary morphology [41], resulting in marked decreased coronary blood flow [42] and persistently decreased regional myocardial perfusion [41]. Because regional hypoperfusion is one of the first steps in the ischemic cascade, symptoms of chest discomfort are often a late clinical manifestation, so that regional hypoperfusion will frequently be present even in the absence of symptoms. Suboptimal flow frequently persists despite prolonged treatment with newer pharmacologic treatments, such as glycoprotein IIb/IIIa antagonists [43,44].

Perfusion defects may also result from distal embolization of a proximal thrombus leading to downstream microvascular obstruction [45]. In a study of 75 patients who underwent sestamibi injection during rotational atherectomy, a procedure in which distal embolization of microparticles is frequent, perfusion defects were present in 65% of patients [45].

Finally, a third potential mechanism was reported in an interesting study of 40 patients who had a percutaneous intervention. Fram and colleagues [46] found that perfusion abnormalities persisted in patients injected with Tc-99m sestamibi at varying intervals after balloon inflation, although the size of the perfusion defect decreased as the interval after the procedure increased. One explanation is that the pharmacodynamics of sestamibi are dependent on membrane and mitochondrial functional integrity, which may be depressed as a result of lingering metabolic alterations, especially in high-energy metabolites that occur after transient ischemia.

All of these findings strongly support the conclusion that the sensitivity of acute MPI will be dependent on the extent, duration, severity, and reperfusion status of the ischemic insult. It must be kept in mind that chest pain is not the gold standard for myocardial ischemia and that silent ischemia is common. In patients who have been pain-free for prolonged periods, acute MPI will have a lower sensitivity for detection of the presence of coronary disease, but persistent abnormality suggests a more complex and possibly unstable condition associated with higher risk.

Special populations

Although not normally considered candidates for acute MPI because of their higher pretest likelihood of ischemia, rest MPIs can provide useful additional diagnostic information in selected subgroups of patients who have known coronary artery disease. This group includes patients who have a nonischemic ECG and atypical symptoms (particularly if they are different from their typical angina), those who have had a recent negative cardiac evaluation, or those in whom the risk for coronary angiography is increased, such as patients who have significant renal disease. In patients who have multivessel disease, such as those who have had prior bypass surgery, the ability to determine risk area can be used to delineate the culprit lesion.

It should be recognized that patients who have prior MI, especially those who have Q waves, are likely to have perfusion defects, and that subsequent repeat rest-imaging after a pain-free period is required to differentiate new ischemia from old infarction. Alternatively, if prior images are available, they can be used for comparison to determine the significance of perfusion defects. When deciding whether to pursue further invasive or noninvasive treatment, it has been our experience that minor differences in images when compared with prior studies are unlikely to be of clinical significance.

Another group of patients in whom ED rest MPI can be useful are those presenting with cocaine-associated chest pain. In the absence of ischemic ECG changes or known coronary disease, the risk for ACS is low [47]. Rather than admitting the patient, an alternative evaluation process is to perform rest MPI, with discharge if images are negative. We found that in 216 consecutive patients who had chest pain after recent cocaine use who underwent ED MPI, only five (2.3%) patients had abnormal studies, including two who had acute MI [48]. None of the 38 patients who had normal MPI had subsequently acute MI by biomarkers after admission to the CCU, and only 7% of the 67 patients undergoing subsequent stress MPI had reversible myocardial perfusion defects. At 30-day follow-up there were no cardiac events in patients who had normal rest MPI. This finding indicates that hospital admission can be avoided in this subgroup of patients who have a history of cocaine use if rest MPI is negative.

Cost-effectiveness

The ability to discharge patients directly from the ED has obvious cost implications. Despite the application of complex and expensive technology, ED MPI can be cost-effective if the number of patients admitted is decreased [16,49–51]. Several observational studies have confirmed that cost reductions occur when rest MPI is used as an integral part of patient management. Costs are reduced in two ways. One obvious mechanism is by discharging more patients directly from the ED, with an increase in the admission of more appropriate patients. A second mechanism is by more appropriate selection of diagnostic procedures, as the rate of coronary angiography in low-risk patients is reduced [39,49]. A preliminary analysis from the ERASE study confirms that using ED MPI as a key part of the initial diagnostic strategy was cost-effective, with costs reduced to an average of $70 per patient [52].

Incorporation into chest pain evaluation

Recent updated guidelines for the clinical use of cardiac radionuclide imaging indicate that acute ED MPI has a Class IA indication for assessing myocardial risk in patients who have possible ACS and have nondiagnostic ECGs and negative initial serum markers and enzymes, if available [53].

In addition, recommendations for using MPI in the ED have been published [54]. The recommended patient selection criteria are similar to those used for admission to a chest pain evaluation unit. Patients should be low risk (no ischemic ECG changes or history of coronary disease) and hemodynamically stable. The optimal use of MPI as a triage tool is in patients who will be discharged home and have stress testing as an outpatient if imaging is negative.

One of the first programs to incorporate rest MPI as a strategy was at Virginia Commonwealth University Medical Center (formerly Medical College of Virginia). In contrast to most chest pain programs, the systematic chest pain protocol developed and implemented is designed for all chest pain patients, with MPI used for evaluation of lower-risk patients (Table 2) [14]. All patients presenting to the ED with chest pain or other symptoms consistent with myocardial ischemia undergo rapid evaluation with assignment to a triage level, which is based on the probability of having MI or myocardial ischemia derived from clinical and ECG variables. After the initial evaluation, patients thought to be at high risk (those who have ischemic ECG changes and those who have known coronary disease experiencing typical symptoms) and characterized as levels 1 and 2 are admitted directly to the CCU. Patients considered low to moderate risk for ACS (eg, absence of ischemic ECG changes or history of coronary disease) undergo further risk stratification using acute rest MPI [14]. Level 3 patients are admitted as observation patients and undergo a rapid rule-in protocol. Level 4 patients are evaluated in the ED. If images are either negative or unchanged from previous studies, patients are discharged home and scheduled for outpatient stress testing. If MPI is positive, they are admitted and advanced to the level 2 treatment protocol.

It is important to appreciate the difference in the role of acute rest MPI between level 3 and level 4 patients. In level 3 patients, the presence of a significant perfusion defect identifies a high-risk patient in whom early initiation of aggressive treatment is indicated, with the potential for early intervention. Negative MPI and negative markers, on the other hand, identify patients who can safely undergo early stress testing and discharge. Although the identification of higher-risk patients is the focus of much interest, the ability to better risk-stratify intermediate-risk patients into low-risk who can be stressed safely is an important advantage. In contrast, the role of MPI in patients

Table 2
Acute chest pain diagnostic treatment pathways at Medical College of Virginia/Virginia Commonwealth University Medical Center

Primary risk assignment	Probability of AMI	Probability of ischemia	Diagnostic criteria	Disposition	Secondary risk stratification	Treatment strategy
Level 1: AMI	Very high (>95%)	Very high (>95%)	Ischemic ST elevation; Acute posterior MI	Admit CCU	Serial ECGs; Cardiac markers every 6–8 h until peak	Fibrinolytics within 30 min; Primary PCI within 90 min
Level 2: Definite or highly probable ACS	Moderate (10%–50%)	High (20%–50%)	Ischemic ECG; Acute CHF; Known CAD with typical symptoms	Admit CCU; Fast track rule-in protocol	Serial ECGs; Cardiac Markers at 0, 3, 6, and 8 h; If rule-in for AMI (markers positive) continue every 6–8 h until peak	ASA; IV UFH or SC LMWH; IV and/or topical NTG; IV and/or PO Beta Blocker; Clopidogrel; GP IIb/IIIa inhibitor if TnI positive; Cath/PCI
Level 3: Probable ACS	Low (1%–10%)	Moderate (5%–20%)	Nonischemic ECG and either: Typical symptoms >30 min, no CAD, or Atypical symptoms >30 min, known CAD,	Observation; Fast track rule-in protocol	MPI; Cardiac Markers at 0, 3, 6, and 8 h; Serial ECGs	ASA; If cardiac markers or MPI positive: treat per level 2 protocol; If negative: stress
Level 4: Possible UA	Very low (<1%)	Low (<5%)	Nonischemic ECG and either: Typical symptoms <30 min, or Atypical symptoms,	ED evaluation	MPI	MPI positive: admit to level 2 treatment protocol; MPI negative: discharge; schedule out patient stress
Level 5: Very low suspicion for AMI or UA	Very low (<1%)	Very low (<1%)	Evaluation must clearly document a noncardiac etiology for the symptoms	ED evaluation as deemed necessary	As appropriate for the clinical condition	As appropriate for the clinical condition

Abbreviations: ACS, acute coronary syndrome; AMI, acute myocardial infarction; ASA, aspirin; CAD, coronary artery disease; CCU, coronary care unit; CHF, congestive heart failure; ED, emergency department; GP, glycoprotein; IV, intravenous; LMWH, low molecular weight heparin; MPI, myocardial perfusion imaging; NTG, nitroglycerin; PCI, percutaneous intervention; TnI, troponin I; UA, unstable angina; UFH, unfractionated heparin.

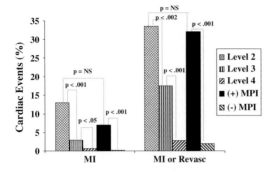

Fig. 6. Cardiac outcomes compared with the initial triage level assignment and the MPI results. The incidence of MI or MI or revascularization was significantly different among level 2 (*hatched bars*), level 3 (*vertical bars*), and level 4 (*diagonal bars*) patients. Patients who had positive imaging (*dark bars*) had an incidence of MI or MI or revascularization similar to the level 2 patients. (*Adapted from* Tatum JL, Jesse RL, Kontos MC, et al. Comprehensive strategy for the evaluation and triage of the chest pain patient. Ann Emerg Med 1997; 29:116–23; with permission.)

who are considered level 4 is to diagnose unsuspected ACS and prevent the inadvertent discharge of these patients from the ED. Follow-up stress testing is used to exclude significant coronary disease.

This simple risk stratification scheme accurately separates patients into high-, intermediate-, and low-risk groups. The ability of MPI to further risk stratify lower-risk patients is also obvious, as outcomes in patients who have positive MPI are similar to those in the patients considered high-risk level 2 (Fig. 6) [14]. Close collaboration of the CCU and nuclear medicine staff has resulted in the ability to successfully triage patients who do not have known coronary disease and have large perfusion defects at the time of imaging directly to coronary angiography and revascularization.

Patients presenting with chest pain are evaluated similarly to the Medical College of Virginia protocol. Patients who present without chest pain undergo rest SPECT thallium imaging. If images are negative, subsequent stress SPECT Tc-99m sestamibi imaging is immediately performed. If rest images are abnormal, the patient is re-evaluated for possible ACS before stress testing.

Summary

The rapid triage of the patient who has suspected ACS continues to be a challenge. Chest pain and other symptoms suggestive of ischemia remain nonspecific and frequent presentations to the ED. The ECG appropriately remains the first triage tool and is essential for identifying the patient who requires admission; however, numerous studies have demonstrated that it is inadequate for triaging most of the remaining patients. Acute MPI has been shown to have a high NPV and is a powerful risk stratification tool. When MPI is used in conjunction with the newer biomarkers such as troponin, the combination provides an impressive risk profile.

The inherent success of acute MPI in the ACS population is not serendipitous but rather based on the knowledge of the pathophysiology of ACS and the ischemic cascade that has been elucidated through the work of many investigators. The fact that one of the earliest events in the cascade is a marked reduction in absolute blood flow, leading to metabolic ischemia and its functional consequences, led researchers decades ago to attempt to noninvasively detect this early signature of ACS. However, as is often the case, these early investigators were limited by available technology. With the development of technological advances such as SPECT imaging and the introduction of Tc-99m–labeled MPI agents, it became possible to translate basic science observations into meeting a recognized patient need. Importantly, the ability to noninvasively assess perfusion acutely in combination with a quantitative measurement of function has important prognostic power. The studies that followed have confirmed that when this information is applied to the appropriate population in a timely manner it has significant clinical impact. A key aspect of the clinical success of nuclear cardiology techniques in this and other settings has been the ability to standardize all aspects of this process, from image acquisition to computer-assisted diagnosis. As new techniques are applied to the ACS population, the same questions posed earlier will need to be answered for each new technique.

References

[1] Faroghi A, Kontos MC, Jesse RL, et al. Are cardiac risk factors predictive in low risk emergency department chest pain patients who have chest pain? J Am Coll Cardiol 2000;35:379A.
[2] Lee TH, Goldman L. Evaluation of the patient with acute chest pain. N Engl J Med 2000;342:1187–95.

[3] Wackers FJ, Lie KI, Liem KL, et al. Potential value of thallium-201 scintigraphy as a means of selecting patients for the coronary care unit. Br Heart J 1979; 41:111–7.

[4] van der Wieken LR, Kan G, Belfer AJ, et al. Thallium-201 scanning to decide CCU admission in patients with non-diagnostic electrocardiograms. Int J Cardiol 1983;4:285–99.

[5] Henneman PL, Mena IG, Rothstein RJ, et al. Evaluation of patients with chest pain and nondiagnostic ECG using thallium-201 myocardial planar imaging and technetium-99m first-pass radionuclide angiography in the emergency department. Ann Emerg Med 1992;21:545–50.

[6] Mace SE. Thallium myocardial scanning in the emergency department evaluation of chest pain. Am J Emerg Med 1989;7:321–8.

[7] Okada RD, Glover D, Gaffney T, et al. Myocardial kinetics of technetium-99m-hexakis-2-methoxy-2-methylpropyl-isonitrile. Circulation 1988;77:491–8.

[8] Mannting F, Morgan-Mannting MG. Gated SPECT with technetium-99m-sestamibi for assessment of myocardial perfusion abnormalities. J Nucl Med 1993;34:601–8.

[9] Bilodeau L, Theroux P, Gregoire J, et al. Technetium-99m sestamibi tomography in patients with spontaneous chest pain: correlations with clinical, electrocardiographic and angiographic findings. J Am Coll Cardiol 1991;18:1684–91.

[10] Nicholson CS, Tatum JL, Jesse RL, et al. The value of gated tomographic Tc-99m-sestamibi perfusion imaging in acute ischemic syndromes. J Nucl Cardiol 1995;2:S57.

[11] Kaul S, Senior R, Firschke C, et al. Incremental value of cardiac imaging in patients presenting to the emergency department with chest pain and without ST-segment elevation: a multicenter study. Am Heart J 2004;148:129–36.

[12] Varetto T, Cantalupi D, Altieri A, et al. Emergency room technetium-99m sestamibi imaging to rule out acute myocardial ischemic events in patients with nondiagnostic electrocardiograms. J Am Coll Cardiol 1993;22:1804–8.

[13] Hilton TC, Thompson RC, Williams HJ, et al. Technetium-99m sestamibi myocardial perfusion imaging in the emergency room evaluation of chest pain. J Am Coll Cardiol 1994;23:1016–22.

[14] Tatum JL, Jesse RL, Kontos MC, et al. Comprehensive strategy for the evaluation and triage of the chest pain patient. Ann Emerg Med 1997;29:116–23.

[15] Kontos MC, Jesse RL, Schmidt KL, et al. Value of acute rest sestamibi perfusion imaging for evaluation of patients admitted to the emergency department with chest pain. J Am Coll Cardiol 1997;30:976–82.

[16] Heller GV, Stowers SA, Hendel RC, et al. Clinical value of acute rest technetium-99m tetrofosmin tomographic myocardial perfusion imaging in patients with acute chest pain and nondiagnostic electrocardiograms. J Am Coll Cardiol 1998;31:1011–7.

[17] Kontos MC, Jesse RL, Anderson FP, et al. Comparison of myocardial perfusion imaging and cardiac troponin I in patients admitted to the emergency department with chest pain. Circulation 1999;99: 2073–8.

[18] Udelson JE, Beshansky JR, Ballin DS, et al. Myocardial perfusion imaging for evaluation and triage of patients with suspected acute cardiac ischemia: a randomized controlled trial. JAMA 2002;288:2693–700.

[19] Kontos MC, Kurdziel K, McQueen R, et al. Comparison of 2-dimensional echocardiography and myocardial perfusion imaging for diagnosing myocardial infarction in emergency department patients. Am Heart J 2002;143:659–67.

[20] Cohen M, Demers C, Gurfinkel EP, et al. A comparison of low-molecular-weight heparin with unfractionated heparin for unstable coronary artery disease. N Engl J Med 1997;337:447–52.

[21] Lindahl B, Venge P, Wallentin L. Relation between troponin T and the risk of subsequent cardiac events in unstable coronary artery disease. The FRISC study group. Circulation 1996;93:1651–7.

[22] Alpert JS, Thygesen K, Bassand JP, et al. Myocardial infarction redefined–a consensus document of the Joint European Society of Cardiology/American College of Cardiology Committee for the redefinition of myocardial infarction. J Am Coll Cardiol 2000;36:959–69.

[23] O'Connor MK, Hammell T, Gibbons RJ. In vitro validation of a simple tomographic technique for estimation of percentage myocardium at risk using methoxyisobutyl isonitrile technetium 99m (sestamibi). Eur J Nucl Med 1990;17:69–76.

[24] Duca MD, Giri S, Wu AH, et al. Comparison of acute rest myocardial perfusion imaging and serum markers of myocardial injury in patients with chest pain syndromes. J Nucl Cardiol 1999;6:570–6.

[25] Kontos MC, Fratkin MJ, Jesse RL, et al. Sensitivity of acute rest myocardial perfusion imaging for identifying patients with myocardial infarction based on a troponin definition. J Nucl Cardiol 2004;11:12–9.

[26] Hilton TC, Fulmer H, Abuan T, et al. Ninety-day follow-up of patients in the emergency department with chest pain who undergo initial single-photon emission computed tomography perfusion scintigraphy with technetium 99m-labeled sestamibi. J Nucl Cardiol 1996;3:308–11.

[27] Miller TD, Christian TF, Hopfenspirger MR, et al. Infarct size after acute myocardial infarction measured by quantitative tomographic 99mTc sestamibi imaging predicts subsequent mortality. Circulation 1995;92:334–41.

[28] Miller TD, Hodge DO, Sutton JM, et al. Usefulness of technetium-99m sestamibi infarct size in predicting posthospital mortality following acute myocardial infarction. Am J Cardiol 1998;81: 1491–3.

[29] Reimer KA, Jennings RB, Cobb FR, et al. Animal models for protecting ischemic myocardium: results

of the NHLBI Cooperative Study. Comparison of unconscious and conscious dog models. Circ Res 1985;56:651–65.

[30] De Coster PM, Wijns W, Cauwe F, et al. Area-at-risk determination by technetium-99m-hexakis-2-methoxyisobutyl isonitrile in experimental reperfused myocardial infarction. Circulation 1990; 82:2152–62.

[31] Sinusas AJ, Trautman KA, Bergin JD, et al. Quantification of area at risk during coronary occlusion and degree of myocardial salvage after reperfusion with technetium-99m methoxyisobutyl isonitrile. Circulation 1990;82:1424–37.

[32] Christian TF, Behrenbeck T, Gersh BJ, et al. Relation of left ventricular volume and function over one year after acute myocardial infarction to infarct size determined by technetium-99m sestamibi. Am J Cardiol 1991;68:21–6.

[33] Christian TF, Behrenbeck T, Pellikka PA, et al. Mismatch of left ventricular function and infarct size demonstrated by technetium-99m isonitrile imaging after reperfusion therapy for acute myocardial infarction: identification of myocardial stunning and hyperkinesia. J Am Coll Cardiol 1990;16:1632–8.

[34] Behrenbeck T, Pellikka PA, Huber KC, et al. Primary angioplasty in myocardial infarction: assessment of improved myocardial perfusion with technetium-99m isonitrile. J Am Coll Cardiol 1991; 17:365–72.

[35] Kontos MC, Kurdziel KA, Ornato JP, et al. A non-ischemic electrocardiogram does not always predict a small myocardial infarction: results with acute myocardial perfusion imaging. Am Heart J 2001; 141:360–6.

[36] Huey BL, Beller GA, Kaiser DL, et al. A comprehensive analysis of myocardial infarction due to left circumflex artery occlusion: comparison with infarction due to right coronary artery and left anterior descending artery occlusion. J Am Coll Cardiol 1988;12:1156–66.

[37] Christian TF, Clements IP, Gibbons RJ. Noninvasive identification of myocardium at risk in patients with acute myocardial infarction and nondiagnostic electrocardiograms with technetium-99m-Sestamibi. Circulation 1991;83:1615–20.

[38] O'Keefe JH Jr, Sayed-Taha K, Gibson W, et al. Do patients with left circumflex coronary artery-related acute myocardial infarction without ST-segment elevation benefit from reperfusion therapy? Am J Cardiol 1995;75:718–20.

[39] Knott JC, Baldey AC, Grigg LE, et al. Impact of acute chest pain Tc-99m sestamibi myocardial perfusion imaging on clinical management. J Nucl Cardiol 2002;9:257–62.

[40] de Winter RJ, Koster RW, Sturk A, et al. Value of myoglobin, troponin T, and CK-MBmass in ruling out an acute myocardial infarction in the emergency room. Circulation 1995;92:3401–7.

[41] Emre A, Ersek B, Gursurer M, et al. Angiographic and scintigraphic (perfusion and electrocardiogram-gated SPECT) correlates of clinical presentation in unstable angina. Clin Cardiol 2000;23:495–500.

[42] Topol EJ, Weiss JL, Brinker JA, et al. Regional wall motion improvement after coronary thrombolysis with recombinant tissue plasminogen activator: importance of coronary angioplasty. J Am Coll Cardiol 1985;6:426–33.

[43] Heeschen C, van den Brand MJ, Hamm CW, et al. Angiographic findings in patients with refractory unstable angina according to troponin T status. Circulation 1999;100:1509–14.

[44] Zhao X-Q, Theroux P, Snapinn SM, et al. Intracoronary thrombus and platelet glycoprotein IIb/IIIa receptor blockade with Tirofiban in unstable angina or non-Q-wave myocardial infarction. Angiographic results from the PRISM-PLUS trail (platelet receptor inhibition for ischemic syndrome management in patients limited by unstable signs and symptoms). Circulation 1999;100:1609–15.

[45] Koch KC, vom Dahl J, Kleinhans E, et al. Influence of a platelet GPIIb/IIIa receptor antagonist on myocardial hypoperfusion during rotational atherectomy as assessed by myocardial Tc-99m sestamibi scintigraphy. J Am Coll Cardiol 1999;33:998–1004.

[46] Fram DB, Azar RR, Ahlberg AW, et al. Duration of abnormal SPECT myocardial perfusion imaging following resolution of acute ischemia: an angioplasty model. J Am Coll Cardiol 2003;41:452–9.

[47] Hollander JE, Hoffman RS, Gennis P, et al. Prospective multicenter evaluation of cocaine-associated chest pain. Cocaine Associated Chest Pain (COCHPA) Study Group. Acad Emerg Med 1994; 1:330–9.

[48] Kontos MC, Schmidt KL, Nicholson CS, et al. Myocardial perfusion imaging with technetium-99m sestamibi in patients with cocaine-associated chest pain. Ann Emerg Med 1999;33:639–45.

[49] Kontos MC, Schmidt KL, McCue M, et al. A comprehensive strategy for the evaluation and triage of the chest pain patient: a cost comparison study. J Nucl Cardiol 2003;10:284–90.

[50] Radensky PW, Hilton TC, Fulmer H, et al. Potential cost effectiveness of initial myocardial perfusion imaging for assessment of emergency department patients with chest pain. Am J Cardiol 1997;79:595–9.

[51] Weissman IA, Dickinson CZ, Dworkin HJ, et al. Cost-effectiveness of myocardial perfusion imaging with SPECT in the emergency department evaluation of patients with unexplained chest pain. Radiology 1996;199:353–7.

[52] McGuire DK, Hudson MP, East MA, et al. Highlights from the American Heart Association 72nd Scientific Sessions: November 6 to 10, 1999. Am Heart J 2000;139:359–70.

[53] Klocke FJ, Baird MG, Lorell BH, et al. ACC/AHA/ASNC guidelines for the clinical use of cardiac radionuclide imaging–executive summary: a report of

the American College of Cardiology/American
Heart Association Task Force on Practice Guidelines (ACC/AHA/ASNC Committee to Revise the
1995 Guidelines for the Clinical Use of Cardiac Radionuclide Imaging). J Am Coll Cardiol 2003;42:
1318–33.

[54] Wackers FJ, Brown K, Heller G, et al. American Society of Nuclear Cardiology position statement on
radionuclide imaging in patients with suspected
acute ischemic syndromes in the emergency department or chest pain center. J Nucl Cardiol 2002;9:
246–50.

ELSEVIER
SAUNDERS

CARDIOLOGY
CLINICS

Cardiol Clin 23 (2005) 531–539

Echocardiography in the Evaluation of Patients in Chest Pain Units

William R. Lewis, MD

4860 Y Street, Suite 2820, Sacramento, CA 95864, USA

In experimental models, impairment of left ventricular segmental wall motion is apparent almost immediately after the onset of myocardial ischemia, preceding symptoms and ST-segment alterations (Fig. 1). Using percutaneous angioplasty to induce the ischemic cascade in the cardiac catheterization laboratory, echocardiographic wall motion abnormalities have been documented to precede electrocardiographic abnormalities and angina [1]. Therefore, detection of cardiac wall motion abnormalities is potentially more sensitive than the history, physical examination, and ECG for identification of myocardial ischemia. Echocardiography is highly reliable for assessing cardiac wall motion and, thus, it has been used for diagnosis and risk assessment in patients presenting to the emergency department (ED) with symptoms suggestive of myocardial ischemia. In patients who have acute ST-elevation myocardial infarction (MI), echocardiography is comparable to invasive left ventriculography for detecting wall motion abnormalities [2]. However, the usefulness of echocardiography in the low-risk population that has chest pain of uncertain origin and a nondiagnostic initial presentation is less well established.

Table 1 depicts the results of nine studies in patients presenting to the ED with chest pain in which resting echocardiography was used to predict cardiac events during the initial presentation by detection of resting wall motion abnormalities [3–11]. The events defined by the authors ranged from hard events, such as MI [4], to a combination of hard and soft end points, such as MI, revascularization, angiographic coronary disease, and abnormal perfusion imaging studies [11]. Although

six of these reports indicated a high positive predictive value (PPV) for this technique, the overall event rate in these studies was approximately 51%. In these high-risk populations, the positive predictive value of a test for ischemia/infarction will be augmented compared with that in typical low-risk, rule-out MI (ROMI) patients. Thus, in the study of Sabia and colleagues [4] in which the cardiac event rate was 17%, the PPV of a resting wall motion abnormality was only 31%. When comparing resting ECG with resting echocardiography in a similarly low-risk population, Kontos and colleagues [5] demonstrated similar positive and negative predictive values for predicting cardiac events: 60% and 88% for ECG versus 44% and 98% for echocardiography. In another report with a similarly low cardiac event rate, echocardiography did not add to a 3-hour evaluation consisting of clinical assessment and cardiac serum enzymes [12]. Furthermore, in all the aforementioned investigations, the patients who had false-negative echocardiographic findings had non–ST elevation MI (NSTEMI) or unstable angina, reflecting the limited sensitivity of wall motion abnormalities for identification of this population. Unstable angina (with or without small troponin elevation) is the more common event in the low-risk patients who have ischemic events.

Typical of a high-risk ST-elevation MI population, Mohler and colleagues [11] studied 92 patients who had a 60% cardiac event rate. The echocardiogram was abnormal in 15 of the 18 patients who had MI, and in 12 of the 37 patients who had unstable angina. Five patients who had unstable angina had wall motion abnormalities unchanged from prior echocardiographic studies, and they were therefore considered to be echocardiographically negative. Two of the three patients

E-mail address: william.lewis@ucdmc.ucdavis.edu

0733-8651/05/$ - see front matter © 2005 Elsevier Inc. All rights reserved.
doi:10.1016/j.ccl.2005.08.009

Ischemic Cascade

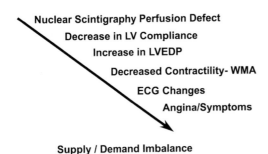

Nuclear Scintigraphy Perfusion Defect
Decrease in LV Compliance
Increase in LVEDP
Decreased Contractility- WMA
ECG Changes
Angina/Symptoms

Supply / Demand Imbalance

Fig. 1. The ischemic cascade as seen in the cardiac catheterization laboratory during controlled coronary occlusion. LV, left ventricle; LVEDP, left ventricular end-diastolic pressure; WMA, wall motion abnormality.

who had MI that were not detected by echocardiography had been given thrombolytic therapy. All patients who had a new wall motion abnormality had an event, leading to a PPV of 100%. The negative predictive value was 57%, demonstrating that MIs in 43% of patients who had events were not detected by echocardiography. These events were predominantly unstable angina diagnosed by typical chest pain lasting more than 30 minutes without ECG or enzymatic changes.

All of these studies were performed in the 1980s and 1990s using older echocardiographic machinery. For example, the study by Kontos and colleagues [11] used Hewlett-Packard 500, 1000, and 1500 machines (Hewlett-Packard, Palo Alto, California). Newer equipment with improved imaging techniques could improve wall motion imaging and improve the predictive value of resting echocardiography for detecting ischemia. Fundamental echocardiography receives echocardiographic signals at the same frequency at which they were transmitted, usually in the 2- to 3-MHz range for adult imaging. Fundamental echocardiography has difficulty imaging structures nearest the transducer because of artifact generated by the chest wall. Artifacts can also be generated from the side of the transducer, causing "side lobes." As echocardiographic sound waves travel through the heart, the tissues start to oscillate and can produce harmonics. Tissue harmonic echocardiography sends signals at the 2- to 3-MHz fundamental, but uses the 4- to 6-MHz harmonic signals received for imaging. This technique reduces the near-field artifact, as near-field signals don't usually produce harmonic signals. Harmonic signals also travel in a narrower beam, reducing the side lobe artifact.

Table 1
Predictive accuracy of echocardiography in patients presenting with acute chest pain

	N	Event+	Event−	PPV (%)	NPV (%)
Kontos et al [3]	130	RWA+ 15	29	34	
		RWA− 6	80		93
Sabia et al [4]	169	RWA+ 27	60	31	
		RWA− 2	80		98
Kontos et al [5]	260	RWA+ 41	53	44	
		RWA− 4	162		98
Korosoglou et al [6]	98	RWA+ 19	2	90	
		RWA− 18	59		77
Saeian et al [7]	60	RWA+ 22	3	88	
		RWA+ 2	33		94
Sasaki et al [8]	46	RWA+ 17	1	94	
		RWA− 6	22		79
Horowitz et al [9]	65	RWA+ 34	2	94	
		RWA− 2	27		93
Peels et al [10]	35	RWA+ 22	4	85	
		RWA− 3	14		82
Mohler et al [11]	92	RWA+ 27	0	100	
		RWA− 28	37		57

Abbreviations: N, number of patients; RWA+, regional wall motion abnormality present; RWA−, no regional wall motion abnormality; Event+, Coronary event present; Event−, no coronary event; PPV, positive predictive value; NPV, negative predictive value.
Adapted from Lewis W. Evaluation of the patient with "rule out myocardial infarction". Arch Intern Med 1996;156:41–5; with permission.

Hickman and colleagues [13] studied 80 patients presenting to the ED with chest pain of suspected cardiac origin that lasted at least 30 minutes within the previous 6 hours. The population studied was typical of the ROMI population in that 13 of the 80 patients (16%) were subsequently diagnosed as having had an event. An HDI 3000 (ATL, Bothell, Washington) machine with tissue harmonics was used for echocardiographic imaging. Tissue harmonic imaging was significantly better than fundamental imaging and allowed for adequate visualization of all segments in all patients, compared with fundamental imaging in which 11% of segments could not be visualized (Fig. 2). The positive and negative

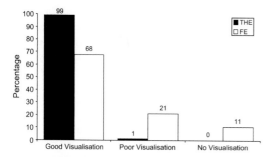

Fig. 2. Bar graph comparing quality of segmental visualization with echocardiography using fundamental (FE) and tissue harmonics (THE) imaging. (*Adapted from* Hickman M. Wall thickening assessment with tissue harmonic echocardiography results in improved risk stratification for patients with non-ST-segment elevation acute chest pain. Eur J Echocardiogr 2004;5(2):142–8; with permission.)

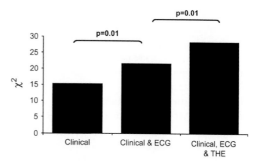

Fig. 3. Bar graph showing incremental value of clinical, ECG, and echocardiographic (THE) variables for the prediction index acute MI or a subsequent cardiac event. (*Adapted from* Hickman M. Wall thickening assessment with tissue harmonic echocardiography results in improved risk stratification for patients with non-ST-segment elevation acute chest pain. Eur J Echocardiogr 2004;5(2):142–8; with permission.)

predictive value of fundamental echocardiography for an event (elevated creatine kinase-myocardial band [CK-MB], coronary revascularization, and cardiac death) was 21% and 90%, respectively. Using tissue harmonic echocardiography, the positive and negative predictive values improved to 26% and 97%, respectively. This predictive accuracy was nearly identical to electrocardiography with a positive and negative predictive value of 24% and 97%, respectively (Table 2). However, tissue harmonic echocardiography provided added ability to predict future cardiac events when compared with clinical history and the electrocardiogram (Fig. 3). This added benefit was not seen using fundamental echocardiography.

There are several factors that limit the value of echocardiography for detecting patients in the

Table 2
Accuracy of clinical, ECG and echocardiographic variables for prediction of myocardial infarction as the presenting event

	PPV (%)	NPV (%)	P
Diabetes	5	80	.09
Abnormal ECG	24	97	>.1
Abnormal fundamental ECG	21	90	>.1
Abnormal tissue harmonic ECG	26	97	.007

Abbreviations: PPV, positive predictive value. NPV, negative predictive value. P, probability.

Adapted from Hickman M. Wall thickening assessment with tissue harmonic echocardiography results in improved risk stratification for patients with non-ST-segment elevation acute chest pain. Eur J Echocardiogr 2004;5(2):142–8; with permission.

ROMI population who are at risk for a cardiac event. The examination is highly dependent on skilled, experienced personnel for adequate data acquisition and reliable interpretation. According to the Task Force on Echocardiography in Emergency Medicine of the American Society of Echocardiography and Technology and Practice Executive Committees of the American College of Cardiology, a minimum of 6 months of training and performance of 300 echocardiographic studies are required to become a competent reader [14]. Therefore, highly specialized physicians, technical personnel, and equipment are required for dedicated use in the ED. Furthermore, although ventricular wall motion abnormalities associated with ischemia may persist for prolonged periods, they may also resolve in as little as 2 hours [15]. Studies in animals have demonstrated that wall motion abnormalities may not be detected when infarction involves less than 20% of ventricular wall thickness [16] or less than 12% of left ventricular circumference [17]. Therefore, patients who have NSTEMI and unstable angina may have no discernible abnormalities of wall motion. Echocardiography provides no information on the age of a wall motion abnormality, reducing its usefulness in patients who have known CAD or other cardiac disease. Finally, wall motion abnormalities may be seen in patients who have left bundle branch block and right ventricular volume or pressure overload that complicate interpretation of the echocardiogram for ischemic wall motion abnormalities.

Newer echocardiographic approaches may overcome some of these limitations. A technique under investigation is analysis of variation in the scatter of acoustic signals during ischemia (ultrasonic tissue characterization). Acute myocardial ischemia results in increased integrated backscatter of ultrasound signals and decreased variability of scatter during systole and diastole. When compared with wall motion analysis for the detection of MI in the coronary care unit, Saeian and colleagues [7] found ultrasonic tissue characterization had comparable sensitivity, specificity, and accuracy. Ultrasonic tissue characterization had difficulty detecting apical infarcts, whereas wall motion analysis had difficulty detecting ischemia in the presence of left bundle branch block. It is possible that a combination of the two techniques would be complementary.

A second strategy that may be useful for identification of myocardial ischemia is contrast echocardiography [18]. In standard contrast imaging, the ultrasonic properties of the myocardium and ventricular cavity can be enhanced by intravenous injection of myocardial contrast agents. The current agents used are microbubbles formed by encapsulated gases that are small enough to traverse the pulmonary capillary bed, access the systemic circulation, and perfuse not only the left ventricular cavity but also the myocardium. When echocardiographic ultrasound strikes these microbubbles, the bubbles vibrate in a nonlinear fashion and give off enhanced echocardiographic signals. When using these agents to assess myocardial perfusion, a pulse of high-intensity ultrasound is given that is strong enough to burst the bubbles in the myocardium. The myocardium is visualized over the next 10 to 15 cycles and analyzed for wash-in of myocardial contrast agent (Table 3). Normally, the myocardium reperfuses within five to ten cardiac cycles. The intensity of the signal in the myocardium at steady state is related to blood volume in the myocardium and can be normalized to the ventricular cavity. Variability in steady state opacification is related to myocardial viability. Delay in regional myocardial reperfusion is related to coronary flow rates and coronary disease (Fig. 4) [19].

Korosoglou and colleagues, [6] studied myocardial contrast echocardiography in 100 patients presenting to the ED with chest pain. Of these patients, 37 were ultimately given the diagnosis of acute coronary syndrome, resulting in a high event rate of 37%; 12 were diagnosed with unstable angina by Braunwald criteria and found to have greater than 70% stenosis in a coronary artery at arteriography; and 25 were diagnosed as having NSTEMI with troponin T elevation. Two patients were excluded from analysis because of poor echocardiographic images. Of the remaining 61 patients diagnosed as having noncardiac chest pain, 21 underwent angiography that showed no high-grade ($\geq 75\%$) lesions and 40 patients underwent stress testing that resulted in normal findings. As shown in Table 3, the presence of resting echocardiographic wall motion abnormalities had a 90% PPV and a 77% negative predictive value (NPV) for acute coronary syndrome. Myocardial contrast echocardiography had an 89% PPV and a 91% NPV for acute coronary event. Using resting wall motion abnormalities plus myocardial contrast echocardiography yielded an 89% PPV and a 93% NPV. Because troponin assays can be rapidly performed in the ED, the group of patients that remain a diagnostic dilemma are those who have unstable angina without troponin elevation or electrocardiographic abnormalities. Focusing on the group diagnosed as having unstable angina without troponin elevation in this current study, the sensitivity of resting wall motion abnormality was 17% and the sensitivity of myocardial contrast

Table 3
Detection of unstable angina and non–ST-elevation myocardial infarction by myocardial contrast echocardiography

Visual assessment	Sensitivity	Specificity	PPV	NPV	Accuracy
Wall motion (2D-echo)	51%	97%	90%	77%	80%
Perfusion (MCE)	84%	93%	89%	91%	90%
Perfusion (MCE), single-vessel CAD	71%	93%	71%	93%	89%
Perfusion (MCE), multivessel CAD	92%	93%	85%	93%	93%
Wall motion and perfusion	89%	93%	89%	93%	92%

Abbreviations: 2D-Echo, two-dimensional echocardiography; CAD, coronary artery disease; MCE, myocardial contrast echocardiography; NPV, negative predictive value; PPV, positive predictive value; $P < .05$, myocardial perfusion versus wall motion.

From Korosoglou G. Usefulness of real-time myocardial perfusion imaging in the evaluation of patients with first time chest pain. Am J Cardiol 2004;94(10):1225–31; with permission.

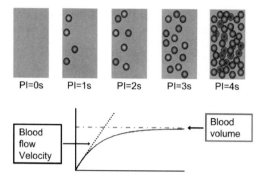

Fig. 4. Method of assessing mean blood flow velocity and myocardial blood volume using myocardial contrast echocardiography. (*From* Lepper W, Belcik T, Wei K, et al. Myocardial contrast echocardiography. Circulation 2004;109:3132–5; with permission.)

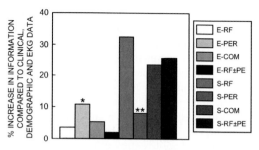

Fig. 5. Percent incremental value of tests performed in hierarchical order after clinical, demographic, and electrocardiographic variables are known. Values were significantly higher (*) ($P<.05$) compared with other CE variables, and significantly lower (**) compared with other SPECT variables. E-RF, echocardiographic regional function; E-PER, echocardiographic perfusion; E-COM, combination of echocardiographic perfusion and function; S-RF, regional function by SPECT; S-PER, perfusion by SPECT; S-COM, combination of perfusion and function by SPECT. (*From* Kaul S. Incremental value of cardiac imaging in patients with chest pain and without ST-segment elevation: a multicenter study. Am Heart J 2004;148(1):129–36; with permission.)

echocardiography was 66%. This means that one of three patients who has unstable angina without troponin elevation will go undetected using myocardial contrast echocardiography, compared with five out of six patients undetected using only resting wall motion as the detection criterion.

From the above data, it is clear that myocardial contrast echocardiography yields greater diagnostic accuracy compared with wall motion analysis in the detection of acute coronary syndromes. Kaul and colleagues [20] compared myocardial contrast echocardiography to resting single photon emission computed tomography (SPECT) in 203 patients. All patients underwent myocardial contrast echocardiography, but only 163 patients underwent SPECT. Thirty-eight patients (19%) had an event, consistent with this being a moderate risk group for a coronary event. When comparing myocardial contrast echocardiography to SPECT, myocardial contrast echocardiography perfusion was superior to SPECT myocardial perfusion in predicting events. However, SPECT myocardial regional function was superior to echocardiographic regional function in predicting events, resulting in SPECT having a greater overall predictive value compared with myocardial contrast echocardiography. The incremental value of tests performed in hierarchical order after clinical, demographic, and electrocardiographic variables are known is shown in Fig. 5.

All of the studies reviewed to this point used resting echocardiographic studies. As with the ECG, resting echocardiographic studies provide information regarding only the presence of resting ischemia within a narrow time frame. When the resting study is normal, then a stress study may

yield further diagnostic information regarding the presence of significant coronary disease that is not producing active ischemia at the time of examination. Geleijnse and colleagues [21] studied dobutamine stress echocardiography in 102 patients presenting to the ED with chest pain of suspected cardiac origin. Of these patients, 59 had known coronary artery disease and 43 did not. The patients who did not have known coronary artery disease underwent stress testing after a minimum 12-hour observation period, whereas patients who had known coronary artery disease underwent a minimum 24-hour observation period. As a result, 13 patients were diagnosed as having events based on abnormal resting electrocardiograms and serum cardiac enzymes, and 89 patients were then referred for dobutamine stress testing. Patients who had resting wall motion abnormalities were not excluded from stress testing. Dobutamine was administered in 10 μg/kg/min increments at 3-minute intervals up to a maximum of 40 μg/kg/min. Atropine, up to 1 mg, was administered to patients failing to reach 85% maximal predicted heart rate with dobutamine infusion alone. The test was terminated for the usual end points of attaining target heart rate, stress-induced wall motion abnormalities, electrocardiographic changes, arrhythmias, severe chest pain, hypertension, or intolerable side effects. The echocardiograms were interpreted using the standard 16-segment model [22]. Three patients had poor acoustic windows precluding stress testing, and six patients failed to reach 85% maximal predicted heart rate. Of the 80 remaining patients, 44 had normal stress echocardiograms and 36 had stress-induced wall motion abnormalities. Results of the stress test were conveyed to the attending physician and could be used to manage the patient. Seven patients who had positive stress echocardiograms underwent coronary revascularization during the index event, and seven patients had unstable angina during the 6-month follow-up period, with three of these patients having coronary revascularization procedures. Two patients who had normal stress studies had events (one MI and one unstable angina). The positive and negative predictive accuracy for dobutamine stress echocardiography was 25% and 95.5% (Table 4). Seven patients had significant dobutamine stress testing–related adverse events. Two patients had stress-induced nonsustained ventricular tachycardia, four patients had stress-induced supraventricular tachycardia, and one patient had stress-induced atrial flutter.

In the largest study to date, Bholasingh and colleagues [23] studied 577 patients admitted to the ED who had suspected acute coronary disease. During a 12-hour observation period, 119 patients were diagnosed with acute coronary syndrome and 34 were given other diagnoses, such as aortic stenosis or atrial fibrillation. Following this period, 404 patients were then referred for dobutamine stress

echocardiography using 3-minute stages and dobutamine at 10 µg/kg/min increments to a maximum of 40 µg/kg/min. Atropine, 1 mg, was given for patients failing to reach 85% maximal predicted heart rate. The test was terminated for the usual end points. This testing determined that 23 patients had poor acoustic windows precluding stress testing, 4 patients had resting wall motion abnormalities and did not undergo stress testing, 377 patients completed the dobutamine stress protocol, and 26 patients had stress-induced wall motion abnormalities in at least one segment of a 16-segment model. The attending physicians were blinded to the results of the dobutamine stress tests and patient management was determined by use of other diagnostic protocols. Over the 6-month follow-up period, eight patients who had positive dobutamine stress echocardiography had events, including one cardiac death (Table 5). Of the 351 patients who had negative dobutamine stress echocardiography studies, 14 patients had events during the follow-up period, including one cardiac death (see Table 5). The PPV for stress-induced wall motion abnormalities was 31% and the NPV was 96% (see Table 4). In 75 (19.9%) patients, the protocol was not completed because of the prespecified criteria: extensive new wall motion abnormality (1 patient), electrocardiographic changes (7 patients), chest pain (28 patients), and intolerable

Table 4
Predictive accuracy of dobutamine stress echocardiography in patients presenting with acute chest pain and good quality images

	N		Event+	Event−	PPV (%)	NPV (%)
Geleijnse et al [21]	80	RWA+	9	27	25	
		RWA−	2	42		95.5
Bholasingh et al [23]	377	RWA+	8	18	31	
		RWA−	14	337		96
Trippi et al [24]	137	RWA+	7	0	100	
		RWA−	2	128		98.5

Abbreviations: N, number of patients; RWA+, regional wall motion abnormality present; RWA−, no regional wall motion abnormality; Event+, coronary event present; Event−, no coronary event; PPV, positive predictive value; NPV, negative predictive value.

Table 5
Clinical outcomes at 6 months according to dobutamine stress echocardiography results

	Positive DSE (n – 26)	Negative DSE (n – 351)
Cardiac death	1	1
Nonfatal AMI	2	0
Rehosp UA	2	6
Primary end point	5	7
PTCA	2	4
CABG	1	3
Combined end point	8	14

Abbreviations: AMI, acute myocardial infarction; CABG, coronary artery bypass grafting; DSE, dobutamine stress echocardiography; PTCA, percutaneous transluminal coronary angioplasty; Rehosp-UA, rehospitalization for unstable angina. Primary end point, cardiac death, AMI + rehosp-UA. Combined end point, primary end point + PTCA + CABG.

From Bholasingh R, Cornel JH, Kamp O, et al. Prognostic value of predischarge obutamine stress echocardiography in chest pain patients with a negative cardiac troponin T. J Am Coll Cardiol 2003;41(4):596–602; with permission.

side effects (39 patients) such as arrhythmia and severe hypertension or hypotension.

Stress echocardiography requires experienced personnel to perform and interpret the test results. Cardiologists may not be available at off hours for the performance or interpretation of dobutamine stress testing. To circumvent these limitations, Trippi and colleagues [24] developed a protocol in which dobutamine stress echocardiography was performed by trained nurses and sonography technicians and then transmitted through telemedicine for interpretation by cardiologists. The authors studied 163 patients admitted to the hospital for chest pain with negative cardiac enzymes and electrocardiogram. Overall, 57% of the studies were performed after regular hours or on weekends. Of this population, 26 patients had resting wall motion abnormalities and were excluded from stress testing. Dobutamine was administered in 3-minute stages of 5, 10, 20, 30, 40, and 50 μg/kg/min infusions. Stress testing was terminated prematurely in 9 patients because of chest pain or arrhythmias. The symptoms resolved in less than 10 minutes and required no specific therapy. There were no major complications of dobutamine stress testing. The study showed that 7 patients had stress-induced wall motion abnormalities and were found to have greater than 50% coronary stenoses on arteriography (100% PPV), 130 patients had normal dobutamine stress tests, and 2 patients were subsequently found to have coronary disease during the 3-month follow-up period (one inferior wall MI and one unstable angina, 98.5% NPV). Two patients were not described as either positive or negative by the authors. In patients who had normal resting echocardiograms, overall PPV and NPV for combined rest and subsequent dobutamine stress echocardiography was 51.5% and 98.5%, respectively (see Table 4). The authors have subsequently reported over 4 years of experience in 734 patients being managed by this protocol [25]. In this larger group of patients, the test was discontinued prematurely in only 3.1% of patients, 12.5% of patients had abnormal stress echocardiograms, and 70% of patients were discharged after negative stress echocardiograms.

Although none of the patients suffered an MI with dobutamine stress testing in these papers, MI has been reported with dobutamine stress echocardiography in outpatients [26]. Dobutamine has also been shown to tremendously activate platelets, independent of circulating catecholamines [27]. Platelet activation was not seen with exercise testing. Caution is therefore warranted when using dobutamine stress echocardiography in evaluating these patients, and none of the published guidelines yet include dobutamine stress testing as part of the evaluation of patients who have chest pain in the ED.

The NPV is uniformly good when comparing the three dobutamine stress studies, whereas the PPV varies greatly. The low PPV seen in the study by Geleijnse and colleagues [21] may be caused by the inclusion of a large number of patients who have pre-existing disease and resting wall motion abnormalities. A true positive study was also defined as one in which the patient had a hard event. One could argue that in patients who have known coronary disease, a positive stress echocardiogram is by definition a true positive. This assertion would result in a greatly increased PPV in this study. In the study by Bholasingh and colleagues [23], the attending physicians were blinded to the results of the dobutamine stress test and therefore not all patients underwent coronary arteriography. Again, a true positive test was defined as one with a hard event in the follow-up period. The true predictive value may be much greater and the other diagnostic modalities, which were unreported by the authors, may not have detected the disease in these patients. In the study by Trippi and colleagues [24], all patients who had abnormal stress echocardiograms underwent coronary arteriography and the true PPV was known and found to be 100% for the detection of more than 50% coronary stenoses.

In summary, resting echocardiography may lack sufficient sensitivity to be of clinical usefulness in the patient who has low-risk chest pain in the ED, and the role of resting echocardiography is debatable. The National Heart Attack Alert Program Working Group concluded that "false negative rates in the prospective studies are too high to be safe" [28]. In addition, the American College of Cardiology/American Heart Association 2002 Guideline Update for the Management of Patients with Unstable Angina and Non-ST-Segment Elevation Myocardial Infarction does not include echocardiography in the initial evaluation and management of patients [29]. In contrast, another viewpoint is offered by the American College of Cardiology/American Heart Association/American Society of Echocardiography that states that "early echocardiography is particularly useful in patients with a high clinical suspicion of acute myocardial infarction but a non diagnostic ECG" [30].

One of the aims in evaluating patients in the ED who have suspected acute coronary syndrome is to identify patients who are at low enough risk to be discharged home and those who are at high risk and require admission. Inclusion of myocardial contrast echocardiography or stress echocardiography can significantly improve the diagnostic accuracy of echocardiography in the detection of ischemia. Therefore, a rational use of echocardiography in this schema would be to evaluate patients for resting wall motion abnormalities in whom serial electrocardiograms and serum cardiac markers were negative. Patients who have resting wall motion abnormalities could be admitted to the hospital for further evaluation. Patients who do not have resting wall motion abnormalities could be scheduled for exercise or dobutamine stress testing, myocardial perfusion imaging, or other diagnostic modalities as part of their accelerated diagnostic protocol.

References

[1] Hauser AM, Gangadharan V, Ramos RG, et al. Sequence of mechanical, electrocardiographic and clinical effects of repeated coronary artery occlusion in human beings: echocardiographic observations during coronary angioplasty. J Am Coll Cardiol 1985;5:193–7.

[2] Lundgren C, Bourdillon PD, Dillon JC, et al. Comparison of contrast angiography and two-dimensional echocardiography for the evaluation of left ventricular regional wall motion abnormalities after acute myocardial infarction. Am J Cardiol 1990;65: 1071–7.

[3] Kontos MC, Arrowood JA, Jesse RL, et al. Comparison between 2-dimensional echocardiography and myocardial imaging in the emergency department in patients with possible myocardial ischemia. Am Heart J 1998;136(4 Pt 1):724–33.

[4] Sabia P, Afrookteh A, Touchstone DA, et al. Value of regional wall motion abnormality in the emergency room diagnosis of acute myocardial infarction. A prospective study using two-dimensional echocardiography. Circulation 1991;84:I85–92.

[5] Kontos MC, Arrowood JA, Paulsen WH, et al. Early echocardiography can predict cardiac events in emergency department patients with chest pain. Ann Emerg Med 1998;31(5):550–7.

[6] Korosoglou G, Labadze N, Hansen A, et al. Usefulness of real-time myocardial perfusion imaging in the evaluation of patients with first time chest pain. Am J Cardiol 2004;94(10):1225–31.

[7] Saeian K, Rhyne TL, Sagar KB. Ultrasonic tissue characterization for diagnosis of acute myocardial infarction in the coronary care unit. Am J Cardiol 1994;74:1211–5.

[8] Sasaki H, Charuzi Y, Beeder C, et al. Utility of echocardiography for the early assessment of patients with nondiagnostic chest pain. Am Heart J 1986; 112:494–7.

[9] Horowitz RS, Morganroth J, Parrotto C, et al. Immediate diagnosis of acute myocardial infarction by two-dimensional echocardiography. Circulation 1982;65:323–9.

[10] Peels CH, Visser CA, Kupper AJ, et al. Value of two dimensional echocardiography for immediate detection of myocardial ischemia in the emergency room. Am J Cardiol 1990;65:687–91.

[11] Mohler ER, Ryan T, Segar DS, et al. Clinical utility of troponin T levels and echocardiography in the emergency department. Am Heart J 1998;135 (2 Pt 1):253–60.

[12] Levitt MA, Promes SB, Bullock S, et al. Combined cardiac marker approach with adjunct two-dimensional echocardiography to diagnose acute myocardial infarction in the emergency department. Ann Emerg Med 1996;27:1–7.

[13] Hickman M, Swinburn JM, Senior R. Wall thickening assessment with tissue harmonic echocardiography results in improved risk stratification for patients with non-ST-segment elevation acute chest pain. Eur J Echocardiogr 2004;5(2): 142–8.

[14] Stewart WJ, Douglas PS, Sagar K, et al. Echocardiography in emergency medicine: a policy statement by the American Society of Echocardiography and the American College of Cardiology. J Am Soc Echocardiogr 1999;12:82–4.

[15] Jeroudi MO, Cheirif J, Habib G, et al. Prolonged wall motion abnormalities after chest pain at rest in patients with unstable angina: a possible manifestation of myocardial stunning. Am Heart J 1994;127: 1241–50.

[16] Lieberman AN, Weiss JL, Jugdutt BL, et al. Two-dimensional echocardiography and infarct size: relationship of regional wall motion and thickening to the extent of myocardial infarction in the dog. Circulation 1981;63:739.

[17] Kaul S. Echocardiography in coronary artery disease. Curr Probl Cardiol 1990;15:233.

[18] Sakuma T, Hayashi Y, Shimohara A, et al. Usefulness of myocardial contrast echocardiography for the assessment of serial changes in risk area in patients with acute myocardial infarction. Am J Cardiol 1996;78:1273–7.

[19] Lepper W, Belcik T, Wei K, et al. Myocardial contrast echocardiography. Circulation 2004;109: 3132–5.

[20] Kaul S, Senior R, Firschke C, et al. Incremental value of cardiac imaging in patients with chest pain and without ST-segment elevation: a multicenter study. Am Heart J 2004;148(1):129–36.

[21] Geleijnse ML, Elhendy A, Kasprzak JD, et al. Safety and prognostic value of early dobutamine-atropine stress echocardiography in patients with

spontaneous chest pain and a non-diagnostic electrocardiogram. Eur Heart J 2000;21(5):344–5.

[22] Schiller NB, Shah PM, Crawford M, et al. Recommendations for quantitation of the left ventricle by two-dimensional echocardiography: American Society of Echocardiography Committee on Standards, Subcommittee on Quantitation of Two-Dimensional Echocardiograms. J Am Soc Echocardiogr 1989;2:358–67.

[23] Bholasingh R, Cornel JH, Kamp O, et al. Prognostic value of predischarge dobutamine stress echocardiography in chest pain patients with a negative cardiac troponin T. J Am Coll Cardiol 2003;41(4): 596–602.

[24] Trippi JA, Lee KS, Kopp G, et al. Dobutamine stress tele-echocardiography for the evaluation of emergency department patients with chest pain. J Am Coll Cardiol 1997;30(3):627–32.

[25] Trippi JA, Lee KS. Dobutamine stress tele-echocardiography as a service in the emergency department to evaluate patients with chest pain. Echocardiography 1999;16(2):179–85.

[26] Lewis WR, Arena FJ, Galloway MT, et al. Acute myocardial infarction associated with dobutamine stress echocardiography. J Am Soc Echocardiogr 1997;10(5):576–8.

[27] Galloway MT, Paglieroni TG, Wun T, et al. Platelet activation during dobutamine stress echocardiography. Am Heart J 1998;135:888–900.

[28] Selker HP, Zalenski RJ, Antman EM, et al. An evaluation of technologies for identifying acute cardiac ischemia in the emergency department: a report from a National Heart Attack Alert Program Working Group. Ann Emerg Med 1997;29:13–87.

[29] ACC/AHA 2002 Guideline Update for the Management of Patients with Unstable Angina and Non-St-Segment Elevation Myocardial Infarction. A report of the American College Of Cardiology/American Heart Association Task Force on Practice Guidelines (Committee on the Management of Patients with Unstable Angina). Available at www.acc.org/clinical/guidelines/unstable/incorporated/index.htm. Accessed September 15, 2005.

[30] Cheitlin MD, Armstrong WF, Aurigemma GP, et al. ACC/AHA/ASE 2003 Guideline Update for the Clinical Application of Echocardiography. A report of the American College of Cardiology/American Heart Association Task Force on Practice Guidelines (ACC/AHA/ASE Committee to Update the 1997 Guidelines for the Clinical Application of Echocardiography). J Am Coll Cardiol 2003;42: 954–70.

ELSEVIER
SAUNDERS

Cardiol Clin 23 (2005) 541–548

CARDIOLOGY
CLINICS

Newer Imaging Methods for Triaging Patients Presenting to the Emergency Department with Chest Pain

James McCord, MD[a,*], Ezra A. Amsterdam, MD[b]

[a]Henry Ford Health System, Heart & Vascular Institute, 2799 West Grand Boulevard,
K-14, Detroit, MI 48202-2689, USA
[b]Department of Internal Medicine, University of California School of Medicine (Davis)
and Medical Center, 4860 Y Street, Suite 200, Sacramento, CA 95817, USA

Electron beam computed tomography (EBCT), also known as ultrafast CT, is highly sensitive for detecting and quantifying coronary artery calcium. Coronary artery calcium is absent in the normal vessel and occurs almost exclusively in the arteries with atherosclerosis [1–3]. The degree of coronary calcium is strongly associated with the total atherosclerotic burden [4–6]. Patients who have more coronary artery calcium are more likely to have significant angiographic obstructions and, more importantly, are known to suffer more adverse cardiac events [7–13]. These findings, and the procedure's noninvasive methodology and low cost, have provided the rationale for the use of EBCT for risk stratification of patients in the emergency department (ED) who have possible acute coronary syndrome (ACS) [14–16].

Technology considerations

EBCT involves an electron emitter rather than a standard radiograph that allows for rapid screening times. Transaxial images are obtained at 100 ms with 3-mm to 6-mm slices during one to two breath holds. Scanning is triggered near end-diastole to minimize motion artifact. No intravenous or oral contrast is required and the entire scan can be completed in 10 to 15 minutes. Multislice CT (MSCT) is another CT modality that can assess coronary calcium, and studies have shown that this technology correlates well with EBCT for the detection of coronary calcium [17,18]. Many institutions employ MSCT for coronary calcium scoring as this CT modality can also be used for scanning other organs, and EBCT is only useful for coronary calcium quantification. However, most clinical studies have employed EBCT for cardiac risk stratification. The cost of an EBCT is approximately $400.

Histologic studies have shown that tissue densities greater than 130 Hounsfield units (a measurement that characterizes the relative density of a substance) are associated with calcified plaque. A coronary calcium score, also called the Agatston score, is calculated as a product of the area of calcification and a factor based on the maximal calcium density. A composite score to indicate the quantity of calcium detected in the entire coronary artery system is typically used: a score of 0 is considered normal, 1 to 99 is mild, 100 to 400 is moderate, and more than 400 is severe. Coronary calcium scores have also been age- and sex-adjusted as coronary calcium is more extensive in older and male patients [19]. A more recently developed calcium volume score may offer more precision as compared with the traditional Agatston score [20,21].

Coronary calcium score and cardiac risk assessment

Numerous studies have shown that that the coronary calcium score has prognostic value

---

* Corresponding author.
E-mail address: jmcord1@hfhs.org (J. McCord).

significance in symptomatic and asymptomatic individuals [22–31]. A study of 5365 asymptomatic individuals demonstrated 224 adverse events (death, nonfatal myocardial infarction (MI), coronary bypass surgery, or percutaneous intervention) over 3 years [23]. Individuals who have a score of more than zero had a significantly higher event rate compared with those who do not have calcium (6.1% versus 0.4% in men; 3.3% versus 1.0% in women). The magnitude of cardiac risk is directly related to the extent of calcification [24]. However, controversy has arisen concerning the additional prognostic significance of coronary calcium after accounting for traditional risk factors. In 2000, the American College of Cardiology/American Heart Association published a consensus document concerning EBCT that states, "Importantly, the incremental value of EBCT over traditional multivariate risk assessment models has yet to be established" [32].

Some early studies suggest that coronary calcium scores do not offer additional prognostic information after accounting for the Framingham risk score [9], which predicts cardiac risk based on age; sex; low-density lipoprotein and high-density lipoprotein cholesterol; hypertension; cigarette smoking; and diabetes mellitus [33]. The consensus document published in 2000 was written after a literature review through 1998. However, since that time publications have shown that coronary calcium scores give additional independent prognostic information. A recent meta-analysis of four studies demonstrated that an elevated coronary calcium score was associated with an increased risk for adverse cardiac events after accounting for classic cardiac risk factors [26]. Across the categories of the Framingham risk score, a study of 1461 asymptomatic individuals showed at a median of 7 years at follow-up that coronary calcium was predictive of cardiac risk among patients who had a Framingham risk score higher than 10%, but not among patients who had a score less than 10% [34]. Thus, more recent studies suggest that coronary calcium scores are independently predictive of cardiac risk even after accounting for traditional risk factors.

Electron beam CT in patients who present to the emergency department with chest pain

Between 1999 and 2001, there have been three published studies evaluating the diagnostic usefulness of EBCT in patients evaluated in the ED who had chest pain [14–16]. The first study by McLaughlin and colleagues [14] evaluated 181 patients who were admitted to the hospital from the ED with chest pain of presumed cardiac origin. Patients were included if they had a normal or nondiagnostic ECG at presentation. Exclusion criteria were history of coronary artery disease (CAD) (MI, coronary bypass surgery, or percutaneous intervention), diagnostic ST changes or Q waves on electrocardiogram, weight more than 250 lb, initial elevated creatine kinase-myocardial band (CK-MB), and known or suspected pregnancy. Among those evaluated, 44 patients did not meet entry criteria and 4 patients did not give consent, yielding 133 patients in the final analysis. An EBCT was considered positive if the score was more than one; the results of the scan were blinded to the responsible clinician.

Patients had 30-day follow-up by phone call for adverse events such as MI (as defined by World Health Organization criteria), coronary artery bypass surgery, percutaneous intervention, or sudden cardiac death. The population was 71% African-American, Hispanic 19%, 19% White, and 1% Asian, and comprised 84 (63%) women and 50 (37%) men. The mean age was 53 ± 2 years. There were 86 (64%) patients who had a positive scan and 48 (36%) patients who had a negative scan. In the entire group there were seven (5%) adverse cardiac events, including four MIs, two coronary artery bypass surgeries, and one percutaneous intervention. Among the 48 patients who had normal coronary calcium scores, there was one (2%) adverse event. This patient was a 45-year-old man who suffered a MI after cocaine use. Of the patients who had an abnormal coronary calcium scan, there were six (12%) adverse events. These findings indicated the low event rate associated with the absence of elevated coronary calcium, and the higher adverse event rate in patients who had elevated coronary calcium. However, most patients who had increased coronary calcium did not experience an adverse cardiac event.

The second study by Laudon and colleagues [15] evaluated 105 patients who had chest pain in the ED. Inclusion criteria were women between 40 and 65 years and men between 30 and 55 years; normal initial cardiac marker; and a normal or indeterminate ECG. Exclusion criteria included history of CAD; ECG with ST-segment elevation, Q waves, or left bundle-branch pattern; elevated cardiac marker at presentation, hemodynamic instability; and pregnancy. Patients had follow-up at 4 months and a coronary calcium score more than zero was considered abnormal. The need and type of stress testing was left to the discretion of the physicians who were blinded to the results of the scan.

Of these 105 patients, 54 (51%) were admitted to an inpatient cardiology service and 51 (49%) were admitted to the ED chest pain observation unit. The patient population consisted of 98 Whites, 4 African-Americans, 1 Southeast Asian, 1 Arab, and 1 Hispanic. There were 57 (54%) men and 48 (46%) women. Mean age for men was 45 years and for women 51 years. All patients underwent EBCT and 100 underwent other cardiac testing, including 58 who underwent regular stress testing; 19 who underwent exercise or pharmacologic radionuclide testing; 25 who underwent coronary angiography; and 11 who underwent rest, exercise, or pharmacologic echocardiography. Of the 100 patients who had EBCT and other cardiac testing, 46 patients had an abnormal EBCT and 54 patients had a normal EBCT. There were no patients who had a normal EBCT and abnormal other cardiac test. EBCT had 100% sensitivity, 63% specificity, 100% negative predictive value, and 30% positive predictive value for an abnormal cardiac test. At 4 months there were no adverse events in patients who had a normal EBCT.

The third study by Georgiou and colleagues [16] considered 192 patients who were evaluated in the ED and were believed to require admission to exclude MI. Patients were included if they were aged 30 years or older, had chest pain lasting at least 20 minutes in the last 12 hours, and had a nondiagnostic ECG. Patients were excluded if they had a history of CAD (coronary artery bypass surgery or percutaneous intervention), ECG findings of Q waves, ST-segment elevation more than 1 mm in two consecutive leads, T-wave inversion of 5 mm or more, hemodynamic instability, or pregnancy. There were 221 patients screened. Of these, 13 patients were excluded because of an acute cardiac event at presentation and 16 were excluded because of lack of follow-up data, yielding 192 patients for final analysis.

Of the 192 patients, 69 (36%) were White, 49 (26%) were Hispanic, 48 (25%) were African-American, and 26 (14%) were Asian-American. Prevalence of coronary calcium was significantly lower in Hispanics compared with Whites (47% versus 73%, $P = .004$). There were 104 (54%) men and 88 (46%) women. The average follow-up was 50 months $\pm$ 10. Of the total group, 116 (60%) had some level of calcium detected. There were 58 (30%) patients who had an adverse cardiac event, 30 (16%) who had "hard" events (11 cardiac deaths and 19 nonfatal MIs), and 28 (15%) who had other cardiac events, including nine coronary artery bypass surgeries, four percutaneous interventions, 11 hospitalizations for angina, and four ischemic strokes. Patients who had higher coronary artery calcium scores had significantly more adverse cardiovascular events (Fig. 1). Dividing patients into quartiles of coronary calcium scores, there were no "hard" cardiac events in the first quartile, one in the second quartile, ten in the third quartile, and 19 in the fourth quartile. In a multivariate analysis, coronary calcium scores were more predictive of adverse cardiac events as compared with traditional cardiac risk factors.

Considerations regarding the potential role of electron beam CT in the emergency department

Are we ready to start using EBCT in the ED for the routine evaluation of patients who have possible ACS? Use of an ECG, followed by serial cardiac markers and then a rapid, easily performed, and inexpensive EBCT is an attractive strategy for risk stratification in this setting. For many institutions it is a major logistic challenge to provide timely stress tests, which may include imaging modalities, before discharge of low- to intermediate-risk patients from chest pain observation units. However, there are certain patients who should not have an EBCT in this setting. Patients who have known CAD, which was rightly an exclusion criterion for all three studies, are known to have high coronary calcium scores and therefore EBCT would be unlikely to aid in risk stratification. This exception is a relevant issue as

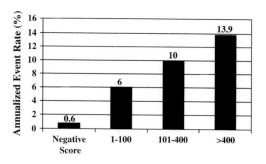

Fig. 1. Patients who have chest pain screened using electron beam tomography in the emergency department. (*Adapted from* Georgiou D, Budoff MJ, Kaufer E, et al. Screening patients with chest pain in the emergency department using electron beam tomography: a follow-up study. J Am Coll Cardiol 2001;38:105–10; with permission.)

more patients who have atypical symptoms and a history of CAD are being managed in chest pain units [35]. One study demonstrated that 38% of patients evaluated in a chest pain unit had known CAD (history of MI, percutaneous intervention, or coronary artery bypass surgery) [36]. In addition, older patients are known to have a higher degree of coronary calcium even without known coronary disease. Thus, if EBCT is to have some role in risk stratification of patients in the ED who have chest pain, it would likely involve a younger population.

Although the low adverse event rates in patients who have normal EBCT scans in these three studies are impressive (Laudon, 0%; McLaughlin, 0% [excluding the one patient who had cocaine-induced MI]; Georgiou, 0.6% per year), these studies do have some significant limitations. These studies include a small number of patients. More unusual cases of adverse cardiac events, such as the patient who has MI secondary to cocaine, may become apparent if a larger number of patients were studied. Also, all three of these studies only involved a single center. Moreover, in two of the studies, the patients who were entered represented a convenience sample that may have led to selection bias. In the study by Georgiou and colleagues [16], the EBCT scanner was available 5 days per week from 7 AM to 11 PM, whereas the study by Laudon and colleagues was "limited at times in the enrollment of patients by the availability of the EBCT scanner" [14]. The thought-provoking results of these small studies will hopefully lead the way to a larger multicenter study of consecutive patients.

A further concern of these three studies is the large proportion of positive EBCT scans: 49%, 64%, and 60% (Table 1). If an EBCT is positive, what should the next step be in patient management? All of these patients likely would not benefit from coronary angiography, as many patients would not have obstructive coronary disease as a cause of their symptoms. These patients would at least require some form of stress testing, which would make the difficult process of risk stratification even more cumbersome. In addition, the need for "double-testing" would likely make the strategy less cost-effective. Instead of using any degree of calcium as defining an abnormal EBCT, certain levels of calcium may be used to assist in risk stratification that may obviate the need for holding the patient for stress testing in the chest pain unit. However, the extent of coronary calcium is affected by age, sex, and race. The optimal degrees of calcium distinguished by age and gender would need to be determined to discriminate a low-risk patient who has chest pain in the ED. The ongoing Multi-Ethnic Study of Atherosclerosis (MESA) is following 6500 individuals over 10 years and will provide additional data concerning EBCT and cardiac risk assessment in a large diverse population.

Finally, although coronary artery calcium is associated with atherosclerosis, EBCT does not detect vulnerable plaques that are the most likely to lead to ACS. In fact, some vulnerable plaques may contain no calcium. A large degree of coronary calcium is associated with more extensive overall atherosclerotic burden, and therefore more stable and unstable plaques. Although more coronary calcium makes developing ACS more likely, the absence of coronary calcium does not preclude the possibility of ACS. In a study of 118 patients who had ACS (101 who had acute MI and 17 who had unstable angina), 12 (10%) had no coronary calcium detected by EBCT [37]. Patients who had ACS and a normal EBCT were significantly younger and more likely to be active

Table 1
Electron beam CT for risk-stratification in patients who have chest pain in the emergency department

Study	Number of patients	Age inclusion criteria in years	Number (%) positive test	Number (%) negative test	Follow-up	Number (%) adverse events in patients who have negative test
Laudon et al 1999 [14]	105	Men aged 30–55 Women aged 40–65	51 (49)	54 (51)	4 m	0 (0)
McLaughlin et al 1999 [15]	134	All ages	86 (64)	48 (36)	30 d	0 (0)
Georgion et al 2001 [16]	192	≥30	116 (60)	76 (40)	50 m	1 (2)

cigarette smokers. Thus, there may be certain groups of patients that are more prone to developing ACS in the setting of a normal EBCT.

Cardiac MRI

Cardiac MRI has diagnostic usefulness for myocardial perfusion and regional wall motion abnormalities. Wall motion abnormalities may not only be detected in MI, but transient ischemia in unstable angina may lead to stunning, which in turn can be detected by MRI. An MRI scan may be more sensitive for stunning as compared with radionuclide imaging. Kwong and colleagues [38] studied 161 consecutive patients who were evaluated in the ED for possible ACS. Inclusion criteria were 30 minutes or more of chest pain within 12 hours of presentation, age over 21 years, and weight less than 270 lb. Exclusion criteria were ST-segment elevation MI, pregnancy, significant heart failure such that patient could not lie flat, and metal prosthesis precluding MRI. Of the 161 patients, 25 (16%) had ACS, 10 had NSTEMI, and 15 had unstable angina. The sensitivity and specificity of MRI for ACS were 84% and 85%, respectively. In a multivariate regression analysis, MRI was independently associated with the diagnosis of ACS and was of greater diagnostic usefulness when compared with ECG and peak troponin-I. Considerable research is presently in progress with MRI in identifying coronary atherosclerotic lesions, including vulnerable plaques, which may prove to be of diagnostic value for patients in the ED who have chest pain of unclear origin [39].

CT coronary angiography

Major advances in noninvasive imaging of the coronary arteries by contrast-enhanced CT have stimulated considerable interest in the potential of this technique to rapidly confirm or exclude CAD in low-intermediate risk patients presenting to the ED with chest pain. Contemporary 64 slice CT scanners [40–42] have overcome many of the limitations of earlier 16 slice devices [43], resulting in recently cited gantry rotation times of 330 msec, spatial resolution of 0.4 mm and temporal resolution of 83–165 msec. Although these values are less than those of conventional coronary angiography (~0.15 mm and 0.33 sec), they are sufficient to yield diagnostic data in a large proportion of patients (Fig. 2). The accuracy of CT coronary angiography with 64 slice scanners is based on limited comparative studies with invasive coronary

angiography in elective patients. In their evaluation of 59 patients, Leber et al reported the following sensitivities of CT angiography for detecting coronary stenoses of various degrees: stenosis <50%, sensitivity 79%; stenosis >50%, sensitivity 73%; stenosis >75%, sensitivity 80% [41]. Specificity was 97%, indicating the utility of the method in identifying absence of CAD. Raff and colleagues compared invasive and CT coronary angiography in 70 patients in whom they analyzed 1,065 coronary artery segments and found a mean difference in percent stenosis of 1.3 $\pm$ 14.2% [42]. Specificity, sensitivity, positive and negative predictive values of CT angiography for significant stenoses were: 86%, 95%, 66% and 98%, respectively. The latter value again indicates the reliability of a negative CT coronary angiogram in excluding CAD. However, there have been no reports of CT coronary angiography in the ED setting in patients presenting with chest pain.

Visualization of the coronary arteries by CT has important advantages that include its noninvasive methodology, rapidity, reliability in excluding severe CAD and simultaneous acquisition of other chest structures such as the aorta and pulmonary arteries. However, limitations of the technique are significant. A low heart rate (optimally, <70/min) is required to avert blurring of the images of the moving coronary arteries. Administration of a beta blocker or rate-limiting calcium channel blocker is often necessary for this purpose. Regular rhythm is also necessary precluding CT angiography in patients with atrial fibrillation or frequent ectopic beats. Even with the currently enhanced resolution, the method cannot precisely assess the severity of coronary stenoses, which has resulted in diagnostic categories such as no CAD, <50% stenosis, >50% stenosis and uninterpretable due to calcification or artifact. A dose of 60–100 cc of iodinated contrast is required, which may be a relative contraindication in patients with renal insufficieny. Finally, the radiation dose is higher than that with invasive coronary angiography and has led to methods for reducing the exposure of the patient [43].

Summary

Three small single-center studies using EBCT in the ED to risk stratify patients who have chest pain and nondiagnostic ECGs show promising results, but limitations of this approach are apparent. Although patients who did not have

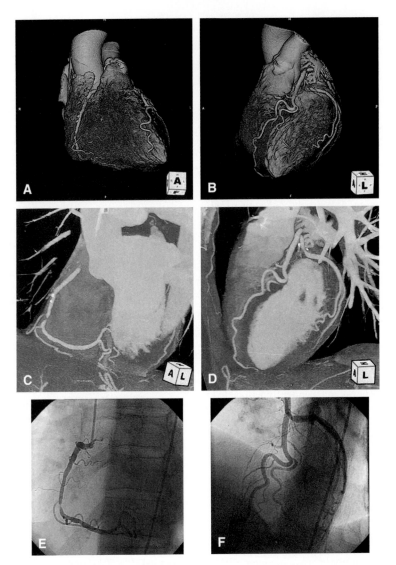

Fig. 2. Noninvasive visualization of coronary artery anatomy by 64-slice multislice computed tomography (CT). (*A,B*) Volume rendering technique depicts a severe stenosis of the right coronary artery (RCA) distal to the marginal branch, nodular coronary calcifications mainly extrinsic to the RCA lumen and normal left coronary artery. (*C,D*) Maximum-intensity projection demonstrates severe soft plaque of the RCA and superficial calcific plaques of the RCA and proximal left circumflex artery. (*E,F*) Invasive coronary angiography confirms the major stenosis of the RCA and absence of significant lesions in the left coronary artery. (*From* Raff GL, Gallagher MJ, O'Neill WW, et al. Diagnostic accuracy of noninvasive coronary angiography using 64-slice spiral computed tomography. J Am Coll Cardiol 2005;46:552–7; with permission.)

coronary calcium detected by EBCT had very low adverse event rates, EBCT in this setting can be associated with poor positive predictive value that would lead to at least the need for another cardiac test, such as stress testing, or even unnecessary hospital admission. Before EBCT is adopted as routine practice in this patient population, a large multicenter study of consecutive patients is required to better ascertain for which subset of patients this would be an effective strategy. This subset would likely include a younger population that does not have a history of CAD. Ideally this would lead to a randomized diagnostic trial comparing EBCT in this population with some form of stress testing. Other imaging technologies, including cardiac MRI and MSCT, are even less well studied in this patient population, but may prove to be of value in this setting in the future.

Limited data with 64 slice scanners indicate diagnostic quality coronary imaging in many patients and a high degree of reliability of a negative study. However, although the technique has important potential, significant limitations remain and there are currently no reported studies of its utility in the ED setting.

References

[1] Ross R. The pathogenesis of atherosclerosis: a perspective for the 1990s. Nature 1993;362:801–9.

[2] Stary HC. Composition and classification of human atherosclerotic lesions. Virchows Arch A Pathol Anat Histopathol 1992;421:277–90.

[3] Stary HC, Chandler AB, Dinsmore RE, et al. A definition of advanced types of atherosclerotic lesions and a histological classification of atherosclerosis: a report from the Committee on Vascular Lesions of the Council on Arteriosclerosis, American Heart Association. Circulation 1995;92:1355–74.

[4] Simons DB, Schwartz RS, Edwards WD, et al. Noninvasive definition of anatomic coronary artery disease by ultrafast computed tomographic scanning: a quantitive pathologic comparison study. J Am Coll Cardiol 1992;20:1118–26.

[5] Mautner SL, Mautner GC, Froehlich J, et al. Coronary artery calcification: assessment with electron beam CT and histomorphometric correlation. Radiology 1994;192:619–23.

[6] Rumberger JA, Simons DB, Fitzpatrick LA, et al. Coronary artery calcium area by electron-beam computed tomography and coronary atherosclerotic plaque area: a histopathologic correlative study. Circulation 1995;15:2157–62.

[7] Sangiorgi G, Rumberger JA, Severson A, et al. Arterial calcification and not lumen stenosis is highly correlated with atherosclerotic plaque burden in humans: a histologic study of 723 coronary artery segments using non-decalcifying methodology: electron beam computed tomography and coronary artery disease: scanning for coronary artery calcification. J Am Coll Cardiol 1998;31:126–33.

[8] Kennedy J, Shavelle R, Wang S, et al. Coronary calcium and standard risk factors in symptomatic patients referred for coronary angiography. Am Heart J 1998;135:696–702.

[9] Secci A, Wong N, Tang W, et al. Electron beam computed tomographic coronary calcium as a predictor of coronary events: comparison of two protocols. Circulation 1997;96:1122–9.

[10] Wexler L, Brundage B, Crouse J, et al. Coronary artery calcification: pathophysiology, epidemiology, imaging methods, and clinical implications: a statement for health professionals from the American Heart Association Writing Group. Circulation 1996;94:1175–92.

[11] Schwartz RS. Coronary artery calcification and prognosis: same song, second verse? J Am Coll Cardiol 1994;24:359–61.

[12] Wong ND, Detrano RC, Abrahamson D, et al. Coronary artery screening by electron beam computed tomography: facts, controversy, and future. Circulation 1995;92:632–6.

[13] Detrano R, Hsiai T, Wang S, et al. Prognostic value of coronary calcification and angiographic stenoses in patients undergoing coronary angiography. J Am Coll Cardiol 1996;27:285–90.

[14] McLaughlin VV, Balogh T, Rich S. Utility of electron beam computed tomography to stratify patients presenting to the emergency room with chest pain. Am J Cardiol 1999;84:327–8.

[15] Laudon DA, Vukov LF, Breen JF, et al. Use of electron-beam computer tomography in the evaluation of chest pain patients in the emergency department. Ann Emerg Med 1999;33:15–21.

[16] Georgiou D, Budoff MJ, Kauger E, et al. Screening patients with chest pain in the emergency department using electron beam tomography. J Am Coll Cardiol 2001;38:105–10.

[17] Stanford W, Thompson BH, Burns TL, et al. Coronary artery calcium quantification at multi-detector row helical CT versus electron-beam tomography. Am J Cardiol 2001;87:210.

[18] Carr JJ, Crouse JR, Goff DC, et al. Evaluation of subsecond gated helical CT for quantification of coronary artery calcium and comparison with electron beam CT. AJR Am J Roentgenol 2000;174:915–21.

[19] Rumberger JA, Brundage BH, Rader DJ, et al. Electron beam computed tomographic coronary calcium scanning: a review and guidelines for use in asymptomatic persons. Mayo Clin Proc 1999;74:243–52.

[20] Nasir K, Raggi P, Rumberger JA, et al. Coronary artery calcium volume scores on electron beam tomography in 12,936 asymptomatic adults. Am J Cardiol 2004;93:1146–9.

[21] Callister TQ, Cooil B, Raya SP, et al. Coronary artery disease: improved reproducibility of calcium scoring with an electron-beam CT volumetric method. Radiology 1998;208:807.

[22] Achenbach S, Ropers D, Mohlenkamp S, et al. Variability of repeated coronary artery calcium measurements by electron beam tomography. Am J Cardiol 2001;87:210.

[23] Kondos GT, Hoff JA, Sevrukov A, et al. Electron-beam tomography coronary artery calcium and cardiac events: a 37-month follow-up of 5635 initially asymptomatic low- to intermediate-risk adults. Circulation 2003;107:2571–6.

[24] Arad Y, Spadaro LA, Goodman K, et al. Predictive value of electron beam computed tomography of the coronary arteries: 19-month follow-up of 1173 asymptomatic subjects. Circulation 1996;93: 1951.

[25] Arad Y, Spadaro LA, Goodman K, et al. Prediction of coronary events with electron beam computed tomography. J Am Coll Cardiol 2000;36:1253.

[26] Pletcher MJ, Tice JA, Pignone M, et al. Using the coronary artery calcium score to predict coronary heart disease events: a systematic review and meta-analysis. Arch Intern Med 2004;164:1285.

[27] Park R, Detrano R, Xiang M, et al. Combined use of computed tomography coronary calcium scores and C-reactive protein levels in predicting cardiovascular events in nondiabetic individuals. Circulation 2002; 106:2073.

[28] Yang T, Doherty TM, Wong ND, et al. Alcohol consumption, coronary calcium, and coronary heart disease events. Am J Cardiol 1999;84:802.

[29] Raggi P, Cooil B, Callister TQ. Use of electron beam tomography data to develop models for predictor of coronary events: comparison of two protocols. Circulation 1997;96:1122.

[30] Wong ND, Hsu JC, Detrano RC, et al. Coronary artery calcium evaluation by electron beam computed tomography and its relation to new cardiovascular events. Am J Cardiol 2000;86:495.

[31] O'Malley PG, Taylor AJ, Jackson JL, et al. Prognostic value of coronary electron-beam computed tomography for coronary heart disease events in asymptomatic populations. Am J Cardiol 2000;85: 945.

[32] O'Rourke RA, Brundage BH, Froelicker VF, et al. American College of Cardiology/American Heart Association expert consensus document of electron beam computed tomography for the diagnosis and prognosis of coronary artery disease. Circulation 2000;102:126–40.

[33] Wilson PWF, D'Agostino RB, Levy D, et al. Prediction of coronary heart disease using risk factor categories. Circulation 1998;97(18):1837–47.

[34] Greenland P, LaBree L, Azen SP, et al. Coronary Artery calcium score combined with Framingham score for risk prediction in asymptomatic individuals. JAMA 2004;291(2):210–5.

[35] Amsterdam EA, Kirk JD, Dierks DB, et al. Early exercise testing in the management of low risk patients in chest pain centers. Prog Cardiovasc Dis 2004;46: 438–52.

[36] McCord J, Nowak RM, McCullough PA, et al. Ninety-minute exclusion of acute myocardial infarction by use of quantitative point-of-care testing of myoglobin and troponin I. Circulation 2001;104: 1483–8.

[37] Schmermund A, Baumgart D, Gunter G, et al. Coronary artery calcium in acute coronary syndromes: a comparative study of electron-beam computed tomography, coronary angiography, and intracoronary ultrasound in survivors of acute myocardial infarction and unstable angina. Circulation 1997; 96:1461–9.

[38] Kwong RY, Schussheim AE, Rekhraj S, et al. Detecting acute coronary syndrome in the emergency department with cardiac magnetic resonance imaging. Circulation 2003;107:531–7.

[39] Fayad ZA. MR imaging for the noninvasive assessment of atherothrombotic plaques. Magn Reson Imaging Clin N Am 2003;11(1):101–13.

[40] Leber AW, Knez A, Becker A, et al. Accuracy of multidetector spiral computed tomography in identifying and differentiating the composition of coronary atherosclerotic plaques: a comparative study with intracoronary ultrasound. J Am Coll Cardiol 2004;43:1241–7.

[41] Budhoff MJ, Cohen MC, Garcia MJ, et al. ACCF/ AHA Clinical competence statement on cardiac imaging with computed tomography and magnetic resonance. J Am Coll Cardiol 2005;46:383–402.

[42] Leber AW, Knez A, von Ziegler F, et al. Quantification of obstructive and nonobstructive coronary lesions by 64-slice computed tomography. J Am Coll Cardiol 2005;46:147–54.

[43] Raff GL, Gallagher MJ, O'Neill WW, et al. Diagnostic accuracy of noninvasive coronary angiography using 64-slice spiral computed tomography. J Am Coll Cardiol 2005;46:552–7.

ELSEVIER
SAUNDERS

Cardiol Clin 23 (2005) 549–557

CARDIOLOGY
CLINICS

Chest Pain Units: Management of Special Populations

Deborah B. Diercks, MD[a],*, J. Douglas Kirk, MD, FACEP[a],
Ezra A. Amsterdam, MD, FACC[b]

[a]Department of Emergency Medicine, University of California School of Medicine (Davis) and Medical Center,
4150 V Street, PSSB Suite 2100, Sacramento, CA 95817, USA
[b]Department of Internal Medicine, University of California, Davis Medical Center,
2315 Stockton Boulevard, Sacramento, CA 95817, USA

Chest pain evaluation units provide a safe and cost-effective means for risk stratification of patients who present to the emergency department (ED) with chest pain and no evidence of myocardial infarction (MI) or ischemia on initial evaluation. A standardized protocol is often used that combines serial measurements of cardiac injury markers, repeat electrocardiograms (ECG), and telemetry monitoring followed by secondary risk stratification by additional diagnostic testing for coronary artery disease (CAD). The latter usually comprises provocative testing with exercise or pharmacologic stress. Although these units rely heavily on a protocol-driven approach, appreciation of the limitations of this method in certain patient populations is essential. In particular, the inclusion of women, diabetics, patients with a history of CAD, and those with chest pain after stimulant use (eg, cocaine, methamphetamine) may necessitate additional consideration in the choice of diagnostic testing. Some would suggest that these patients should be excluded from chest pain unit evaluation based solely on their presumed high risk of cardiac disease and adverse events. Additionally, exercise stress, the most common provocative test used in chest pain units, has important limitations in these patients. However, the clinical presentations of many of these patients often lack high-risk features associated with adverse cardiac events, making them appropriate candidates for a chest pain unit. This article reviews the evaluation of these special populations

by accelerated diagnostic protocols, focusing on the value and limitations of this strategy for assessment of these unique patients.

Women

Cardiovascular disease is the leading cause of death in women, accounting for nearly half of all deaths in this population. Timely diagnosis early in the course of the disease is essential. Thirty-eight percent of women who have MI die within a year, compared with 25% of men. This staggering variation is in part because MI occurs at a significantly older age in women than in men. In addition, within 6 years of MI, as many as one third of women will have another heart attack, 15% will develop angina, 13% will have a stroke, and 30% will be disabled with heart failure [1]. These alarming numbers have led to an increased interest in cardiovascular health in women. Recent studies have revealed unique aspects of pathophysiology, diagnosis, prognosis, and treatment of CAD in women. The lower age-specific risk of CAD and prevalence of acute coronary syndrome (ACS) in women leads to decreased accuracy of diagnostic tools commonly used in a chest pain unit (Box 1).

In addition, there are important gender-specific physiologic responses to exercise stress [2]. Challenges to diagnostic testing in women include variable ability to reach target heart rate and baseline ECG changes that may decrease accuracy of treadmill testing [3–5]. Women also have labile ST-segment alterations and body habitus attributes that may result in false-positive exercise ECG interpretation. Despite these unique

* Corresponding author.

E-mail address: dbdiercks@ucdavis.edu
(D.B. Diercks).

Box 1. Unique factors in women
affecting exercise test results

Decreased exercise capacity
Baseline electrocardiographic
   abnormalities
Body habitus
Lower age-specific risk of coronary
   artery disease
High rate of single vessel disease

physiologic issues, the chest pain unit provides an important option for the evaluation of women. Their exclusion would result in the costly use of traditional hospital beds to evaluate these patients with a low rate of CAD, especially those of pre-menopausal age, no diabetes, and absence of a smoking history. Nevertheless, understanding these limitations is important for the prudent selection of diagnostic modalities when evaluating women in a chest pain unit.

Several approaches to risk stratification in women in the nonacute setting have been published. A recent review of the evaluation of chest pain in women suggests that it is possible to risk stratify them into low, moderate, and high likelihood of CAD solely by the presence or absence of traditional cardiac risk factors. Based on this scheme, recommendations for diagnostic testing were presented to improve the cost-effectiveness of the evaluation [6]. However, these recommendations have not been validated in any published clinical trials. Wilson and colleagues [7,8] developed a risk prediction model based on blood pressure, cholesterol level, history of diabetes or smoking, and age. This model was derived from Framingham data; information on estrogen use was not available. The risk score was very effective in stratifying remaining lifetime risk for coronary heart disease in women, with 1.5- to 3-fold higher absolute risk in the highest versus lowest tertile of risk score at all ages. Despite initial promise, risk stratification based on simple tools such as these has not gained general clinical use and outcome data are limited. In part, this may be due to the lack of utility of such models in the acute setting.

Exercise stress testing, a cornerstone of the evaluation of patients with chest pain, has a diagnostic accuracy as low as 52% in women, with a false-positive rate as high as 40% [9,10]. Thus, its utility in women has been questioned, especially in those considered low risk for CAD. Despite

these criticisms, the ED-based exercise stress test has provided useful prognostic information for adverse cardiac events in low- to moderate-risk chest pain patients that have included women [10,11]. Diercks and colleagues have evaluated the use of treadmill exercise testing in 666 women who underwent evaluation in our chest pain unit. Using Agency for Health Care Policy and Research classification, 38 (5.7%) women were retrospectively identified as high risk, 136 (20.4%) were intermediate risk and 492 (73.9%) were low risk for CAD. Of these, 465 (70%) had negative exercise testing, 145 (22%) had nondiagnostic tests, and 56 (8%) had positive tests. Thirty-day clinical follow-up or confirmatory cardiac evaluation was achieved in 512 of 666 (77%) patients. The sensitivity, specificity, and negative and positive predictive values of the treadmill test are shown for patients with a positive or abnormal test result (positive or nondiagnostic) in Table 1. Compared with a negative exercise test, the relative risk of CAD for a positive test was 19 (95% CI 6–56) and for a nondiagnostic test it was 8 (95% CI 3–22) [12]. Despite the poor positive predictive value of exercise testing in the women, positive tests were relatively infrequent and the negative predictive value affords excellent accuracy in identifying those patients who do not require hospital admission. As recommended in the American College of Cardiology/American Heart Association guidelines, treadmill testing should be applied as a first-line diagnostic method only in those women with a normal baseline ECG and ability to exercise [13].

Imaging techniques such as myocardial stress perfusion scintigraphy have higher sensitivity and specificity than treadmill testing, but gender-

Table 1
Diagnostic accuracy of positive or abnormal exercise treadmill testing in women evaluated in a chest pain observation unit

	Sensitivity	Specificity	Negative predictive value	Positive predictive value
Positive exercise treadmill testing (N = 56)	41%	91%	96%	22%
Abnormal exercise treadmill testing (N = 201)	82%	70%	99%	14%

specific confounders still exist. Breast attenuation, small left ventricular size, and a high rate of single vessel disease may affect the diagnostic utility of this modality [14]. Despite these limitations, myocardial perfusion imaging has been established as a safe, noninvasive, cost-effective and accurate method to identify CAD in women [15]. After injection of thallium-201, areas of decreased uptake by the myocardium are seen as a negative scintigraphic image, indicating regions of ischemic or infarcted myocardium. Gated single photon emission CT radionuclide imaging with thallium or technetium99 sestamibi has been used in the ED to improve the diagnostic accuracy and risk stratification of patients presenting with chest pain and a nondiagnostic ECG [16–18].

Cardiac stress imaging methods provide several advantages in women. They allow for pharmacologic stress, which alleviates the problem of decreased exercise capacity and failure to reach target heart rate that limits the value of traditional exercise stress testing. In addition, the use of gated images allows differentiation of breast tissue attenuation from a true perfusion defect. Studies that have evaluated the benefit of gated images, which included 170 women, report an improved specificity for the detection of CAD from 67% to 91% [19,20].

The prognostic value of myocardial perfusion imaging has also been evaluated in women. Pooled data from more than 7500 women demonstrated an annual cardiac event rate of < 1% in those with a normal perfusion scan [14]. These results were also found in women with a high pretest probability of CAD [21]. Hachamovitch and colleagues [22] evaluated the determinants of risk and prognosis in patients with a normal myocardial perfusion scan. Diabetic women had the highest rate of cardiac-related death or MI at 1 year after adjusting for confounders. The lowest 1-year event rate was in nondiabetic women (< 1%). The results of these trials have led the American Society of Nuclear Cardiology Task Force on Women and Heart Disease to incorporate the use of myocardial scintigraphy into an algorithm for the initial evaluation of women with chest pain. These guidelines recommend the use of exercise or pharmacologic gated single photon emission CT as a first line test in intermediate- to high-risk women with diabetes, an abnormal resting ECG, or inability to exercise. In addition, they recommend this modality as a second-line diagnostic adjunct or confirmatory test in patients who have an intermediate risk exercise ECG.

These recommendations are based on the high sensitivity and specificity and prognostic utility of scintigraphy [23].

History of coronary artery disease

Patients with a history of CAD compose a high-risk subgroup whose inclusion in the standard chest pain unit strategy is controversial. These patients are often complex and frequently have undergone prior myocardial revascularization. In general, their suitability for chest pain unit management should primarily depend on the immediate risk of ACS based on symptoms, ECG features, and cardiac serum markers rather than their past history and risk factors (Box 2) [24,25]. Other considerations should include review of prior evaluations and management goals of the patient's cardiologist.

The Chest Pain Evaluation in the Emergency Room (CHEER) trial examined the utility of a chest pain observation unit in a group of patients with suspected unstable angina and intermediate risk for adverse cardiac events based on AHCPR guidelines [26]. This cohort of patients included 27% with known CAD, defined by history of prior MI or prior percutaneous coronary intervention. After adjustment for comorbid conditions, the investigators observed no difference in cardiac events at 6 months in those patients randomized to the chest pain unit and those receiving traditional hospital admission [26]. Our group evaluated the use of immediate exercise testing of 100 patients with a history of CAD evaluated in a chest pain unit. These patients had a normal or nondiagnostic ECG at presentation and were pain free at the time of evaluation. A negative exercise treadmill test was found in 38% of patients and 39% had nondiagnostic tests, with two-thirds discharged home immediately from the ED. An additional 19

Box 2. Unique factors in patients with a history of coronary artery disease that affect stress test results

Multiple co-morbidities
Prior myocardial revascularization
Baseline left ventricular wall motion
  abnormalities
Baseline fixed myocardial perfusion
  deficits
Use of anti-anginal medications

patients were discharged within 24 hours of presentation. Of the 23% who had a positive exercise test, uncomplicated non-ST segment elevation MI was diagnosed in two patients. No adverse events occurred during the 6-month follow-up period. Despite a slightly higher incidence of abnormal tests and adverse events than the typical chest pain unit patient population, this strategy was quite effective in risk stratification and prompt disposition of patients [27].

Diercks and colleagues [28] have also evaluated the utility of an accelerated diagnostic protocol in patients with a history of CAD evaluated in their chest pain unit from 1/94 to 10/01. A diagnosis of ACS was based on clinical presentation and cardiac testing consistent with myocardial ischemia, MI, or the need for revascularization within 30 days of presentation. Of the 6839 patients evaluated, 1153 (17%) had a history of CAD. MI was detected in 12 patients (1%) during their chest pain unit evaluation. Initial diagnostic testing was performed in 639/1153 (55%), yielding positive results in 191. Testing included 371 (58%) exercise treadmill tests, 208 (32%) myocardial scintigrams, 54 (8%) exercise echocardiograms, and 51 (7%) cardiac catheterizations. Subsequent testing was done in 77 patients who had no initial diagnostic test during their chest pain unit stay. During the follow-up period there were two deaths, three MIs, and revascularization was performed in 46 patients. A final diagnosis of ACS was made in 238 patients (22%). The data indicate that although the frequency of ACS in patients with a history of CAD is higher than that in typical low-risk patients presenting with chest pain, evaluation in a chest pain unit is appropriate.

Studies using myocardial scintigraphy in patients with a history of CAD have reported satisfactory diagnostic and prognostic ability. Zellweger and colleagues [29] evaluated the prognostic value of stress radionuclide imaging in patients with prior MI. In 1143 patients, they reported 118 adverse events during follow-up. The annual rate of adverse events was proportional to the size of the perfusion abnormality. In addition, the size of the infarction was also an independent predictor of adverse events. Elhendy and colleagues [30] studied the use of stress technetium 99 sestamibi in patients with a history of prior MI. In the 383 patients evaluated, there were 48 cardiac events during follow-up. The frequency of events was again directly proportional to the size of the perfusion defect with an event rate of 0.4%, 2.4%, and 4% in patients with

normal perfusion, perfusion deficit consistent with single vessel disease, and that consistent with multi-vessel disease, respectively. Although these studies were not performed in patients in a chest pain unit, they support the use of scintigraphy in this setting for risk stratification of patients with history of CAD.

A further issue complicating chest pain unit management of patients with a history of CAD is the high prevalence of anti-ischemic medications in this group, which may confound the diagnostic utility of stress testing. Beta-blockers and calcium channel-blockers limit the heart rate and blood pressure response during exercise testing and they can avert angina in patients with CAD [31–33]. There are conflicting data regarding the effect of these drugs on the sensitivity of the exercise test in detection of CAD, and patients are often considered ineligible for diagnostic exercise testing if they are taking these agents [31–38]. This potential problem may exclude patients from an accelerated assessment in a chest pain unit, cause a delay in diagnosis, or require hospital admission for further management.

Diercks and colleagues [39] have evaluated the use of beta-blockers and calcium channel-blockers in patients undergoing immediate stress testing in their chest pain unit. Of 176 patients on one of these agents who underwent exercise testing, 50 (28.6%) were taking a beta-blocker only, 116 (66.6%) a calcium channel-blocker only, and 10 (5.7%) were being treated with both classes of drugs. After adjusting for age, gender, cardiac risk factors, and presenting complaint, those patients on beta-blockers or calcium channel-blockers (study group) were more likely to have nondiagnostic tests 69 of 176 (39%) (OR 2.1, 95% CI 1.5–3.1) compared with patients in the cohort who were not taking these agents. The proportion of patients with a nondiagnostic exercise test was higher in the group on antianginal drugs, and beta-blockers were more problematic in this regard than calcium channel-blockers. However, the majority of patients on one or both of these drugs had a diagnostic test 107 of 176 (61%) (negative or positive), confirming the utility of exercise testing in these patients. Thus, despite a higher rate of nondiagnostic tests, inclusion of these patients in a chest pain unit protocol did afford timely disposition of a substantial proportion that would have otherwise been admitted to the hospital [39].

Taillefer and colleagues [40] evaluated the influence of beta-blockers in patients undergoing dypridamole Tc-99 sestamibi myocardial scintigraphy. They randomly assigned patients with known CAD to receive placebo, low-dose metoprolol, or high-dose metoprolol. Of the 21 patients completing the study, the sensitivity for detection of CAD was 85.7% in the placebo group versus approximately 71.0% in both the low- and high-dose beta-blocker group. In addition, the beta-blocker appeared to decrease the ability to assess severity of CAD based on the size of the perfusion deficit compared with placebo [39]. Although the rate of nondiagnostic tests is higher and sensitivity lower for detecting CAD in patients on beta-blockers, these medications should not be considered an absolute contraindication to chest pain unit management. Although patients with a history of CAD, including those on antianginal medications, pose a challenge to traditional chest pain unit protocols, their inclusion in this diagnostic strategy appears to be safe and effective if appropriate selection criteria are used.

Diabetics

Diabetic patients represent a group with increased risk and a high rate of atypical symptoms for CAD. Cardiovascular disease is the leading cause of death in diabetic patients, and the prevalence of CAD in some diabetic populations is over 50% [23]. Detection of CAD and risk stratification is often confounded by several unique features, including the markedly increased risk in female diabetics, lower predictive value of LDL cholesterol, and high rate of silent myocardial ischemia. In addition, diabetic patients often have poor exercise tolerance and nonspecific ST segment alterations that can result in nondiagnostic or false-positive exercise testing (Box 3) [41].

Despite the foregoing confounders, the value of exercise testing for detection of CAD in asymptomatic patients with type 2 diabetes was demonstrated by Bacci and colleagues [42]. They studied 141 patients who also had peripheral arterial disease or atherogenic risk factors, 71 of whom underwent coronary angiography. The diagnostic accuracy of exercise treadmill testing was 79%. In patients with a positive exercise test, 20 of 27 (74%) had a stenotic lesion > 70%. Marwick and colleagues [41] evaluated the use of stress echocardiography in 937 patients with diabetes and confirmed CAD or symptoms of CAD and observed that a positive stress echocardiogram was an independent predictor of death. Elective stress myocardial perfusion imaging has

---

Box 3. Unique factors in diabetics that affect stress test results

Increased risk of cardiac events in females with diabetes
Lower predictability of traditional cardiac risk factors
High rate of silent myocardial ischemia
Limited exercise capacity
Nonspecific baseline ST segment alterations

---

also been an acceptable tool for detection of CAD in diabetic patients. A retrospective review of diabetic patients who underwent myocardial perfusion imaging followed by cardiac catheterization reported a sensitivity of 97% and positive predictive value of 88% for CAD [43]. Kang and colleagues [44] reported a similarly high sensitivity (86%) but a specificity of 56% in a similar patient population. These studies support a detection rate for CAD by stress scintigraphy, but specificity of the method may be limited in diabetic patients.

Myocardial stress scintigraphy has also provided prognostic information. Berman and colleagues [45] evaluated 2826 patients who underwent adenosine myocardial perfusion imaging. They noted that diabetics who had an abnormal perfusion scan were at a significantly increased risk of death compared with nondiabetics and that perfusion imaging data was an independent predictor of events. Including diabetic patients in an accelerated protocol that involves stress scintigraphy is a potentially important tool for safe, expedient diagnosis and risk stratification in these often difficult to manage patients.

The studies in diabetics cited previously were performed largely in stable outpatients. Diabetic patients are frequently excluded from chest pain unit evaluation due to their presumed high risk [7]. As in patients with a prior history of CAD, the suitability of diabetics for chest pain unit management is controversial, but it should primarily depend on the immediate risk of ACS rather than the likelihood of underlying CAD. However, the safety and efficacy of including diabetics in a rapid diagnostic protocol are not well documented in the literature. Diercks and colleagues [46] have assessed the use of immediate exercise treadmill testing in diabetic patients evaluated in a chest pain unit. Their findings demonstrated that, whereas diabetics had more frequent evidence of CAD at 30-day follow-up than nondiabetics (12% versus 5%, RR 2.6, CI 1.7–4.1, $P < .0001$) and required more subsequent diagnostic studies (26% versus 14%, RR 2.0, CI 1.5–2.6, $P < .001$), there was no significant difference in acute cardiac events or length of stay in the chest pain unit between the two populations. Immediate exercise treadmill testing was also equally sensitive in detecting CAD in diabetics as in nondiabetics. Hence, exercise testing in diabetics with a normal baseline ECG and negative cardiac injury markers is a safe, efficacious, and cost-effective method for risk stratification and improves quality of care in this patient population.

Further evidence in support of the safety of this strategy was presented by Sanchez and colleagues [47] who evaluated the 30-day outcomes, resource use, and severity of CAD in patients with and without diabetes admitted to a chest pain unit, who comprised a subgroup of the Chest pain Evaluation and Creatinine Kinase-MB, Myoglobin, and Troponin I (CHECK-MATE) study. The study included 772 patients, of whom 109 had diabetes. All patients were assigned to a chest pain unit or evaluated in the ED for more than 6 hours. In accord with the author's aforementioned findings, the investigators reported an increase in adverse cardiac events (death/MI) in the diabetic patients (8.3% versus 3.2%, $P = .027$). In addition, they reported higher rates of the following events in the diabetic group: admission from the chest pain unit, incidence of elevated cardiac markers, and rate of multivessel disease, especially in patients with > 2 cardiac risk factors. However, there were no safety issues related to assignment to the accelerated diagnostic protocol. Indeed, even the higher adverse event rate in the diabetic group was well within that expected in a typical chest pain unit population.

These studies indicate that chest pain unit observation is appropriate in the foregoing populations if it is predicated on recognition of the higher prevalence of CAD in these patients and appreciation of the limitations of the diagnostic tools. Rigorous patient selection and firm adherence to protocol standards cannot be overemphasized to enhance safe evaluation of in the chest pain unit.

Chest pain related to stimulant use

The use of stimulants such as cocaine and methamphetamines is of epidemic proportions.

According to recent data, 25 million people in the United States have reported using cocaine [48,49], and it is likely that these numbers are similar for methamphetamine. The cardiovascular complications of cocaine have been well studied. It has been reported that the risk of MI is 24 times baseline risk in the hour after cocaine use [50]. In patients under the age of 45 years with acute MI, approximately 25% are cocaine related [51]. Of patients who present to the ED with cocaine-related chest pain, 6% have MI and the rate of cardiac arrhythmia has been reported to be over 2% [52]. Because there are no prospective studies in the methamphetamine patient population, data for cocaine are often extrapolated to the methamphetamine patients. A small study of patients admitted to the hospital with a positive screen for methamphetamine reported an in-hospital event rate of 8%, and in this selected group of patients ACS was diagnosed in 25% [53]. Because this rate of ACS is similar to that in the typical chest pain unit population, it is important to examine the potential utility of this strategy in patients with chest pain during stimulant use. Important considerations include defining the optimal time of observation and the need for specific diagnostic testing after an initial negative evaluation that included cardiac injury markers and ECG on presentation to ED.

Weber and colleagues [48] performed a prospective study to determine the safety of a 9- to 12-hour period of observation in patients who were at low to moderate risk for coronary events. The patient cohort consisted of 347 patients presenting with acute chest pain associated with cocaine use. A total of 42 patients (12%) were admitted to the hospital, of whom 20 had a final diagnosis of ACS, three had congestive heart failure, and two had ventricular tachycardia. Of the remaining 305 patients discharged home after a negative 9- to 12-hour observation period, including exercise testing, there were four nonfatal MIs (1.6%) in patients who continued to use cocaine. The investigators concluded that a 9- to 12-hour period of observation that included cardiac monitoring, serial cardiac biomarkers, and stress testing based on physician discretion was safe.

These results support prior retrospective studies that evaluated the use of an observation unit for the management of cocaine related chest pain. Kushman and colleagues [54] reported a similarly low rate of complications in a retrospective study of 197 consecutive patients admitted to a chest pain unit. Their protocol included cardiac bio-markers at hours 0, 3, and 6 and consultation by a cardiology fellow with selective use of stress evaluation by treadmill testing. Of the entire group, 22 (11.2%) were admitted to the hospital from the observation unit, one of whom had MI. In the remaining patients who were discharged, there was one (0.6%) cardiac complication during follow-up. However, the implications of provocative testing could not be assessed, because it was performed in only 40.6% of patients.

Current studies on the inclusion of patients with cocaine-related chest pain in a chest pain unit have concluded that a 6- to12-hour observation period is safe. In both studies mentioned previously, approximately 10% of patients were admitted to the hospital from the observation unit. This result substantiates the utility of inclusion of these patients in a chest pain unit, despite the overall low risk of ACS and arrhythmia. Because of the general lack of provocative testing in these studies, it is difficult to determine the overall cardiac risk of these patients and therefore difficult to compare the prevalence of CAD in these patients with that in a more typical chest pain unit population.

Summary

Chest pain units provide an important alternative to traditional hospital admission for patients who present to the ED with symptoms compatible with ACS and a normal or inconclusive initial evaluation. Although patient subgroups such as women, diabetics, those with established CAD, and those with symptoms related to stimulant use present unique challenges, management in a chest pain unit appears to be appropriate in these populations. Judicious application of accelerated diagnostic protocols and current testing methods can promote safe, accurate, and cost-effective risk stratification of special populations to identify patients who can be safely discharged and patients who require hospital admission for further evaluation.

References

[1] American Heart Association. Heart disease and stroke statistics—2005 update. Dallas, TX: American Heart Association; 2005.

[2] Daida H, Allison TG, Johnson BD, et al. Comparison of peak exercise oxygen uptake in men versus women in chronic heart failure secondary to ischemic or idiopathic dilated cardiomyopathy. Am J Cardiol 1997;80:85–8.

[3] Cummings GR, Dufrense C, Kich L, Sann J. Exercise electrocardiogram patterns in normal women. Br Heart J 1973;35:1055–61.

[4] Weiner DA, Ryan TJ, Parsons L, et al. Long-term prognostic value of exercise testing in men and women from the Coronary Artery Surgery Study (CASS) registry. Am J Cardiol 1995;75:865–70.

[5] Barolsky SM, Gilbert CA, Faruqui A, et al. Differences in electrocardiographic response to exercise of women and men: a non-Bayesian factor. Circulation 1979;60:1021–7.

[6] Douglas PS, Ginsburg GS. The evaluation of chest pain in women. N Engl J Med 1996;334:1311–5.

[7] Wilson PW, D'Agostino RB, Levy D, et al. Prediction of coronary heart disease using risk factor categories. Circulation 1998;97:1837–47.

[8] Lloyd-Jones, Wilson PW, Larson MG, et al. Framingham risk score and prediction of lifetime risk for coronary heart disease. Am J Cardiol 2004;94: 20–4.

[9] Bartel AG, Behar VS, Peter RH, et al. Graded exercise stress tests in angiographically documented coronary artery disease. Circulation 1974;49: 348–56.

[10] Diercks DB, Gibler WB, Liu T, et al. Identification of patients at risk by graded exercise testing in an emergency department chest pain center. Am J Cardiol 2000;86:289–92.

[11] Amsterdam EA, Kirk JD, Diercks DB, et al. Immediate exercise testing to evaluate low risk patients presenting to the emergency department with chest pain. J Am Coll Cardiol 2002;40:251–6.

[12] Diercks DB, Kirk JD, Turnipseed SD, Amsterdam EA. Exercise treadmill testing in women evaluated in a chest pain evaluation unit [abstract]. Acad Emerg Med 2000;8(5):565.

[13] Gibbons RJ, Balady GJ, Beasley JW. ACC/AHA guidelines for exercise testing: executive summary. A report of the American College of Cardiology/ American Heart Association Task Force on Practice Guidelines (Committee on Exercise Testing). J Am Coll Cardiol 1997;30:260–311.

[14] Mieres JH, Rosman DR, Shaw LJ. The role of myocardial perfusion imaging in special populations: women, diabetics, and heart failure. Semin Nucl Med 2005;35:52–81.

[15] Radensky PW, Hilton TC, Fulmer H, et al. Potential cost effectiveness of initial myocardial perfusion imaging for assessment of emergency department patients with chest pain. Am J Cardiol 1997;79: 595–9.

[16] Fesmire FM, Hughes AD, Stout PK, et al. Selective dual nuclear scanning in low-risk patients with chest pain to reliably identify and exclude acute coronary syndromes. Ann Emerg Med 2001;38: 207–15.

[17] Kontos MC, Jesse RL, Schmidt KL, et al. Value of acute rest sestamibi perfusion imaging for evaluation of patients admitted to the emergency department with chest pain. J Am Coll Cardiol 1997;30: 976–82.

[18] Kontos MC, Jesse RL, Anderson FP, et al. Comparison of myocardial perfusion imaging and cardiac troponin I in patients admitted to the emergency department with chest pain. Circulation 1999;99: 2073–8.

[19] Santana-Boado C, Candell-Riera J, Castell-Conesa J. Diagnostic accuracy of technetium-99m-MIBI myocardial SPECT in women and men. J Nucl Med 1998;39:751–5.

[20] Taillefer R, DePuey EG, Udelson JE. Comparative diagnostic accuracy of Tl-201 and Tc-99m sestamibi SPECT imaging (perfusion and ECG-gated SPECT) in detecting coronary artery disease in women. J Am Coll Cardiol 1997;29:69–77.

[21] Hachamovitch R, Berman DS, Kiat H, et al. Effective risk stratification using exercise myocardial perfusion SPECT in women: gender-related differences in prognostic nuclear testing. J Am Coll Cardiol 1996;28:34–44.

[22] Hachamovitch R, Hayes S, Friedman JD, et al. Determinants of risk and its temporal variation in patients with normal stress myocardial perfusion scans: what is the warranty period of a normal scan? J Am Coll Cardiol 2003;41:1329–40.

[23] Mieres JH, Shaw LJ, Hendel RC, et al. American Society of Nuclear Cardiology consensus statement: Task Force on Women and Coronary Artery Disease—the role of myocardial perfusion imaging in the clinical evaluation of coronary artery disease in women [correction]. J Nucl Cardiol 2003;10:95–101.

[24] Brush JE Jr, Brand DA, Acampora D, et al. Use of the initial electrocardiogram to predict in-hospital complications of acute myocardial infarction. N Engl J Med 1985;312:1137–41.

[25] Goldman L, Cook EF, Brand DA, et al. A computer protocol to predict myocardial infarction in emergency department patients with chest pain. N Engl J Med 1988;318:797–803.

[26] Farkouh ME, Smars PA, Reeder GS, et al. A clinical trial of a chest-pain observation unit for patients with unstable angina. Chest Pain Evaluation in the Emergency Room (CHEER) Investigators. N Engl J Med 1998;339:1882–8.

[27] Lewis WR, Amsterdam EA, Turnipseed S, Kirk JD. Immediate exercise testing of low risk patients with known coronary artery disease presenting to the emergency department with chest pain. J Am Coll Cardiol 1999;33:1843–7.

[28] Diercks DB, Kirk JD, Amsterdam EA. Evaluations of patients with a history of coronary artery disease in a chest pain unit [abstract]. 5th National Congress, Society of Chest Pain Centers and Providers. New Haven, Connecticut, 2002.

[29] Zellweger MJ, Dubois EA, Lai S, et al. Risk stratification in patients with remote prior myocardial infarction using rest-stress myocardial perfusion SPECT: prognostic value and impact on referral to early catheterization. J Nucl Cardiol 2002;9: 23–32.

[30] Elhendy A, Mahoney DW, Khandheria BK. Prognostic significance of impairment of heart rate response to exercise: impact of left ventricular function and myocardial ischemia. J Am Coll Cardiol 2003;42:823–30.

[31] Wander GS, Pasricha S, Aslam N, et al. Should beta-blockers be withdrawn in post-myocardial infarction patients before treadmill test? Indian Heart J 1997; 49:503–6.

[32] Ades PA, Thomas JD, Hanson JS, et al. Effect of metoprolol on the submaximal stress test performed early after acute myocardial infarction. Am J Cardiol 1987;60:963–6.

[33] Ashmore RC, Corkadel LK, Green CL, Horwitz LD. Verapamil but not nifedipine impairs left ventricular function during exercise in hypertensive patients. Am Heart J 1990;119:636–41.

[34] Ho SW, McComish MJ, Taylor RR. Effect of beta-adrenergic blockade on the results of exercise testing related to the extent of coronary artery disease. Am J Cardiol 1985;55:258–62.

[35] Pellinen TJ, Virtanen KS, Valle M, Frick MH. Studies on ergometer exercise testing. II. Effect of previous myocardial infarction, digoxin, and beta-blockade on exercise electrocardiography. Clin Cardiol 1986;9:499–507.

[36] Herbert WG, Dubach P, Lehmann KG, Froelicher VF. Effect of beta-blockade on the interpretation of the exercise ECG: ST level versus delta ST/HR index. Am Heart J 1991;122:993–1000.

[37] Martin GJ, Henkin RE, Scanlon PJ. Beta blockers and the sensitivity of the thallium treadmill test. Chest 1987;92:486–7.

[38] Sweeney ME, Fletcher BJ, Fletcher GF. Exercise testing and training with beta-adrenergic blockade: role of the drug washout period in "unmasking" a training effect. Am Heart J 1989;118: 941–6.

[39] Diercks DB, Kirk JD, Turnipseed SD, Amsterdam EA. Utility of immediate exercise treadmill testing in patients taking beta-blockers or calcium channel blockers. Am J Cardiol 2002;90:882–5.

[40] Taillefer R, Ahlberg AW, Masood Y, et al. Acute beta-blockade reduces the extent and severity of myocardial perfusion defects with dipyridamole Tc-99m sestamibi SPECT imaging. J Am Coll Cardiol 2003;42:1475–83.

[41] Marwick TH, Case C, Sawada S. Use of stress echocardiography to predict mortality in patients with diabetes and known or suspected coronary artery disease. Diabetes Care 2002;25:1042–8.

[42] Bacci S, Villella M, Villella A, et al. Screening for silent myocardial ischemia in type 2 diabetic patients

with additional atherogenic risk factors: applicability and accuracy of the exercise stress test. Eur J Endocrinol 2002;147:649–54.

[43] Bell DS, Yumuk VD. Low incidence of false-positive exercise thallium-201 scintigraphy in a diabetic population. Diabetes Care 1996;19:183–6.

[44] Kang X, Berman DS, Lewin H, et al. Comparative ability of myocardial perfusion single-photon emission computed tomography to detect coronary artery disease in patients with and without diabetes. Am Heart J 1999;137:949–57.

[45] Berman DS, Kang X, Hayes SW, et al. Adenosine myocardial perfusion single photon emission computed tomography in women compared to men. Impact of diabetes in incremental prognostic value and effect on patient management. J Am Coll Cardiol 2003;41:1125–33.

[46] Diercks DB, Kirk JD, Onesko N, Amsterdam EA. Patients with diabetes can undergo immediate exercise treadmill testing in a chest pain evaluation unit. Acad Emerg Med 2003;10:540A.

[47] Sanchez CD, Newby LK, Hasselblad V, et al. Comparison of 30-day outcome, resource use, and coronary artery disease severity in patients with suspected coronary artery disease with and without diabetes mellitus assigned to chest pain units. Am J Cardiol 2003;91:1228–30.

[48] Weber JE, Shofer FS, Larkin GL, et al. Validation of a brief observation period for patients with cocaine-associated chest pain. N Engl J Med 2003; 348:510–7.

[49] Lange RA, Hillis RD. Cardiovascular complications of cocaine use. N Engl J Med 2001;345:351–8 [Erratum: N Engl J Med 2001;345:1432].

[50] Mittleman MA, Mintzer D, Maclure M, et al. Triggering of myocardial infarction by cocaine. Circulation 1999;99:2737–41.

[51] Quershi AI, Suri MF, Guterman LR, et al. Cocaine use and the likelihood of nonfatal myocardial infarction and stroke: data from the Third National Health and Nutrition Examination Survey. Circulation 2001;103:502–6.

[52] Weber JE, Chudnofsky CR, Boczar M, et al. Cocaine-associated chest pain: how common is myocardial infarction? Acad Emerg Med 2000;7: 873–7.

[53] Turnipseed SD, Richards JR, Kirk JD, et al. Frequency of acute coronary syndrome in patients presenting to the emergency department with chest pain after methamphetamine use. J Emerg Med 2003;24: 369–73.

[54] Kushman SO, Storrow AB, Liu T, Gibler WB, et al. Cocaine-associated chest pain in a chest pain center. Am J Cardiol 2000;85:394–6.

CARDIOLOGY CLINICS

Cardiol Clin 23 (2005) 559–568

Management of the Patient with Chest Pain and a Normal Coronary Angiogram

Eric H. Yang, MD, Amir Lerman, MD*

The Center of Coronary Physiology and Imaging, Division of Cardiovascular Diseases, Mayo College of Medicine, 200 First Street Southwest, Rochester, Minnesota 55905, USA

Approximately 20% to 30% of patients undergoing coronary angiography for symptomatic chest pain are found to have normal epicardial coronary arteries [1,2]. When compared with patients who present with obstructive coronary artery disease, these patients are more likely to be women and tend to be younger [3,4]. Several conditions can result in chest pain with a normal coronary angiogram (NOCAD) and a proper diagnosis of the etiology is essential in managing these patients. This article discusses the pathophysiology of NOCAD and provides a systematic diagnostic approach to these patients. Potential therapeutic options and prognosis are also reviewed.

Pathophysiology

Angina occurs when there is a mismatch between myocardial oxygen supply and demand. In the absence of significant coronary artery stenosis, coronary blood flow (CBF) is regulated and limited by two main factors: coronary endothelial function and microvascular function.

Endothelial function

Traditionally, the coronary endothelium has been thought of as a monolayer of endothelial cells that line the lumen of the vascular bed; however, it is now known that the endothelium also extends into the vascular wall and adventitia

[5]. The endothelium plays an important role in the regulation of vasomotor tone and CBF. This regulation occurs by way of the production and release of vasoactive factors. The important vasodilators are:

1. *Nitric oxide:* Nitric oxide (NO) is a potent vasodilator. Its effects are mediated by the secondary messenger cyclic $3'5'$-guanosine monophosphate [6]. It has a short half-life and is synthesized from the oxidation of the N'-terminal of arginine [7]. This reaction is catalyzed by the enzyme endothelial nitric oxide synthase, which is produced by endothelial cells [7].
2. *Prostacyclin I:* Prostacyclin I_2 causes coronary vasodilation by increasing the production of cyclic $3'5'$-adenosine monophosphate in platelets and smooth muscle cells [8]. It is derived from arachidonic acid by the sequential reactions of cyclooxygenase and prostacyclin synthase [9].

The most potent vasoconstricting agents produced by the endothelium are:

1. *Endothelin-1:* Endothelin-1 is produced in endothelial cells from the cleavage of a propeptide by endothelin converting enzymes I and II [10–12]. Vasoconstriction occurs when endothelin-1 binds to the ETA-receptor located on smooth muscle cells [13].
2. *Thromboxane A_2:* Thromboxane A_2 is derived from arachidonic acid by way of a cyclooxygenase catalyzed reaction. It stimulates vasoconstriction by binding to the thromboxane receptor located on vascular smooth muscle cells [14].

Dr. Lerman is supported by NIH grants R01 HL 63911 and K24 HL 69840.

* Corresponding author.

E-mail address: lerman.amir@mayo.edu (A. Lerman).

If the endothelium does not function properly, NOCAD may occur as a result of a mismatch between myocardial oxygen supply and demand. In addition to NOCAD, endothelial dysfunction also promotes atherosclerosis and the eventual development of coronary artery stenosis.

Microvascular function

The coronary microcirculation consists of the small arteriolar vessels that are less than 300 μm in diameter. These vessels determine 80% of the coronary resistance and therefore play an important role in the regulation of CBF. Four factors regulate the microcirculation:

1. *Myogenic control:* The pressure exerted from the surrounding myocardium influences the intraluminal area of the microcirculation. Myogenic control of the microcirculation allows for the optimal transport of metabolic substances across capillary membranes by maintaining intraluminal pressure within a physiologic range [15].
2. *Flow-mediated control:* This process is endothelium-dependent allowing for autoregulation of microvascular blood flow [16]. Flow-mediated control helps to maintain intracoronary pressure and prevent shear stress-mediated injury.
3. *Metabolic control:* The metabolic state of the myocardium plays an important role in the regulation of blood flow. Oxygen consumption is the main regulating factor and mediators, such as adenosine, prostacyclin, norepinephrine, and carbon dioxide are involved [17].
4. *Neurohormonal control:* Sympathetic and parasympathetic innervation of the microcirculation allows for neural regulation of CBF. Neurotransmitters, such as acetylcholine, norepinephrine, and neuropeptide Y, help mediate the response [17].

If these control mechanisms do not function properly, microvascular dysfunction occurs. A reduction in the coronary flow reserve (CFR) in the absence of epicardial coronary artery stenosis indicates the presence of endothelial-independent microvascular dysfunction. CFR is the ratio of the average peak velocity (APV) during maximal hyperemia to the APV at baseline. Intracoronary or intravenous adenosine can be used to achieve hyperemia, and APV can be measured with an intracoronary Doppler wire or by way of transthoracic echocardiography. Patients who present with endothelial-independent microvascular dysfunction have a CFR less than or equal to 2.5.

Differential diagnosis

The differential diagnosis of NOCAD can be classified anatomically into three categories: (1) epicardial disease, (2) coronary microvascular dysfunction, and (3) noncoronary disease (Table 1). Epicardial disease resulting in NOCAD includes endothelial dysfunction, coronary artery spasm, and coronary artery bridging. Microvascular dysfunction may be secondary to endothelial dysfunction, hypertension, cardiomyopathy, infiltrative disease, valvular disease, or idiopathic. Noncoronary artery disease involving other organs systems, such as the pulmonary, gastrointestinal, or musculoskeletal systems, can also result in NOCAD.

Epicardial disease

Endothelial dysfunction

Proper endothelial function is necessary to insure that CBF is adequate to meet myocardial oxygen demand and endothelial dysfunction can result in NOCAD. Intracoronary acetylcholine can be used to assess endothelial function [18,19]. In patients who have normal endothelial function, the smooth muscle contraction mediated by acetylcholine is counterbalanced by its stimulation

Table 1
Differential diagnosis of chest pain in the setting of a normal coronary angiogram

I. Coronary disease
  A. Epicardial disease
    1. Endothelial dysfunction
    2. Coronary spasm
    3. Coronary bridging
  B. Microvascular dysfunction
    1. Microvascular endothelial dysfunction
    2. Hypertension
    3. Cardiomyopathy
    4. Infiltrative disease
    5. Valvular disease
    6. Idiopathic
II. Noncoronary disease
  A. Gastrointestinal
  B. Pulmonary
  C. Musculoskeletal
  D. Psychologic

of NO production in endothelial cells. According to previous studies, epicardial endothelial dysfunction is defined as a reduction in coronary artery diameter greater than 20% in response to acetylcholine [20,21].

Coronary spasm

Angina caused by coronary spasm was first described in 1959 by Prinzmetal and colleagues [22]. The chest pain induced by coronary spasm is similar to the pain caused by coronary artery disease but tends to occur at rest and between midnight and 8:00 AM [23]. Each episode can last from 30 to 60 minutes and may be associated with ischemic changes on the ECG. Although the mechanism of disease is not completely known, it seems to involve endothelial dysfunction and an increased response to vasoconstrictor agents, such as catecholamines and thromboxane A_2 [24,25]. Evidence also exists that an increase in autonomic tone may play a role in coronary spasm [26].

Intracoronary acetylcholine can be used as a provocative test for the diagnosis of coronary spasm [27]. Other direct vasoconstricting agents, such as ergonovine maleate, also can be used [28]. Although many patients have some degree of vasoconstriction to these agents, spasm is defined as a greater than 50% focal reduction in lumen caliber that is reversed with intracoronary nitroglycerin [29].

Myocardial bridging

Systolic compression of a coronary artery by the surrounding myocardium is referred to as myocardial bridging. It was first described in 1737 by Reyman [30] and occurs when a segment of the coronary artery is tunneled in the myocardium. Bridging most frequently occurs in the left anterior descending artery, but reports have shown that it may involve any of the major epicardial coronary arteries. The prevalence of myocardial bridging in autopsy studies has varied from 5% to 86%, but angiographic studies have shown a lower rate of 0.5% to 33% [31]. Although the mechanism is not clear, myocardial bridging can cause NOCAD. Intravascular ultrasound studies have shown that compression can extend into early diastole and reduce CBF [32]. Intracoronary hemodynamic studies have also shown that bridging results in a greater dependence on diastolic CBF [32]. Tachycardia can therefore decrease the diastolic time period and cause a decrease in CBF and ischemia. Endothelial dysfunction and coronary artery spasm also can occur at the site of myocardial bridging and may result in myocardial ischemia and coronary artery thrombosis [33].

Microvascular disease

Microvascular endothelial dysfunction

Impaired microvascular endothelial function can result in NOCAD by disrupting autoregulation of CBF. Previous studies have defined microvascular endothelial dysfunction as an increase in CBF less than 50% in response to acetylcholine [20,21].

Hypertension and microvascular dysfunction

Patients who present with hypertension can present with NOCAD. The mechanism of chest pain in these patients may involve a decrease in CBF caused by an increase in microvascular resistance [34,35]. The increase in resistance may be a result of an increase in myogenic tone caused by elevated diastolic pressures or compression of the microcirculation by the hypertrophied myocardium. A previous study suggests that ventricular hypertrophy plays an important role in microvascular dysfunction because hypertensive patients without ventricular hypertrophy did not have a reduction in CFR [36].

Cardiomyopathy and microvascular dysfunction

NOCAD occurs in approximately 50% of patients who present with dilated cardiomyopathy [37] and studies have shown that these patients have microvascular dysfunction and a reduced CFR [38,39]. The mechanism of microvascular dysfunction most likely involves myogenic compression secondary to elevated filling pressures or microvascular endothelial dysfunction. Patients who present with hypertrophic cardiomyopathy may also have a reduced CFR and NOCAD [40,41]. Histologic studies suggest that microvascular dysfunction in these patients may be caused by a reduction in the number of small arterioles and a narrowing of the luminal area of the microcirculation [42,43]. An alternative mechanism for the reduction in CFR may be that the microcirculation is already near maximally dilated in the basal state to meet the increase in oxygen demand [44]. Because the vessels are already dilated, their ability to further dilate is limited and the CFR is reduced.

Infiltrative disease and microvascular dysfunction

Patients who present with cardiac amyloidosis can present with NOCAD [45] caused by endothelial dysfunction [46] and amyloid deposits in the tunica media [47]. These deposits cause a reduction in the luminal area of the microcirculation [48–50] and the subsequent ischemia may be one of the factors responsible for the sudden cardiac death that occurs in cardiac amyloidosis.

Valvular disease and microvascular dysfunction

NOCAD can occur in patients who develop aortic stenosis, aortic regurgitation, and mitral regurgitation [51–54]. Previous studies have shown that these patients have a reduction in CFR that may be caused by an increase in filling pressures and wall stress [52,55–57]. These factors increase the myogenic tone and the amount of microvascular compression. Surgical treatment of the underlying valvular disease seems to correct the microvascular dysfunction in these patients [52,58,59].

Idiopathic microvascular dysfunction

Patients who present with no apparent etiology for microvascular dysfunction have idiopathic disease. Syndrome X has been used to describe these patients, but the term is not specific and probably should not be used. The mechanism of disease is not known but may involve an impaired vasodilator response as a result of smooth muscle cell dysfunction and primary microvascular endothelial dysfunction [60]. Increased activity of the sodium-hydrogen ion channel also may play a role in idiopathic microvascular disease [61].

Noncoronary etiologies

The noncoronary etiologies of NOCAD are shown in Table 1. Although these causes of NOCAD are not discussed in this review, the clinician should be aware of noncardiac disease when evaluating patients who present with NOCAD.

Systematic approach to diagnosing the etiology of normal coronary angiogram

Functional angiogram

Determination of the etiology of NOCAD is essential in its management. A "functional angiogram" (Fig. 1) involving the invasive assessment of coronary physiology allows for a systematic diagnostic approach to these patients. The protocol

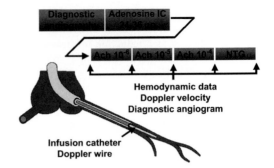

Fig. 1. Functional angiogram protocol to assess coronary endothelial and microvascular function. Ach, acetylcholine; IC, intracoronary; NTG, nitroglycerin.

has been described previously [20,62–64] and a summary is as follows:

After coronary angiography, a guiding catheter is placed into the left main coronary artery. A 0.014-inch Doppler guide wire is placed within a 2.2-F coronary infusion catheter and the system is advanced through the guiding catheter into the middle portion of the left anterior descending coronary artery. The Doppler wire is then positioned 2 to 3 mm distal to the tip of the infusion catheter, and a baseline APV is obtained. Coronary artery diameter is measured 5 mm distal to the tip of the Doppler wire and baseline CBF is calculated with the following equation: $CBF = \pi$ (coronary artery diameter/2) [2] $\times$ (APV/2). Microvascular function is assessed with the use of an intracoronary adenosine (18–42 μg) bolus. CFR is calculated as the ratio of the APV during maximal hyperemia to the APV at baseline. The authors define a normal CFR as greater than 2.5. Endothelial function is then assessed with the use of acetylcholine. Intracoronary acetylcholine is infused through the infusion catheter at three different doses: 10^{-6}, 10^{-5}, and 10^{-4} M for 3 minutes each to achieve intracoronary concentrations of 10^{-8}, 10^{-7}, and 10^{-6} respectively. Two hundred micrograms of intracoronary nitroglycerin is then given at the end of the procedure. APV and coronary diameter is measured before and after each infusion. Based on prior studies, an abnormal response to acetylcholine is an increase in CBF less than or equal to 50% or a reduction in epicardial coronary artery diameter greater than or equal to 20% [20,62].

Interpretation of results

Epicardial stenosis and myocardial bridging can be ruled out by carefully reviewing the diagnostic angiogram. The functional angiogram then can be used to classify patients into one of four groups (Fig. 2). Those patients who experience an abnormal response to acetylcholine but a normal CFR have abnormal endothelial function. If there is a focal greater than 50% reduction in luminal caliber during the infusion of acetylcholine then coronary spasm is present. Patients who present with a normal response to acetylcholine but an abnormal CFR have endothelial-independent microvascular dysfunction. These patients probably should undergo echocardiography to help determine the etiology of their microvascular dysfunction. An abnormal response to acetylcholine and a reduced CFR indicates the presence of endothelial dysfunction and endothelial-independent microvascular dysfunction. Finally, those patients who experience a normal response to acetylcholine and a normal CFR are most likely to have a noncoronary etiology of NOCAD. These patients should be evaluated for other etiologies of chest pain, such as gastrointestinal, pulmonary, or musculoskeletal disease. The distribution of findings from 820 functional angiograms performed at the Mayo Clinic are summarized in Fig. 3.

Prognosis and treatment

Endothelial dysfunction

Coronary endothelial dysfunction is a marker of early coronary atherosclerosis and has been shown to be associated with an increase in myocardial infarction, coronary revascualrization, and cardiac death [20]. Fortunately, endothelial dysfunction is reversible if the proper therapy is initiated. Risk factor modification is the cornerstone of therapy and previous studies have shown improvement in endothelial function with exercise, weight loss, and smoking cessation [65,66]. Blood pressure and cholesterol control are also essential. Angiotensin-converting enzyme inhibitors (Table 2) have been shown to improve endothelial function [67–70]. The mechanisms are unknown but seem to be independent of their blood pressure effects. The benefits of 3-hydroxy-3-methylglutaryl coenzyme A reductase inhibitors (statins) on endothelial function seem to be independent of their cholesterol lowering effects and may involve their antioxidant and anti-inflammatory properties [71]. Initial studies with peroxisome-activated receptor-γ agonists, such as rosiglitazone, have shown some beneficial effects on endothelial function [72]. Finally, other therapies, such as L-arginine and folic acid, have also been shown to improve endothelial function [73,74].

Coronary spasm

During the initial active phase (first 6 months) patients experience frequent episodes of angina and are at increased risk for adverse cardiac events; however, long-term studies have shown

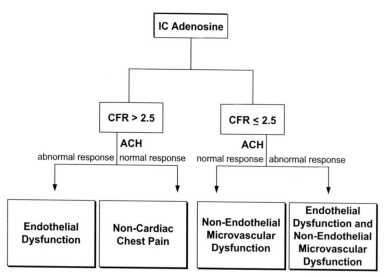

Fig. 2. Algorithm for a systematic diagnostic approach to patients who present with chest pain and NOCAD. An abnormal response to acetylcholine is defined as an increase in CBF less than 50% (microvascular endothelial dysfunction) or less than a 20% increase in coronary artery diameter (epicardial endothelial dysfunction). Ach, acetylcholine; CFR, coronary flow reserve; IC, intracoronary. (*Data from* Al Suwaidi J, Higano ST, Holmes DR Jr, et al. Pathophysiology, diagnosis, and current management strategies for chest pain in patients with normal findings on angiography. Mayo Clin Proc 2001;76:813.)

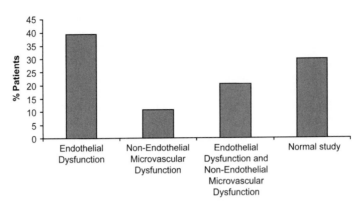

Fig. 3. Distribution of results from 820 functional angiograms performed at the Mayo Clinic.

that after the active phase, the 5-year survival is excellent and there is no increase in cardiac events [75,76]. The first line of therapy for patients who present with coronary spasm (see Table 2) is nondihydropyridine calcium channel blockers and long-acting nitrates [77]. Nonselective beta-blocking agents, such as propranolol, should be avoided because of their potential to exacerbate spasm by way of unopposed alpha-1 action [78]. Aspirin also should be used with caution because of its potential to inhibit the production of vasodilating prostacyclin derivatives [79]. Additional therapy with nifedipine and alpha-blocking agents can be used in patients refractory to first-line therapy [80,81]. Finally, when medical therapy becomes unsuccessful, placement of coronary artery stents or bypass surgery can be considered [82].

Myocardial bridging

Patients who present with myocardial bridging have been shown to have a good long-term prognosis [83]. Pediatric patients who present with hypertrophic obstructive cardiomyopathy and myocardial bridging, however, may have an increased risk for death and adverse cardiac events [84]. This increased risk does not seem to occur in adult patients who have developed hypertrophic obstructive cardiomyopathy and myocardial bridging [85].

All patients who develop NOCAD as a result of myocardial bridging should be treated with beta-blockers [86]. Those patients who do not improve with medical therapy can be treated with more invasive procedures, such as surgical

Table 2
Treatment strategies for patients with chest pain and a normal coronary angiogram

Etiology	First Line Therapy	Second Line Therapy	Comments
Endothelial Dysfunction	Life style modification, ACEI, Statins	L-arginine, folate	PPAR-γ agents may offer benefit
Coronary Spasm	Non-dihydropyridine calcium channel blockers, long-acting nitrates	Nifedipine, alpha-blockers, coronary artery stenting, bypass surgery	Non-selective beta blockers should be avoided, aspirin may exacerbate spasm
Myocardial Bridging	Beta-blockers	Coronary artery stenting, surgical myotomy, bypass surgery	Higher rates of in-stent restenosis occurs in bridging segment
Endothelial-Independent Microvascular Dysfunction	Treatment of underlying etiology of microvascular dysfunction	Beta-blockers, Statins	Imipramine may offer benefits in idiopathic microvascular dysfunction

Abbreviations: ACEI, angiotensin converting enzyme inhibitor; PPAR-γ, peroxisome-activated receptor-γ agonist.

myotomy, coronary artery stenting, and bypass surgery [87–89]. Stents placed in coronary segments with bridging have a higher restenosis rate than those placed in segments without bridging [90].

Microvascular dysfunction

Little is known about the long-term prognosis of patients who experience microvascular dysfunction and otherwise normal coronary arteries. Patients who develop hypertrophic cardiomyopathy and microvascular dysfunction seem to have an increase in adverse clinical events [91]. The interaction between microvascular dysfunction and dilated cardiomyopathy is not known. Treatment of the underlying etiology of microvascular dysfunction is the focus of therapy. Blood pressure control in those with hypertension and reduction of filling pressures and wall stress in patients who present with dilated cardiomyopathy improves microvascular function. Valvular replacement or repair has been shown to improve microvascular function in patients who have valvular disease [52,58,59]. In patients who develop hypertrophic obstructive cardiomyopathy, the effect of myectomy and septal ablation on microvascular function is not known.

Numerous therapies have been investigated for the treatment of patients who present with idiopathic microvascular dysfunction (see Table 2). The efficacy of these therapies is difficult to determine because of the heterogeneous population of patients. Beta-blockade seems to reduce angina symptoms, but no large randomized studies have been performed. Treatment with angiotensin converting enzyme inhibitors and HMG-CoA reductase inhibitors also result in some benefit [92,93]. Imipramine, a tricyclic antidepressant, has been shown to reduce anginal pain in patients who develop idiopathic microvascular dysfunction [94]. The mechanism is not understood completely but may involve inhibition of pain-modulating neurons by blockade of norepinephrine reuptake [95].

Summary

Approximately 20% to 30% of patients who experience chest pain who undergo coronary angiography are found to have normal epicardial coronary arteries. The management of these patients can be challenging and a correct diagnosis of the etiology is essential. A systematic approach to diagnosing the cause of chest pain can be accomplished with a functional angiogram to assess endothelial and microvascular function. Once the etiology of chest pain is determined, the appropriate therapy can be initiated.

References

[1] Kemp H Jr, Vokonas P, Cohn P, et al. The anginal syndrome associated with normal coronary arteriograms. Report of a six year experience. Am J Med 1973;54:735–42.

[2] Proudfit W, Shirey E, Sones FJ. Selective cine coronary arteriography. Correlation with clinical findings in 1,000 patients. Circulation 1966;33:901–10.

[3] Hasdai DH, Higano DR Jr, Burnett ST, et al. Prevalence of coronary blood flow reserve abnormalities among patients with nonobstructive coronary artery disease and chest pain. Mayo Clin Proc 1998;73: 1133–40.

[4] Papanicolaou MN, Califf RM, Hlatky MA, et al. Prognostic implications of angiographically normal and insignificantly narrowed coronary arteries. Am J Cardiol 1986;58:1181–7.

[5] Herrmann J, Lerman LO, Rodriguez-Porcel M, et al. Coronary vasa vasorum neovascularization precedes epicardial endothelial dysfunction in experimental hypercholesterolemia. Cardiovasc Res 2001;51: 762–6.

[6] Rapoport RM, Draznin MB, Murad F. Endothelium-dependent relaxation in rat aorta may be mediated through cyclic GMP-dependent protein phosphorylation. Nature 1983;306:174–6.

[7] Palmer RMJ, Ashton DS, Moncada S. Vascular endothelial cells synthesize nitric oxide from L-arginine. Nature 1988;333:664–6.

[8] Moncada S, Vane VR. Pharmacology and endogenous roles of prostaglandin endoperoxides, thromboxane A2 and prostacyclin. Pharmacol Rev 1979; 30:293.

[9] Vane JR, Botting RM. Pharmacodynamic profile of prostacyclin. Am J Cardiol 1995;75:3A–10A.

[10] Yanagisawa M, Kurihara H, Kimura S, et al. A novel potent vasoconstrictor peptide produced by vascular endothelial cells. Nature 1988;332:411–5.

[11] Ohnaka K, Takayanagi R, Nishikawa M, et al. Purification and characterization of a phosphoramidon-sensitive endothelin-converting enzyme in porcine aortic endothelium. J Biol Chem 1993;268: 26759–66.

[12] Xu D, Emoto N, Giaid A, et al. ECE-1: a membrane-bound metalloprotease that catalyzes the proteolytic activation of big endothelin-1. Cell 1994;78:473–85.

[13] Arai H, Hori S, Aramori I, et al. Cloning and expression of a cDNA encoding an endothelin receptor. Nature 1990;348:730–2.

[14] Luscher TF, Noll G. The pathogenesis of cardiovascular disease: role of the endothelium as a target and mediator. Atherosclerosis 1995;118:S81–90.

[15] Davis MJ. Microvascular control of capillary pressure during increases in local arterial and venous pressure. Am J Physiol 1988;254:H772–84.

[16] Pohl U, Holtz J, Busse R, et al. Crucial role of endothelium in the vasodilator response to increased flow in vivo. Hypertension 1986;8:37–44.

[17] Komaru T, Kanatsuka H, Shirato K. Coronary microcirculation: physiology and pharmacology. Pharmacol Ther 2000;86:217–61.

[18] el-Tamimi H, Mansour M, Wargovich T, et al. Constrictor and dilator responses to intracoronary acetylcholine in adjacent segments of the same coronary artery in patients with coronary artery disease. Endothelial function revisited. Circulation 1994;89:45–51.

[19] Egashira KIT, Hirooka Y, Yamada A, et al. Impaired coronary blood flow response to acetylcholine in patients with coronary risk factors and proximal atherosclerotic lesions. J Clin Invest 1993; 91:29–37.

[20] Suwaidi JA, Hamasaki S, Higano ST, et al. Long-term follow-up of patients with mild coronary artery disease and endothelial dysfunction. Circulation 2000;101:948–54.

[21] Hasdai D, Holmes DR Jr, Higano ST, et al. Prevalence of coronary blood flow reserve abnormalities among patients with nonobstructive coronary artery disease and chest pain [see comment]. Mayo Clin Proc 1998;73:1133–40.

[22] Prinzmetal M, Kennamer R, Merliss R, et al. Angina pectoris. I. A variant form of angina pectoris: preliminary report. Am J Med 1959;27:375.

[23] Ogawa H, Yasue H, Oshima S, et al. Circadian variation of plasma fibrinopeptide A level in patients with variant angina. Circulation 1989;80:1617–26.

[24] Cox ID, Kaski JC, Clague JR. Endothelial dysfunction in the absence of coronary atheroma causing Prinzmetal's angina. Heart 1997;77:584.

[25] Maseri A, Crea F, Lanza GA. Coronary vasoconstriction: where do we stand in 1999. An important, multifaceted but elusive role. Cardiologia 1999;44: 115–8.

[26] Lanza GA, Pedrotti P, Pasceri V, et al. Autonomic changes associated with spontaneous coronary spasm in patients with variant angina. J Am Coll Cardiol 1996;28:1249–56.

[27] Okumura K, Yasue H, Matsuyama K, et al. Diffuse disorder of coronary artery vasomotility in patients with coronary spastic angina. Hyperreactivity to the constrictor effects of acetylcholine and the dilator effects of nitroglycerin. J Am Coll Cardiol 1996;27:45–52.

[28] Previtali M, Ardissino D, Storti C, et al. Hyperventilation and ergonovine tests in Prinzmetal's variant angina: comparative sensitivity and relation with the activity of the disease. Eur Heart J 1989;10: 101–4.

[29] Scanlon PJ, Faxon DP, Audet AM, et al. ACC/AHA guidelines for coronary angiography: a report of the American College of Cardiology/American Heart Association Task Force on Practice Guidelines (Committee on Coronary Angiography) developed in collaboration with the Society for Cardiac Angiography and Interventions. J Am Coll Cardiol 1999;33:1756–824.

[30] Reyman H. Disertatio de vasis cordis propriis. Med Diss Univ Göttingen 1737;7:1–32.

[31] Mohlenkamp S, Hort W, Ge J, et al. Update on myocardial bridging. Circulation 2002;106:2616–22.

[32] Ge J, Jeremias A, Rupp A, et al. New signs characteristic of myocardial bridging demonstrated by intracoronary ultrasound and Doppler. Eur Heart J 1999;20:1707–16.

[33] Herrmann J, Higano ST, Lenon RJ, et al. Myocardial bridging is associated with alteration in coronary vasoreactivity. Eur Heart J 2004;25:2134–42.

[34] Opherk D, Mall G, Zebe H, et al. Reduction of coronary reserve: a mechanism for angina pectoris in patients with arterial hypertension and normal coronary arteries. Circulation 1984;69:1–7.

[35] Brush J, Cannon R, Schenke W, et al. Angina due to coronary microvascular disease in hypertensive patients without left ventricular hypertrophy. N Engl J Med 1988;319:1302–7.

[36] Hamasaki S, Al Suwaidi J, Higano ST, et al. Attenuated coronary flow reserve and vascular remodeling in patients with hypertension and left ventricular hypertrophy. J Am Coll Cardiol 2000; 35:1654–60.

[37] Abelmann WH, Lorell BH. The challenge of cardiomyopathy. J Am Coll Cardiol 1989;13:1219–39.

[38] Pasternac A, Noble J, Streulens Y, et al. Pathophysiology of chest pain in patients with cardiomyopathies and normal coronary arteries. Circulation 1982;65:778–89.

[39] Cannon RO III, Cunnion RE, Parrillo JE, et al. Dynamic limitation of coronary vasodilator reserve in patients with dilated cardiomyopathy and chest pain. J Am Coll Cardiol 1987;10:1190–200.

[40] Maron B, Epstein S, Roberts W. Hypertrophic cardiomyopathy and transmural myocardial infarction without significant atherosclerosis of the extramural coronary arteries. Am J Cardiol 1979;43: 1086–102.

[41] Cannon RO III, Rosing DR, Maron BJ, Leon MB, et al. Myocardial ischemia in patients with hypertrophic cardiomyopathy: contribution of inadequate vasodilator reserve and elevated left ventricular filling pressures. Circulation 1985;71:234–43.

[42] Schwartzkopff B, Mundhenke M, Strauer B. Alterations of the architecture of subendocardial arterioles in patients with hypertrophic cardiomyopathy and impaired coronary vasodilator reserve: a possible cause for myocardial ischemia. J Am Coll Cardiol 1998;31:1089–96.

[43] Tanaka M, Fujiwara H, Onodera T, et al. Quantitative analysis of narrowings of intramyocardial small arteries in normal hearts, hypertensive hearts, and

hearts with hypertrophic cardiomyopathy. Circulation 1987;75:1130–9.

[44] Yang EH, Yeo TC, Higano ST, et al. Coronary hemodynamics in patients with symptomatic hypertrophic cardiomyopathy. Am J Cardiol 2004;94: 685–7.

[45] Brandt KS, Cathcart ES, Cohen A. A clinical analysis of the course and prognosis of forty-two patients with amyloidosis. Am J Med 1968;44: 955–69.

[46] Suwaidi JA, Velianou JL, Gertz MA, et al. Systemic amyloidosis presenting with angina pectoris. Ann Intern Med 1999;131:838–41.

[47] Hongo M, Yamamoto H, Kohda T, et al. Comparison of electrocardiographic findings in patients with AL (primary) amyloidosis and in familial amyloid polyneuropathy and anginal pain and their relation to histopathologic findings. Am J Cardiol 2000;85: 849–53.

[48] Roberts WC, Waller BF. Cardiac amyloidosis causing cardiac dysfunction: analysis of 54 necropsy patients. Am J Cardiol 1983;52:137–46.

[49] Saffitz JE, Sazama K, Roberts WC. Amyloidosis limited to small arteries causing angina pectoris and sudden death. Am J Cardiol 1983;51:1234–5.

[50] Smith RRL, Hutchins GM. Ischemic heart disease secondary to amyloidosis of intramyocardial arteries. Am J Cardiol 1979;44:413–7.

[51] Basta LL, Raines D, Najjar S, et al. Clinical, haemodynamic, and coronary angiographic correlates of angina pectoris in patients with severe aortic valve disease. Br Heart J 1975;37:150–7.

[52] Akasaka T, Yoshida K, Hozumi T, et al. Restricted coronary flow reserve in patients with mitral regurgitation improves after mitral reconstructive surgery. J Am Coll Cardiol 1998;32:1923–30.

[53] Alexopoulos D, Kolovou G, Kyriakidis M, et al. Angina and coronary artery disease in patients with aortic valve disease. Angiology 1993;44: 707–11.

[54] Hakki AH, Kimbiris D, Iskandrian AS, et al. Angina pectoris and coronary artery disease in patients with severe aortic valvular disease. Am Heart J 1980;100: 441–9.

[55] Nitenberg A, Foult JM, Antony I, et al. Coronary flow and resistance reserve in patients with chronic aortic regurgitation, angina pectoris and normal coronary arteries. J Am Coll Cardiol 1988;11: 478–86.

[56] Marcus ML, Doty DB, Hiratzka LF, et al. Decreased coronary reserve: a mechanism for angina pectoris in patients with aortic stenosis and normal coronary arteries. N Engl J Med 1982;307:1362–6.

[57] Julius BK, Spillmann M, Vassalli G, et al. Angina pectoris in patients with aortic stenosis and normal coronary arteries. Mechanisms and pathophysiological concepts [see comment]. Circulation 1997;95: 892–8.

[58] Hildick-Smith DJR, Shapiro LM. Coronary flow reserve improves after aortic valve replacement for aortic stenosis: an adenosine transthoracic echocardiography study. J Am Coll Cardiol 2000;36: 1889–96.

[59] Nemes A, Forster T, Kovacs Z, et al. The effect of aortic valve replacement on coronary flow reserve in patients with a normal coronary angiogram. Herz 2002;27:780–4.

[60] Chauhan AMP, Taylor G, Petch MC, et al. Both endothelium-dependent and endothelium-independent function is impaired in patients with angina pectoris and normal coronary angiograms. Eur Heart J 1997; 18:60–8.

[61] Gaspardone A, Ferri C, Crea F, et al. Enhanced activity of sodium-lithium countertransport in patients with cardiac syndrome X: a potential link between cardiac and metabolic syndrome X. J Am Coll Cardiol 1998;32:2031–4.

[62] Hasdai D, Gibbons RJ, Holmes DR Jr, et al. Coronary endothelial dysfunction in humans is associated with myocardial perfusion defects. Circulation 1997; 96:3390–5.

[63] Vita J, Treasure C, Nabel E, et al. Coronary vasomotor response to acetylcholine relates to risk factors for coronary artery disease. Circulation 1990;81: 491–7.

[64] Zeiher A, Drexler H, Wollschlager H, et al. Modulation of coronary vasomotor tone in humans. Progressive endothelial dysfunction with different early stages of coronary atherosclerosis. Circulation 1991;83:391–401.

[65] Hambrecht R, Wolf A, Gielen S, et al. Effect of exercise on coronary endothelial function in patients with coronary artery disease. N Engl J Med 2000; 342:454–60.

[66] Celermajer D, Sorensen K, Georgakopoulos D, et al. Cigarette smoking is associated with dose-related and potentially reversible impairment of endothelium-dependent dilation in healthy young adults. Circulation 1993;88:2149–55.

[67] O'Driscoll G, Green D, Rankin J, et al. Improvement in endothelial function by angiotensin converting enzyme inhibition in insulin-dependent diabetes mellitus. J Clin Invest 1997;100:678–84.

[68] O'Driscoll G, Green D, Maiorana A, et al. Improvement in endothelial function by angiotensin-converting enzyme inhibition in non-insulin-dependent diabetes mellitus. J Am Coll Cardiol 1999;33: 1506–11.

[69] Mancini GBJ, Henry GC, Macaya C, et al. Angiotensin-converting enzyme inhibition with quinapril improves endothelial vasomotor dysfunction in patients with coronary artery disease: the TREND (Trial on Reversing Endothelial Dysfunction) Study. Circulation 1996;94:258–65.

[70] Prasad A, Narayanan S, Husain S, et al. Insertion-deletion polymorphism of the ace gene modulates

reversibility of endothelial dysfunction with ACE inhibition. Circulation 2000;102:35–41.

[71] Bonetti PO, Lerman LO, Napoli C, et al. Statin effects beyond lipid lowering—are they clinically relevant? Eur Heart J 2003;24:225–48.

[72] Reusch JE, Regensteiner JG, Watson PA. Novel actions of thiazolidinediones on vascular function and exercise capacity. Am J Med 2003;115:69S–74S.

[73] Lerman A, Burnett JC Jr, Higano ST, et al. Long-term L-arginine supplementation improves small-vessel coronary endothelial function in humans. Circulation 1998;97:2123–8.

[74] Doshi SN, McDowell IFW, Moat SJ, et al. Folate improves endothelial function in coronary artery disease: an effect mediated by reduction of intracellular superoxide? Arterioscler Thromb Vasc Biol 2001;21:1196–202.

[75] Bory M, Pierron F, Panagides D, et al. Coronary artery spasm in patients with normal or near normal coronary arteries. Long-term follow-up of 277 patients [see comment]. Eur Heart J 1996;17: 1015–21.

[76] Mark DB, Califf RM, Morris KG, et al. Clinical characteristics and long-term survival of patients with variant angina. Circulation 1984;69:880–8.

[77] Mayer S, Hillis LD. Prinzmetal's variant angina. Clin Cardiol 1998;21:243–6.

[78] Robertson R, Wood A, Vaughn W, et al. Exacerbation of vasotonic angina pectoris by propranolol. Circulation 1982;65:281–5.

[79] Miwa K, Kambara H, Kawai C. Effect of aspirin in large doses on attacks of variant angina. Am Heart J 1983;105:351–5.

[80] Goldberg S, Reichek N, Wilson J, et al. Nifedipine in the treatment of Prinzmetal's (variant) angina. Am J Cardiol 1979;44:804–10.

[81] Taylor SH. Alpha- and beta-blockade in angina pectoris. Drugs 1984;28:69–87.

[82] Kultursay H, Can L, Payzin S, et al. A rare indication for stenting: persistent coronary artery spasm. Heart Vessels 1996;11:165–8.

[83] Kramer KH Jr, Proudfit WL, Sones FM Jr. Clinical significance of isolated coronary bridges: benign and frequent condition involving the left anterior descending artery. Am Heart J 1992;103:283–8.

[84] Yetman AT, McCrindle BW, MacDonald C, et al. Myocardial bridging in children with hypertrophic cardiomyopathy—a risk factor for sudden death. N Engl J Med 1998;339:1201–9.

[85] Sorajja P, Ommen SR, Nishimura RA, et al. Myocardial bridging in adult patients with hypertrophic cardiomyopathy. J Am Coll Cardiol 2003;42:889–94.

[86] Schwarz ER, Klues HG, vom Dahl J, et al. Functional, angiographic and intracoronary doppler flow characteristics in symptomatic patients with myocardial bridging: effect of short-term intravenous beta-blocker medication. J Am Coll Cardiol 1996;27:1637–45.

[87] Klues HG, Schwarz ER, vom Dahl J, et al. Disturbed intracoronary hemodynamics in myocardial bridging: early normalization by intracoronary stent placement. Circulation 1997;96:2905–13.

[88] Hillman ND, Mavroudis C, Backer CL, et al. Supra-arterial decompression myotomy for myocardial bridging in a child. Ann Thorac Surg 1999;68:244–6.

[89] Iversen SHU, Mayer E, Erbel R, et al. Surgical treatment of myocardial bridging causing coronary artery obstruction. Scand J Thorac Cardiovasc Surg 1992;26:107–11.

[90] Haager PK, Schwarz ER, Dahl JV, et al. Long term angiographic and clinical follow up in patients with stent implantation for symptomatic myocardial bridging. Heart 2000;84:403–8.

[91] Cecchi F, Olivotto I, Gistri R, et al. Coronary microvascular dysfunction and prognosis in hypertrophic cardiomyopathy. N Engl J Med 2003;349:1027–35.

[92] Chen JW, Hsu NW, Wu TC, et al. Long-term angiotensin-converting enzyme inhibition reduces plasma asymmetric dimethylarginine and improves endothelial nitric oxide bioavailability and coronary microvascular function in patients with syndrome X. Am J Cardiol 2002;90:974–82.

[93] Pizzi C, Manfrini O, Fontana F, et al. Angiotensin-converting enzyme inhibitors and 3-hydroxy-3-methylglutaryl coenzyme a reductase in cardiac Syndrome X: role of superoxide dismutase activity. Circulation 2004;109:53–8.

[94] Cannon RO, Quyyumi AA, Mincemoyer R, et al. Imipramine in patients with chest pain despite normal coronary angiograms. N Engl J Med 1994;330: 1411–7.

[95] Dubner R, Bennett GJ. Spinal and trigeminal mechanisms of nociception. Annu Rev Neurosci 1983;6: 381–418.

CARDIOLOGY
CLINICS

Cardiol Clin 23 (2005) 569–588

Using the Emergency Department Clinical Decision Unit for Acute Decompensated Heart Failure

W. Frank Peacock, MD, FACEP

Department of Emergency Medicine, The Cleveland Clinic, 9500 Euclid Avenue, Cleveland, OH 44195, USA

In the United States, heart failure (HF) management costs exceed all other single pathologic entities. Because HF is predominately a disease of the elderly, and demographic trends are expected to double the at-risk cohort over the next 30 years, the consequences of HF will only increase. More efficacious strategies for early diagnosis, better treatment options, and improved clinical outcomes are urgently needed. This article reviews the newest options for HF management with particular emphasis on care in the emergency department (ED) observation unit (OU).

Epidemiology and economics

Disproportionately affecting the elderly, HF is the only cardiovascular pathology that is increasing in both incidence and prevalence [1,2]. If under 50 years of age, less than 1% of the U.S. population is diagnosed with HF, but by age 80, this number rises to 10%. This has huge cost implications for our national health system. Inpatient HF costs are estimated as high as $23.1 billion and outpatient costs at $14.7 billion, annually. Annual HF hospitalization costs exceed the combination of costs for breast and lung cancer [3].

In the United States, patients older than 65 have health insurance provided by the Centers for Medical Studies (CMS). Because most HF patients are elderly, statistics from the CMS drive many of HF management decisions. According to CMS, HF is the most common cause of hospitalization, and it is the most common reason for hospital readmission in patients over 65 years of age [3]. Unfortunately, HF has an extremely poor

prognosis. After becoming symptomatic, 2-year mortality is about 35%, and rises to 80% in men and 65% for women over the next 6 years. After a diagnosis of pulmonary edema, only 50% survive at 1 year. Up to 85% of those with cardiogenic shock are dead within 1 week. Unless new strategies are devised, the HF epidemic will markedly worsen. Management in an OU represents an opportunity to improve the quality of care for HF patients.

HF is a disease of recidivism, characterized by frequent clinical exacerbations that prompt ED visits. Although it may have a pattern of deterioration and improvement, the overall course is that of a steadily deteriorating clinical pattern. As HF slowly progresses, quality of life is eroded by frequent ED visits, hospitalizations, and increasing disability until death. The frequency of recidivism is reflected in the ED HF population: only 21% of patients represent a de novo presentation. The majority of the ED HF population already carries the HF diagnosis when they arrive with acute dyspnea.

Once a patient presents to the ED with acute decompensated HF (ADHF), inpatient admission is the rule, rather than the exception. An ED visit is indicative of either severe disease or the consequence of inadequate social support. In the best of situations, definitive resolution of either is difficult, particularly in the ED environment. Consequently, 80% of HF presentations result in hospitalization.

As discussed previously, CMS provides health insurance to patients older than 65 in the United States. Because most HF patients are older than 65, this creates an unusual economic situation where a specific disease is predominately covered by a single third-party payor, and a hospital's

---

E-mail address: peacocw@ccf.org

economic health may be greatly impacted by their reimbursement rules. Inpatient care of HF falls within the diagnostic related group (DRG) system, with DRG 127 (HF) as the single most expensive diagnosis. In this year alone, there will be more than 1 million HF hospital discharges in the United States.

CMS affects care by reimbursement inducements, where three main parameters drive HF management. These include length of stay (LOS), revisit frequency, and intensity of service. By this method, when a hospital submits patient data, a diagnosis-based algorithm is used to calculate reimbursement and a regionally standardized sum of money is paid. The actual amount received by the hospital is determined by the diagnosis and is independent of the actual cost of care. Therefore, the financial margin on which the hospital must survive is the difference between reimbursement and the true cost of providing care.

The single greatest contributor to cost is LOS. Therefore, significant pressure exists for the institution to control LOS so that costs do not exceed the CMS payment. Ultimately, an excessive average LOS results in an institutional loss. With regard to HF, the breakeven point occurs at approximately 5 days. The average LOS must be maintained closer to 4 days to ensure that a profit margin exists to cover the losses incurred by outliers. In reality, the average hospital in the United States is unable to control cost and sustains a net loss of $1,288 for every HF admission [3].

If the only economic incentive were to shorten LOS, undue discharge pressure on hospitals could adversely impact care. Theoretically, patients could be sent home from the hospital every 3 days, only to immediately return for readmission. Therefore, to balance the early discharge incentive, the 30-day revisit penalty was created. After an initial hospitalization, readmission within 30 days for the same DRG may be considered part of the original visit. In this situation, there is no additional reimbursement, and the hospital receives no additional money for the second admission. This creates an economic pressure to prevent premature discharge and eliminate readmissions within 30 days.

The third pressure impacting HF care comes from the resources required to manage the patient. This represents the true cost of care and is proportionate to the intensity of service provided. Therefore, the more staff or physical resources required to manage a patient, the greater the rate of consumption of the DRG payment. In this manner, the areas with the greatest cost of care (eg, the ICU) must be carefully used to prevent economic loss.

When global resource use is considered, diagnostic and therapeutic interventions represent a small percentage of the cost of HF management. Rather, LOS, 30-day revisit frequency, and the intensity of service occurring within the hospital are the main determinants of institutional financial success.

Role of the observation unit

In 2002 CMS began an ambulatory patient classification (APC) code for the OU. The OU is defined as an outpatient environment providing a longer period of management, far exceeding the usual capabilities of the ED, but not considered hospitalization. This new code allows a non-DRG reimbursement, independent of the 30-day revisit penalty, for treatment with a length of stay up to 48 hours. OU admissions may occur as many times as is required, and the hospital is reimbursed for each individual event. Not only is this economically beneficial to the hospital, but by avoiding inpatient hospitalization, limited intensive management could provide quality-of-life improvements.

The OU is an option for HF care in an environment where a period of short intensive therapy, monitoring, and aggressive management can occur. This definition is important for its success. The OU is not a preadmission testing unit, nor is it a holding area for patients with unclear treatment goals, undefined diagnostic endpoints, or vague disposition plans. Successful HF management is complicated and difficult. Physician involvement, and a dedicated nursing staff armed with clear management protocols, can significantly improve the care in the HF patient. A well-orchestrated OU HF management plan has been shown to decreases revisits, hospitalizations, and LOS [4]. Even if subsequent hospitalization is required, overall LOS, inclusive of the OU visit, decreases [4].

To qualify for the APC code, there are several requirements. First, care must be given for at least 8 hours in the OU environment. Second, there are several clinical parameters that must be met; these include the documentation of pulse oximetry measurement, the performance of a chest radiograph, and obtaining an electrocardiogram (ECG). Finally, the APC allows for care that may not exceed 48 hours. However, the length of stay rule is tempered by an important caveat: although the APC structure allows for hospitalization for up to 48 hours, CMS ceases reimbursement at 24 hours. Therefore, most units plan for disposition within 1 day at which time patients are either admitted to the hospital and converted to a DRG or discharged home.

Although the APC thresholds are easily met, it is important that the OU does not admit every ED patient with HF. Because the requirement of the OU is discharge within 24 hours, populating the unit with patients who exceed the LOS parameter results in decreasing its efficiency. Furthermore, nurse-to-patient ratios are usually lower in the OU than in the ICU (three to four patients per nurse), so that admissions to an OU environment should match its ability to manage appropriately selected patients.

An OU HF management program can provide benefit to the institution and the patient. The hospital benefit is two-fold: (1) by providing care outside of the DRG revisit rule, the average per patient reimbursement rate is higher, and (2) the intensity of service costs are lower, compared with the inpatient unit. For the patient, the OU is able to provide short, intensive therapy without the necessity of several days of hospitalization and allows early return to the home environment. Additionally, the OU can facilitate the performance of procedures that may be difficult. For instance, ejection fraction (EF) measurement is a standard for HF treatment and is requirement of the JCAHO [5]. Transportation limitations in nonambulatory patients (eg, a nursing home resident) can delay or prevent this evaluation. Likewise, multiple outpatient visits required for initiation and optimization of HF medication (eg, beta-blockers or angiotensin-converting enzyme inhibitors) can be accomplished.

As a last point of discussion regarding the fiduciary structure options for a hospital, an institution may benefit financially to a greater extent by the admission of all short-stay HF patients to the higher reimbursed inpatient DRG. Although this is accurate in the short-term, in the long-term this behavior is penalized by the case mix multiplier. The case mix multiplier is the tool by which CMS adjusts DRG reimbursements at the local level. It is based on the average acuity for a given DRG. When a hospital's average acuity of illness is decreased, the case mix multiplier is decreased proportionally so that the hospital receives less average DRG payment per patient. If the average acuity increases, the case mix multiplier is increased proportionally. By admitting short-stay HF patients to the hospital and claiming the DRG, the hospital will realize a short-term gain as they receive the higher acuity DRG, up until time for the case mix multiplier adjustment. After their case mix multiplier is decreased, they will receive a decreased DRG reimbursement for all their DRG 127 (HF) patients. This becomes trading short-term gain for long-term loss and provides the incentive for accurate DRG and APC coding.

Pathophysiology

Wall tension is a product of pressure (afterload) and ventricular radius. Increasing wall tension is a stimulus for cardiac remodeling. With increasing tension, cardiac myocytes either hypertrophy or die (apoptosis) to form scar tissue. The dominant response determines HF type. Many different pathologies may ultimately lead to the clinical presentation of HF (Box 1). The dominating pathway determines the type of HF that results.

HF is divided into systolic dysfunction or preserved systolic function (PSF) types by the EF. A normal EF is defined as 60%, with systolic

---

Box 1. Causes of heart failure

- Acute mitral regurgitation (papillary rupture)
- Acute pulmonary embolus
- Anemia
- Arteriovenous fistula (eg, dialysis)
- Cardiac free wall rupture
- Constrictive pericarditis
- Complications of MI
- Coronary artery disease
- Hyperkinetic states
- Idiopathic cardiomyopathy
- Myocarditis
- Pericardial disease/tamponade/ effusion
- Poorly controlled hypertension
- Postpartum cardiomyopathy
- Sustained cardiac arrhythmia/ tachycardia
- Thyrotoxicosis
- Valvular rupture or disease

dysfunction defined as an EF < 40%. Systolic dysfunction is most commonly the result of ischemic heart disease, although many other causes exist. The pathologic feature of systolic dysfunction is a ventricle that has difficulty ejecting blood. Impaired contractility leads to increased intracardiac volumes and pressure, and increasing afterload sensitivity. Consequently, these patients are sensitive to hypertension, and maintaining blood pressure (BP) to as low as is tolerated becomes an important management goal.

PSF HF is defined by preserved mechanical contractile function. When measured, the EF is normal or higher. The pathologic deficit is a ventricle with impaired relaxation, which results in an abnormal diastolic pressure-volume relationship. In this situation, the left ventricle (LV) has difficulty in receiving blood. Decreased LV compliance necessitates higher atrial pressures to ensure adequate diastolic LV filling. The hemodynamic consequence of a stiffened noncompliant ventricle is preload sensitivity, where excessively lowered preload may result in hypotension because of a lack of ventricular filling. The frequency of diastolic dysfunction increases with age. Chronic hypertension and LV hypertrophy are often responsible for this syndrome. Coronary artery disease (CAD) also contributes, and diastolic dysfunction is an early event in the ischemic cascade. It has been reported that as many as 30% to 50% [6] of HF patients have circulatory congestion on the basis of diastolic dysfunction.

The pathologic distinctions based on EF are less important in the acute care setting of the ED and OU. In these environments, volume overload with excessive filling pressures are the most common ED presentation. Irrespective of the EF, the treatment approach is therefore similar. However, once hemodynamics are stabilized, and volume status approaches euvolemia, recognition of the underlying EF and the etiology of HF should be considered. In patients with PSF, excessive diuresis or venodilation may exacerbate the underlying deficit in ventricular filling and result in hypotension.

Determining HF type is difficult using the history and physical examination; consequently, an ECG becomes necessary. Some differentiate between left- and right-sided HF. Left-sided HF has dyspnea, fatigue, weakness, cough, paroxysmal nocturnal dyspnea, and orthopnea in the absence of peripheral edema, jugular venous distention (JVD), or hepatojugular reflux (HJR). Right-sided HF has peripheral edema, JVD, right upper quadrant pain, and HJR, without pulmonary symptoms. Because the cardiovascular system is mechanistically closed and abnormal pressure and chamber volumes are eventually reflected to the contralateral side, this distinction has greatest applicability when there is suspicion of valvular heart disease.

Role of neurohormones

Before the natriuretic peptides (NPs) were identified, extracellular fluid regulation was believed to be controlled by the kidneys, adrenal glands, and sympathetic nervous system via the renin–angiotensin system and other neuroendocrine mechanisms [7]. When arterial BP declines, renin is released by the kidneys. Renin splits hepatically synthesized angiotensinogen to form angiotensin I. Angiotensin I is a biologically inactive decapeptide that is cleaved by angiotensin-converting enzyme (ACE) to form active angiotensin II (AII). AII, a potent vasoconstrictor, increases peripheral vascular resistance and causes an increase in systolic BP. AII also has direct kidney effects that result in salt and water retention and stimulates adrenal aldosterone release. Increased aldosterone causes renal tubular absorption of sodium and results in water retention. Ultimately, extracellular volume and BP increase [7].

Natriuretic peptides are important in both BP and fluid balance. Physiologically, atrial NP (ANP) and B-type NP (BNP) function as a counter-regulatory arm to the renin–angiotensin system in regard to BP and volume maintenance. Three types of natriuretic peptides are recognized. ANP is primarily secreted from the atria. BNP is secreted mainly from the cardiac ventricle. Finally, C-type natriuretic peptide (CNP) is localized in the endothelium. The clinical effects of NPs are vasodilation, natriuresis, decreasing levels of endothelin, and inhibition of both the renin–angiotensin–aldosterone system and the sympathetic nervous system. BNP is synthesized as a prohormone, which is cleaved to inactive N-terminal pro-BNP, with a half-life of approximately 2 hours, and physiologically active BNP with a half-life of about 20 minutes [8].

Although BNP was named "brain natriuretic peptide" because it was first identified in porcine brain [9], in humans the dominant source is myocardial. BNP is secreted and stored in cardiac ventricular membrane granule [9]. BNP is continuously released from the heart in response to both volume expansion and pressure overload [10].

BNP is cleared by three pathways: a protein receptor, neutral endopeptidases, and to a lesser extent, the kidney [11]. Both ANP and BNP have natriuretic and diuretic characteristics that increase sodium and water excretion by increasing glomerular filtration rate and inhibiting renal sodium resorption [12]. They also decrease aldosterone and renin secretion, causing both a reduction in blood pressure and extracellular fluid volume [8–12]. Circulating BNP levels increase in direct proportion to HF severity, as based on the New York Heart Association (NYHA) classification, and BNP is detectable even with minimal clinical symptoms. Physiologically, there is a correlation between BNP concentrations and LV end diastolic pressure (LVEDP). This suggests that the natriuretic effects, coupled with neurohormonal antagonism, serve to counterbalance fluid overload and elevated ventricular wall tension [12]. There is also an inverse correlation between BNP and LV function after acute MI. Elevated BNP occurs in the setting of raised atrial or pulmonary wedge pressures, or MI [12]. Ultimately, BNP measurement offers an independent assessment of ventricular function without the use of intravascular pressure monitoring.

Clinical features of decompensated heart failure

HF may present after myocardial infarction as the result of acute pump dysfunction. This is the result of the loss of a critical amount of myocardial contractile ability, the consequence of which is immediate symptoms. If there is symptomatic hypotension accompanied by findings of symptoms of inadequate perfusion (eg, mental status change, decreased urine output), cardiogenic shock is diagnosed. Patients with cardiogenic shock require hemodynamic monitoring and arrangements for emergency revascularization. They are therefore inappropriate OU candidates.

HF can present precipitously, as acute pulmonary edema (APE), and also insidiously as the final consequence of a cascade of pathologic events initiated by myocardial injury or stress. After a threat to cardiac output, a cascade of neurohormonally mediated reflexes occurs. These include activation of both the renin–angiotensin–aldosterone system and the sympathetic nervous system. Consequently, the levels of these neurohormones increase and include norepinephrine, vasopressin, endothelin (the most potent vasoconstrictor known), and TNF-alpha. Although not available in routine clinical practice, these

hormone elevations are critical and correlate directly with mortality in HF patients.

Neurohormonal activation results in both sodium and water retention and an increase in systemic vascular resistance. Although these reflexes are initially compensatory and function to maintain systemic BP and perfusion, they occur at a cost of increased myocardial workload and cardiac wall tension. HF can be asymptomatic through these initial neurohormonal and hemodynamic perturbations. However, these reflexes establish the mechanism that initiates the secondary pathologic process of cardiac remodeling. Neurohormonal activation portends a worse prognosis in HF. Its attenuation forms the theoretical basis for nearly all treatments that decrease morbidity and mortality. This includes ACE inhibitors, angiotensin-receptor blockers, aldosterone antagonists, beta-blockers, and nesiritide.

Differential diagnosis

Many diseases mimic HF (Box 2). Because treatment omissions prevent optimal response, and misdirected therapy may have adverse consequences, an accurate diagnosis is important. Acute MI must always be considered as the cause of a HF visit. As many as 14% of ED HF presentations will have a troponin diagnostic for MI [13]. Furthermore, ADHF patients with elevations in troponin have markedly worse acute outcomes [14].

Additionally, because shortness of breath is the most common presenting symptom, other dyspneic conditions must be considered. A common confounder is coexisting chronic obstructive

---

Box 2. Differential diagnosis of acute heart failure

- Acute MI or myocardial ischemia
- Aortic dissection
- Chronic obstructive pulmonary disease exacerbation
- Hypoproteinemias (nephrotic syndrome, liver failure)
- Pericardial effusion
- Pneumonia
- Pneumothorax
- Pulmonary embolism
- Renal failure
- Superior vena cava syndrome
- Thyroid disease

pulmonary disease. Severe hypertension and peripheral vasoconstriction may suggest acute HF, even with audible wheezing. Pneumonia or pulmonary embolus can mimic or exacerbate HF. Finally, edema is common in HF, but is nonspecific because it is found in many hypoproteinemic states, including hepatic or renal failure, and vascular diseases.

Diagnostic evaluation

Effective HF care must begin with accurate diagnosis and be followed by expeditious treatment. Failure with either aspect will have adverse effects on outcome. Despite being common in the ED, HF is frequently misdiagnosed. This is due to the fact that the history and physical, ECG, and radiograph findings are either nonspecific or insensitive [6,15–25]. The ED misdiagnosis rate has been reported as 12%. Of these, half are patients diagnosed with HF, although their symptoms are actually the result of other pathology, and the remainder are HF patients given a different diagnosis (eg, chronic obstructive pulmonary disease) [26]. This occurs not only because of the limitations noted previously but also because the differential diagnosis of the at-risk population is complicated by many other conditions. In individual patients, even experienced physicians disagree on the diagnosis of HF, especially if the patient presents early in the disease course [10].

HF has historically been defined as a syndrome, but even with the advent of the BNP assay, clinical data are still required for an accurate diagnosis. This presents a diagnostic challenge, and various strategies have been constructed to improve diagnostic accuracy. Diagnostic criteria, such as the Framingham HF scoring systems [27], help address the challenge. However, they depend on the presence of symptoms, and so they are insensitive if the patient is asymptomatic. Consequently, the severity of illness is important when attempting to determine the presence of an HF diagnosis. In a study of patients presenting to a primary care environment, the first diagnosis of HF was falsely positive in more than 50% of cases. This misdiagnosis rate was attributed to obesity, unsuspected cardiac ischemia, and pulmonary disease [15]. Diagnostic accuracy was also affected by gender, and the rate of a correct HF diagnosis was surprisingly low at the first encounter—18% for women and 36% for men [15].

With regard to the physical diagnosis of HF, the clinical examination is poor. The best physical findings are jugular venous distention and abdominal jugular reflux (AJR), but their overall accuracy is only 81% for predicting a pulmonary capillary wedge pressure (PCWP) > 18 mm Hg. Alone, AJR has a specificity of 94%, but its sensitivity is only 24% [24]. Rales are common, but their negative predictive value is only 35% [23]. Lung sounds, peripheral edema, jugular venous distention, AJR, and the presence of extra heart sounds help to detect fluid overload, but they are either insensitive or nonspecific in those at risk for HF. Unfortunately, the easily available diagnostic tests (laboratory studies, ECG, and radiographs) are not sufficiently accurate to reliably make a correct diagnosis [16,17].

Many physicians rely on the chest radiograph (CXR) for diagnosis; however, it is an insensitive tool. In chronic HF, CXR signs of congestion have poor sensitivity and specificity for detecting a high PCWP [19]. A radiographically enlarged cardiac silhouette can help, but 20% of echocardiographically proven cardiomegaly is undetectable on radiograph [20]. Pleural effusions can also be missed by CXR, especially if the patient is intubated and the radiograph performed supine. The sensitivity, specificity, and accuracy of the supine CXR are reported as 67%, 70%, and 67%, respectively [21], with the portable CXR having even less sensitivity [22].

The determination of EF has been termed the "single most important measurement in HF" [1] and represents the standard for noninvasive ventricular function assessment. It is indicated in those without an established diagnosis of systolic dysfunction, unless performed within the previous year [1,28–30]. Although defining HF cause and type is important, there is no correlation between symptoms and EF. Consequently, EF measurement is usually unnecessary in the ED. EF may be useful in the OU to help determine treatment strategies at discharge.

B-type natriuretic peptide assays

Although a number of companies manufacture central lab BNP assay, and Roche Diagnostics produces a central lab NT-pro-BNP assay, there is currently only one point-of-care BNP assay available (Triage BNP, Biosite Diagnostics, San Diego, California). This has ramifications in the ED, where time to diagnosis has consequences for disposition decisions, as well as general ED operational efficiency. The only point-of-care assay is a fluorescent immunoassay that quantitatively measures whole blood BNP, or plasma specimens in which EDTA is the anticoagulant. It is rated as a moderately complex assay per Clinical Laboratory Improvement Amendment (1988) regulations. To perform the assay, a sample of whole blood is placed in the device, and within 15 minutes it displays the BNP concentration. Testing should not be delayed more than 30 minutes after the blood has been placed in the device. The analytic sensitivity is 5 pg/mL (95% CI 0.2 to 4.8 pg/mL) (per package insert). When this system was tested against more than 50 commonly used cardiac medications (eg, digoxin, warfarin, nitroglycerin, furosemide) and cardiac neurohormones (eg, renin, aldosterone, angiotensin I, and II, ANP), the assay demonstrated no significant measurement interference or cross-reactivity (per package insert).

B-type natriuretic peptide versus filling pressures

In a study of 72 symptomatic LV dysfunction patients with EF < 50%, BNP was an independent predictor of increased LVEDP, and BNP varied directly with changes in LVEDP [31]. In a second study, the sensitivity and specificity for predicting LVEDP > 18 mm Hg were 81% and 85%, respectively [32]. Others support that an elevated BNP is predictive of elevated end-diastolic pressures [31,33]. In decompensated HF patients, with BNP levels obtained every 2 hours during treatment, there was a correlation between PCWP and BNP changes ($r = 0.79$, $P < .05$). BNP levels dropped in parallel with a falling PCWP in response to treatment [34]. These studies suggest that BNP is an indicator of elevated intracardiac pressures and responds dynamically to ventricular volume and pressure changes.

B-type natriuretic peptide confounders

If the BNP assay is construed as only a test for HF, a number of confounders exist. In one report, approximate median BNP levels were increased two-fold in medically treated essential hypertension, three-fold in cirrhosis, and 25-fold in dialysis patients, although all measurements included significant ranges around the median [35]. Although some describe increased BNP with hypertension [36], others have not duplicated this finding unless there was coexistent LV hypertrophy [37]. Therefore, isolated hypertension is probably not associated with elevated BNP unless

there is coexistent LV hypertrophy. BNP is also elevated in a number of other conditions. The elderly can have elevated BNP, and there is good correlation between BNP, age, and LV mass index [38]. In a study of 72 healthy 85 year olds [37], compared with 105 healthy 40-year-old men, the older cohort had a mean BNP level of 24.8 pg/mL, compared with a level of 4 pg/mL in the younger group ($P < .05$). BNP may be elevated in the elderly because of greater ventricular mass as compared with the young [39].

BNP is also elevated in renal failure. It is unclear if this results from volume overload–related BNP elevation or a decrease in BNP clearance. In a study of 32 hemodialysis patients without overt HF, BNP was markedly increased. The predialysis BNP was 688 pg/mL, decreasing to 617 pg/mL after dialysis, although mean BNP levels were higher if the EF was less than 60% [40]. Studies controlling for creatinine clearance have shown that BNP has predictive utility for the diagnosis of HF, and some have suggested using a higher cutpoint of 200 pg/mL for BNP indicating HF [41].

Other causes of non-HF BNP elevation include conditions that result from predominately right ventricular dysfunction. In these situations, BNP can be elevated and may be helpful for determining both diagnosis and prognosis. BNP appears to be elevated in ventricular dysfunction, irrespective if left or right, and independent of the cause of the dysfunction. Although there are limited data to date, this also suggests that BNP may be elevated in other causes of right-sided heart strain (eg, a large pulmonary embolus).

Recent literature has addressed the potential for false-negative BNP levels. Some have reported a negative relationship between body mass index and BNP levels [42]. In the ambulatory care setting, both symptomatic and asymptomatic patients with chronic, stable systolic HF may present with a wide range of plasma BNP levels [43]. Clinical impression, in addition to confirmatory testing, is necessary to interpret the results of BNP testing accurately.

Diagnosis

BNP is markedly elevated over baseline in symptomatic HF. Data from several studies [10,44,45] indicate that its sensitivity for diagnosing HF is from 85% to 97%, with a specificity of 84% to 92%. The positive predictive value is 70% to 95% [10,26], and the negative predictive value consistently exceeds 90% [26,46]. In 250 Veterans Administration dyspneic urgent care patients, BNP was an accurate predictor of the presence of HF. In this trial, the mean BNP in HF was 1076 ± 138 pg/mL, versus 38 ± 4 pg/mL among non–HF patients. Using a cut point of 100 pg/mL, BNP provided sensitivity, specificity, and positive and negative predictive values of 94%, 94%, 92%, and 96%, respectively [26]. In this study, 30 patients were misdiagnosed clinically. In 15 patients diagnosed as having HF, although later proven to have another diagnosis, the mean BNP was 46 ± 13 pg/mL. In the 15 erroneously given non–HF diagnoses, their mean BNP was 732 ± 337 pg/mL. BNP levels also were indicative of being hospitalized; those requiring hospitalization had a mean levels of 700 pg/mL, compared with those who were discharged who had a mean BNP of 254 pg/mL [26].

Similar results were found in the larger Breathing Not Proper trial, which studied 1586 ED patients short of breath. Using a cut point of 100 pg/mL, BNP had a diagnostic accuracy for HF of 83.4%, and the negative predictive value was 96.0% at a cut point of 50 pg/mL [47].

Although excellent for excluding the diagnosis of HF, BNP is only moderately accurate at determining HF type. It predicts systolic dysfunction with a sensitivity and specificity of 83% and 77%, respectively, compared with PSF, for which the sensitivity and specificity were 85% and 70%, respectively [32]. Compared with PSF, systolic HF had higher levels; 362 pg/mL, as compared with 137 pg/mL ($P = .03$) [48]. The receiver operating characteristic (ROC) AUC for BNP detecting HF was 0.92, ($P < .0001$). Although BNP is a good predictor of the presence of HF, it does not accurately predict EF.

Once a baseline BNP is established, serial measures may suggest therapeutic response. In a study of HF patients receiving carvedilol, there was a correlation ($r = 0.698$, $P < .01$) between improving EF and a declining BNP [49]. In a report of malignant hypertension, therapy-associated LV hypertrophy regression was associated with decreasing BNP levels [50]. Sequential BNP measurements may have an application for monitoring therapeutic response.

Prognosis

In decompensated HF, serial BNP measurement may predict outcomes. In a group who died or was readmitted to the hospital within 30 days after receiving inpatient treatment for HF, 52% had an increasing BNP during hospitalization. This compares to the group without readmission or death, in which 84% had a declining BNP during hospitalization [42]. This suggests that therapy-induced BNP changes can predict outcome in decompensated HF.

In the outpatient setting, BNP can reflect HF severity and prognosis [51]. In 290 NYHA class I or II HF patients, with a mean EF of 37%, followed for 812 days, an initial BNP > 56 pg/mL was an independent predictor of HF progression and mortality [52]. Others corroborate BNP predicting cardiovascular mortality. In a 1-year study, an elevated BNP was a better predictor of cardiovascular mortality than age, ANP, EF, PCWP, gender, HF etiology, or NYHA class [53]. An elevated BNP predicts greater mortality and morbidity for HF patients, and this relation is independent of underlying CAD.

N-terminal pro-B-type natriuretic peptide

N-terminal pro-BNP (pro-BNP) is a synthetic BNP precursor. Like BNP, pro-BNP originates primarily from the ventricular myocardium and is released as a result of ventricular stress from either pressure or volume overload. On a molecular basis, pro-BNP is about twice the size of BNP and has a half-life of 1 to 2 hours. According to manufacturer (Roche Diagnostics, San Diego, California) recommendations, the pro-BNP assay has two diagnostic cut points based on age, 125 pg/mL if <75 years and 450 pg/mL if >75 years of age. Only recently available, there are relatively few data guiding the clinician in the clinical use of pro-BNP. One trial directly compared pro-BNP and BNP for predicting EF [54]. They found that while both assays had similar performance, neither was adequately sensitive or specific for clinical EF prediction. In evaluating the development of HF in post-MI patients, pro-BNP had a 97% sensitivity for predicting an EF < 45%, if levels were determined between 3 and 5 days post-MI. Accuracy of predicting post-MI ventricular dysfunction is similar between pro-BNP and BNP, but the level must be obtained later after presentation if using pre-BNP.

Differences between the two assays include that, unlike BNP, biologically inert pro-BNP is not confounded by concurrent nesiritide infusion and, therefore, pro-BNP measurement can be performed accurately during its infusion. Because four half-lives are needed to reach steady state, pro-BNP levels reflect hemodynamics from 6 to 8 hours prior. To make the same determination with BNP, because of its much shorter half-life, a nesiritide infusion must be withheld for 90 minutes so that endogenous BNP levels reflect the hemodynamic state rather than infused BNP. Finally, while BNP is available on a point-of-care platform, pro-BNP is only currently available on a central lab platform.

Clinical use of B-type natriuretic peptide assays

In ED HF patients, an elevated BNP suggests future adverse cardiac events [55] and, when considered with clinical impression, may help in selecting candidates for OU HF therapy. BNP is most useful for excluding HF in those conditions where the differential would normally suggest HF. This includes undiagnosed patients with any of the classic signs or symptoms of HF (shortness of breath dyspnea on exertion, orthopnea, dependent edema, and physical examination findings of a cardiac S3, jugular venous distention, or basilar rales). In this scenario, a normal BNP should prompt the consideration of an alternative diagnosis.

Because non–HF conditions can result in an elevated BNP, the clinical context of a positive BNP must be considered. A positive BNP suggests the need for routine tests to confirm the diagnosis, as well as evaluation of the cause and definition of the type of HF (eg, ECG, CXR, and echocardiogram). See Box 3 for suggested approach to the use of the BNP assay.

BNP is also used to monitor chronic HF, because levels correlate with treatment efficacy. After HF exacerbation, a declining BNP indicates a good response to therapy and portends a more favorable outcome. A rising BNP suggests a greater risk of adverse outcome, and a more aggressive treatment strategy may be warranted.

Emergency department management

General support

The initial approach is based on the acuity of presentation, volume status, and systemic perfusion. In critical patients, airway management overrides all other interventions. This is in contrast to minimally symptomatic patient whose evaluation may occur in lieu of stabilization procedures. Initial stabilization is aimed at maintaining airway control and adequate ventilation.

Box 3. Interpretation of B-type natriuretic peptide (BNP) assays

- Low BNP (< 100 pg/mL)
- Presenting symptoms are unlikely the result of HF, an alternative diagnosis should be considered (eg, chronic obstructive pulmonary disease).
- Intermediate BNP (100 to 500 pg/mL)
- Consider other diagnoses (Cor pulmonale, pulmonary embolism, primary pulmonary hypertension).
- Compare with prior baseline BNP levels.
- High BNP (> 500 pg/mL)
- HF is the likely diagnosis, although confounders should be considered.

Supplemental oxygen can be given based on pulse oximetry. As the consequences of hypoxia are of greater significance than the potential for hypercarbia, O_2 is not withheld based on CO_2 retention concerns. Arterial blood gases may be helpful in the critically ill or if CO_2 retention is likely.

Because patients with HF do not hemodynamically tolerate hypertension, it is desirable to maintain the BP as low as is consistent with the ability to mentate, urinate, and ambulate. Chronic systolic BPs in the 90 mm Hg range are usually well tolerated by the HF patient. In the hypertensive acute pulmonary edema patient, a controlled lowering of BP may result in a profound improvement of symptoms and dyspnea.

Noninvasive positive pressure ventilation (NPPV) is controversial. Some report it may be used to prevent endotracheal intubation in the properly selected patient while awaiting hemodynamic interventions to become effective. Biphasic positive pressure ventilation (BiPAP) requires the delivery of separately controlled inspiratory and expiratory pressures via facemask. Continuous positive airway pressure (CPAP) provides constant pressure throughout the respiratory cycle. For a trial of NPPV, close cardiac monitoring, relative hemodynamic stability, and patient cooperation are needed. NPPV may provide mortality benefit over invasive mechanical ventilation in chronic obstructive pulmonary disease, but the data are controversial in APE. In APE the use of NPPV may decrease the rate of endotracheal intubation, but mortality is unchanged and CPAP patients may have higher rates of MI than those treated with BiPAP [56]. Patients requiring PPV or more than 2 L per nasal cannula supplemental oxygen are not good OU candidates.

Intravenous (IV) access is needed in all with HF exacerbation. This is because electrolyte abnormalities may occur from aggressive diuretic therapy, and HF patients are at risk for ventricular arrhythmia. In both scenarios, prompt therapy can be needed. Limitations notwithstanding, all suspected HF patients should have a chest radiograph to help exclude other confounding diagnoses and provide confirmatory evidence of HF. Underlying coronary artery disease is the most common cause of HF in the United States; therefore, until stability is determined, all suspected HF patients need initial continuous ECG monitoring, a 12-lead ECG, and cardiac biomarker testing. Additionally, a search for the other HF precipitants is needed (Box 4).

Diuresis causes abnormalities in K+, Na+, blood urea nitrogen, and creatinine, undetectable by history or examination, so these should be evaluated. A complete blood count is needed to check for anemia. With hepatomegaly resulting from passive congestion, liver enzymes can exclude other pathologies. Elevated lactate levels may identify unsuspected cardiogenic shock, and testing for drug levels (eg, digoxin) is guided by presentation. Occasionally ethanol and drug screening may be needed. Assessment of the Mg^{2+} level is considered when there is cardiac arrhythmia and if severe or treatment-resistant hypokalemia occurs. Finally, selective foley catheterization

---

Box 4. Common causes of heart failure decompensation

- Atrial fibrillation
- Acute MI
- Chronic nonsteroidal anti-inflammatory drug use
- Excessive alcohol
- Endocrine abnormalities (eg, diabetes, hyperthyroidism)
- Infection
- Negative inotropic medications
- Noncompliance (diet, medication)
- Suboptimal pharmacologic management
- Obesity
- Uncontrolled hypertension

---

may be used to monitor fluid status or if urine output is sufficient to interfere with the patient's ability to rest.

Benefits of early therapy

All patients not being discharged from the ED should receive therapy while still in the ED. The reasons for this are two-fold. Treatments delayed until inpatient arrival are not received by the patient for many hours Second, optimal ED HF outcomes are directly related to time to treatment.

The Acute Decompensated HF National Registry (ADHERE) is a multicenter database that records data from episodes of hospitalizations in patients discharged after an inpatient stay for acutely decompensated HF. Using data from 46,599 hospitalizations from this registry [57], patients were stratified as to where IV vasoactive therapy was started. Vasoactive therapy was defined as the receipt of an intravenous agent that would be administered to effect a change in hemodynamics (eg, dopamine, dobutamine, nitroglycerin, nesiritide). Of the cohort receiving vasoactives, 4096 received them in the ED, compared with 3499 whose treatment was delayed until arrival on the inpatient unit. Patients treated in the ED received the vasoactive agent much sooner (1.1 versus 22.2 hrs), had reduced lengths of stay (4.5 versus 7.0 days), and lower mortality (4.3 versus 10.9%) than those whose treatment was delayed until arrival on the inpatient unit.

An experienced emergency physician usually knows within minutes which patients will need inhospital admission.. When the requirement for HF admission is identified, the early use of vasoactive therapy is indicated. In the minority of HF patients for whom ED treatment may result in discharge home, a limited trial (2 to 3 hours) of intermittent diuretic bolus therapy may be appropriate.

Identifying candidates for the observation unit

The OU is an effective treatment option for many diseases requiring a short period of intensive therapy or diagnostic evaluation. Patients with a HF exacerbation usually require longer than the short treatment course possible in the ED; consequently, many are OU candidates for additional therapy. Relief of congestion is the most common rate-limiting step preventing discharge. In the past, most HF patients were simply admitted for inpatient therapy. Because most will have insufficient diuresis for relief of congestion in the ED, the OU offers an opportunity for longer therapies and may prevent the necessity of an inpatient admission [58].

The OU provides safe and effective therapy for the appropriately selected HF patients. In a retrospective study of decompensated HF [59], post-discharge revisit rates for OU patients treated for 24 hours, compared with inpatients discharged within 24 hours, were superior in the OU cohort. In the OU group, there were no return visits within 1 week of admission compared with a revisit rate of 8% in the hospitalized group. By 1 month, only 8% of the OU patients had a revisit, versus 16% of the inpatient group. There were no mortality differences between the groups ($P > .05$). This study suggested that OU treatment is at least as safe and effective as a similar period of inpatient hospitalization.

Patient selection before OU consideration is important. If a patient has a high likelihood of HF, with pulmonary or systemic congestion, and meets the entry criteria listed in Box 5, OU admission may be appropriate. Because OU treatment is temporally restricted, with lower nursing–patient staffing ratios, and has limited invasive monitoring capability, careful patient selection is necessary to ensure that admissions are appropriate for the available level of care. Exclusion criteria, designed to prevent admissions in those with needs exceeding OU resources, are listed in Box 6 [58]. Patients with airway instability, a high probability of adverse outcome (eg, acute MI), and those with hemodynamics suggestive of critical underlying pathology should be excluded.

Like acute coronary syndromes, patients with decompensated HF represent a spectrum of presentation that must be sorted to determine appropriate OU admission. Although there are very few analyses to define the best OU candidate, the exclusion of patients with excess risk is important. An analysis of the ADHERE registry [60] provides several mortality predictors that should exclude patients from consideration of OU admission. The most of important of these predictors is the BUN. Patients with a BUN exceeding 43 mg/dL have markedly increased inpatient mortality (8.98%) compared with those with a lower BUN (2.68%). Further refining the risk stratification process, in the cohort of patients

---

Box 5. Heart failure observation unit: inclusion criteria

- Adequate systemic perfusion
- Evidence of hemodynamic stability
-Heart rate > 50 and < 130 beats/min
-Systolic BP > 90 and < 175 mm Hg
-Oxygen saturation > 90%
- No evidence of acute ischemia/ infarction by electrocardiogram or cardiac markers
- Chest radiograph findings compatible with the diagnosis of HF
- B-type natriuretic peptide > 100 pg/mL

Box 6. Heart failure observation unit: exclusion criteria[a]

- Unstable vital signs (despite emergency department therapy):
-Systolic BP > 220, Diastolic BP > 120 mm Hg
-Respiratory rate > 25 /min
-Heart rate > 130 beats/min
-Temperature > 38.5°C

- Electrocardiogram or serum markers diagnostic of myocardial ischemia or infarction
- Unstable airway or oxygen requirement > 4 L/min by nasal cannula
- Evidence of cardiogenic shock or signs of end-organ hypoperfusion
- Require continuous titration of vasoactive medication (eg, nitroglycerin)
- Clinically significant cardiac arrhythmia
- Altered mental status
- Severe electrolyte imbalances
- Chronic renal failure requiring dialysis
- Peak expiratory flow rate < 50% of predicted
- Chest radiograph suggestive of pneumonia

---

[a] These criteria are meant to discourage entry by patients not likely to benefit from an aggressive diuresis and vasodilation management protocol.

with a BUN less than 43, adding systolic BP provides additional prognostic data. In this group, the addition of a systolic BP < 115 mm Hg was associated with a mortality rate of 5.49% compared with those with a higher BP whose mortality was 2.89%.

OU admission candidates should have a BUN < 43 and careful consideration if admitted with a systolic BP < 115 mm Hg.

Other studies have specifically examined OU outcome predictors for HF. In 499 patients, Diercks and colleagues [61] reported that a negative troponin and an initial systolic BP > 160 mm Hg identified a cohort who were successfully discharged within 24 hours of admission and had no death or re-hospitalization within the subsequent 30 days. Burkhardt and colleagues [62] reported in 385 OU patients that successful discharge from the OU within 24 hours of an admission for decompensated HF was predicted by an admission BUN < 30 mg/dL. These parameters may also be considered to assist in the selection of the appropriate OU candidate.

Once admitted to the OU, many different aspects of medical management are needed to assure optimal outcomes and discharge rates. Attention to the many details required for HF management [63,64] can be daunting for a physician already running a busy ED. This not only includes medication intervention and titration, but the diagnostic evaluation, patient education, and the discharge planning required by regulatory agencies. HF protocols drive treatment algorithms and provide superior outcomes, as compared with standard therapy, and ensure that required interventions are accomplished [4,58].

ED OU protocol-driven management has been shown to result in a significant improvement in outcomes, as compared with independent physician-driven care. In a before and after study of 154 decompensated OU HF patients, a prespecified management protocol resulted in significant outcome improvements [4]. Use of the protocol resulted in 90-day ED HF revisit rates declining by 56% (0.90 to 0.51, P = .0000) compared with pre-protocol management. Similarly, 90-day HF rehospitalizations decreased by 64% (0.77 to 0.50, P = .007). Lastly, 90-day mortality and OU HF readmissions decreased from 4% to 1% (P = .096), and 18% to 11% (P = .099), respectively. From a cost perspective, during the same time period, annualized hospital costs declined by nearly $100,000, predominately the result of 30-day readmission avoidance [65].

The only validated OU HF protocol published to date includes an aggressive diuretic algorithm, initiated in the ED, and continued throughout the OU stay [4,58]. In this protocol, additional diuretic use was driven by the patient's urine output. If the urine output was inadequate, inpatient admission for invasive monitoring was suggested. Additionally, ACE inhibitor algorithms encouraged physician initiation and up-titration toward target levels, provided there were no renal function contraindications, systolic blood pressure was adequate, and there was no history of ACE inhibitor intolerance. Unless there are significant contraindications (eg, anaphylaxis), all HF patients should be discharged on an ACE inhibitor [1].

The OU provides an opportunity for more extensive evaluation than can be performed in most EDs. EF measurement may be determined in those without an established diagnosis of systolic HF. This should be repeated if PSF HF was previously diagnosed, and it has been more than 1 year since the last assessment of ventricular function. The OU environment also offers the option of elective multidisciplinary consultations, not available in a busy ED, for those who may have transportation difficulties in getting to an outpatient appointment. While in the OU, the option of HF cardiology specialist consultation may help to evaluate discharge medication dosages, and screen candidates for heart transplantation listing. Other ancillary care staff may consult also. This includes dietetics and home health care. Social workers can ensure that all patients have the ability to obtain their medicines and can arrange a home environment assessment to assess the potential of other psychosocial, cultural, or economic factors that could prevent therapeutic compliance. A home health care consultation serves to ensure post-discharge follow-up care and can help arrange visiting nurse services for home bound or nonambulatory patients.

Because noncompliance causes up to 50% of HF rehospitalizations [63,64,66], patient education is a critical facet in the treatment program. Bedside teaching videotapes on HF may provide detailed education during a teachable moment for the patient. Finally, patients should be provided with HF literature, medication information, and lifestyle modification suggestions at discharge.

OU HF management not only impacts the OU, it results in changes in the inpatient HF population as well. By treating selected patients in the

OU, rather than the inpatient unit, patients are diverted to less intensive levels of care. After implementation of an OU HF management protocol, inpatient acuity as indexed by the mean number of billable procedures per HF patient, increased by 11% [65]. This provides improved resource matching between patients requiring intensive monitoring environments and those who could benefit from less costly OU care.

Therapeutic agents

HF management is a complicated task. It requires the successful interaction of many different medications, individual titration regimens, patient factors (eg, education and compliance issues), and multidisciplinary services. Clearly defined patient care management programs addressing these issues have demonstrated clinical and financial success in both the OU and outpatient environment [4,58,63–67]. A validated management protocol is provided in Box 7.

Very large trials provide evidence-based data for managing stable, systolic HF. The principal drugs are beta-blockers, ACE inhibitors, angiotensin-receptor blockers (ARBs), hydralazine/nitrates, diuretics, digoxin, and spironolactone. In general, the strategy focuses on maintaining the lowest possible BP that allows mentation, ambulation, and urination [1]. All HF patients without contraindications should be on an ACE inhibitor and beta-blocker, even in the setting of stable disease with minimal symptoms. In most diseases, therapy is driven by continuing symptoms; this is not the situation in HF because of the unique neurohormonal antagonism requirements for the treatment of HF.

The emphasis on neurohormonal antagonism in HF represents a major management shift. The relief of congestion by the use of diuretics has been the main thrust of ED therapy. Although diuretics are important for acute symptomatic congestion relief, they do not improve mortality. Very large studies evaluating the role of ACE inhibitors, beta-blockers, and other agents show neurohormonal antagonism is required for the greatest mortality improvement.

Diuretics

Initial OU HF therapeutic goals are directed at the relief of congestion by the use of IV diuretics. Recommended dosing strategies are to use up to twice the daily dose of furosemide (or its equivalent) administered as an IV bolus, to a maximum

---

Box 7. Heart failure observation unit: management protocol

- Standardized orders (algorithm)
- Diuretics
- Neurohormonal antagonist (angiotensin-converting enzym inhibitors or nesiritide)

- Aggressive fluid management monitoring
- Admission weights, input/output
- Fluid restriction, low-sodium diet

- Diagnostic testing
- Standing orders for measurement and correction of potassium and magnesium
- Electrocardiogram and cardiac injury markers
- Echocardiography

- Patient education
- Educational videos (living with HF, smoking cessation)
- Personalized educational material
- Nursing and physician bedside teaching
- Dietetic consultations

- Discharge planning
- Social worker, home health nurse consultation
- HF specialist consultation

---

of 180 mg to promote urine output. If a patient is not currently on a diuretic, 40 mg of furosemide is usually adequate [4,58,59,65,68]. Urine output and serum electrolytes are monitored to track diuresis volume and to screen for treatment-induced hypokalemia. If target urine outputs are not met, the diuretic dose is doubled and repeated at 2 hours. Adequate output should exceed 500 cc within 2 hours, unless the creatinine exceeds 2.5 mg/dL. With elevated creatinine, 2-hour urine output goals are halved. Failure to meet output goals suggests inpatient hospitalization may be needed [4,58,59,65,68].

Diuretics prevent hospitalization and provide symptomatic relief. They are indicated for all patients with congestive findings, but not as chronic monotherapy (diuretics should be combined with ACE inhibitors and beta-blockers) because alone they provide no mortality benefit [1,5,27,29]. With aggressive diuresis, potassium supplementation is frequently required. However, if loop diuretics are used in concert with nesiritide, potassium supplements are less often needed. Standing orders for oral or IV potassium supplementation with the goal of maintaining a K^+ between 4.0 and 5.0 meq/dL may be useful.

Magnesium is an important cofactor for myocardial function and should be supplemented if the patient is deficient. Give magnesium if the creatinine is < 1.5 mg/dL; otherwise, therapy should be individualized. Magnesium may be given as 140 mg magnesium oxide orally once.

Limited data suggest that combining loop diuretics treatment with IV vasoactive agents has benefit. In 1442 patients from 42 hospitals, patients receiving intermittent IV bolus therapy (eg, furosemide bolus) of any type while in the ED had a mean hospitalization LOS of 9.9 days. This compared with an LOS of 6.6 days ($P = .004$) for those treated with IV infusion therapy (eg, nesiritide or nitroglycerin) while still in the ED. In this registry analysis, early infusion therapy with a vasoactive agent, as opposed to intermittent bolus therapy, was associated with a significantly shorter hospital LOS [57].

Vasodilators

Certain vasodilators have the potential to provide both symptomatic improvement and mortality reduction in HF. Although hemodynamic improvements are the direct result of the effect on the vascular tree, mortality improvements in long-term outcomes are not a universal feature of all vasodilators. For mortality reduction to occur, the vasodilator must also have the characteristic of neurohormonal antagonism directed at the pathologic hormonal excesses of HF [69–72]. With regard to specific agents, ACE inhibitors, with both vasodilation and neurohormonal antagonistic effects, represent a class of medications with a mortality reduction benefit of such magnitude that all HF patients deserve a therapeutic trial [1,29,5,69–72]. ARBs, predicted to have similar physiologic effects as ACE inhibitors, may have fewer side effects than ACE inhibitors. However, as the preponderance of the current mortality reduction data uses ACEI, they should be replaced by ARBs only if

significant intolerance or a contraindication to the ACE inhibitor exists [1,29].

Improvement of hemodynamic parameters in the acutely decompensated HF patient, reflected by improvements in vital signs and in the clinical presentation of dyspnea, may be obtained with the use of intravenous vasodilators. The appropriate candidate usually has a blood pressure in excess of 90 mm Hg and no contraindications to vasodilation. Vasodilation can result in hypotension in selected populations, including those conditions where there is either an impediment to outflow (eg, aortic stenosis), situations where cardiac output depends on adequate or elevated pre-load (eg, right ventricular infarct, pericardial tamponade), or when preload is already abnormally decreased (eg, volume depletion).

Because their optimal use in HF requires invasive monitoring, nitroprusside and nitroglycerin are generally discouraged from use in the OU environment. Conversely, nesiritide, which can be used safely and efficaciously without invasive hemodynamic monitoring, is permissible in the OU.

Nesiritide is an IV medication for the treatment of decompensated HF. It provides hemodynamic [73,74] and clinical benefits [75–77] from the combination of vasodilation [78], natriuresis, and neurohormonal antagonism [78]. It has been shown to decrease costs and hospital readmissions [79] and lower 6-month mortality as compared with dobutamine [75,76]. Compared with nitroglycerin, nesiritide improves dyspnea and hemodynamics more rapidly and to a greater extent [77]. Nesiritide is appropriate for use in the ED OU. Once stabilized in the ED, patients on the recommended fixed dose of nesiritide (2 μg/kg IV bolus, then a 0.01 μg/kg infusion) are candidates for OU admission.

The Proaction Trial was a multicenter, double-blind, randomized, placebo-controlled safety and efficacy trial of standard OU therapy, with and without nesiritide [80]. In this trial, OU patients with acute decompensated HF and receiving standard therapy were treated with at least 12 hours of either standard dose-blinded nesiritide or placebo. In the safety analysis, there were no differences in adverse outcomes between the standard care and nesiritide cohorts. NYHA class III or IV HF patients receiving nesiritide had a 29% decrease in revisit rates ($P = .057$). Days in the hospital in the month after study entry were markedly lower in patients receiving nesiritide compared with standard therapy (2.5 versus 6.5, respectively; $P = .03$).

Digoxin

Similar to diuretics, digoxin decreases hospitalizations but does not alter mortality. It is recommended for LV systolic dysfunction and rate control in atrial fibrillation [1,5,29]. Toxicity manifests as cardiac arrhythmia (heart block, ectopy, or re-entrant rhythms), gastrointestinal symptoms, or neurologic complaints (eg, visual disturbances and confusion). Serum levels can suggest toxicity if they exceed 2.0 ng/mL, but toxicity can also occur at lower levels if there is coexistent hypokalemia or hypomagnesemia. Digoxin should be used at a dose of 0.125 to 0.250 mg daily [1,5,29].

Beta-blockers

Beta-blockers prolong life in HF patients [81–85] but should only be initiated if the patient is hemodynamically stable [1,29]. They should not be started in decompensated HF; consequently, this generally precludes OU initiation. Conversely, abruptly stopping a beta-blocker has the potential to worsen hemodynamics. Recommended therapy for decompensated HF patients presenting to the ED while on a beta-blocker is to hold the dose or continue it at one dosing level lower than the maintenance dose. If inotropes are required, the beta-blocker may be withheld [1,29]. Patients at this stage of their disease are not usually ideal OU candidates.

Aldosterone antagonists

The aldosterone antagonist spironolactone decreases the relative risk of mortality in end stage HF [86]. These patients should receive 12.5 to 25.0 mg qid [1,29]. It is not recommend if the creatinine exceeds 2.5 mg/dL or the K+ is > 5.0 mEq/L. If a patient is already on an aldosterone antagonist, it should be continued in OU patients.

Anticoagulants

The risk of thromboembolism in the clinically stable HF outpatient is low, estimated at 1% to 3% per year, and is greatest patients with the lowest EF [87,88]. However, hospitalized HF patients are at significant risk for sustaining deep vein thrombosis (DVT) and its complications. In the MEDENOX (prophylaxis in MEDical patients with ENOXaparin) study of hospitalized patients, subcutaneous enoxaparin decreased venographically documented DVT, from 14.9% in the placebo group to 5.5% in the 40-mg every day enoxaparin prophylaxis group [89]. Empiric

DVT prevention in hospitalized, bedridden HF patients must be balanced against the relatively low risk of complications associated with anticoagulant prophylaxis. The precise value of prophylactic anticoagulation has never been reported in ED OU HF management. However, as it is anticipated that this cohort of patients will be discharged in a relatively limited time frame, anticoagulation is usually not performed.

Other agents

Calcium channel blockers (CCBs) are not routinely recommended in HF [1,90]. This is because short-term use may result in pulmonary edema and cardiogenic shock, whereas in the long-term, they may increase the risk of worsening HF and death [91–94]. These adverse effects have been attributed to the negative inotropic effects of CCBs. If necessary, amlodipine, the CCB with no clear adverse mortality effect, may be used for compelling clinical reasons (eg, as an anti-anginal agent despite maximal therapy with nitrates and beta-blockers).

Nonsteroidal anti-inflammatory drugs should be avoided in HF [1,90]. They inhibit the effects of diuretics and ACE inhibitors and can worsen cardiac and renal function [1].

HF is an important risk factor for sudden cardiac death, and its likelihood increases in proportion to the decrease in EF and HF severity [95]. Premature ventricular contractions occur in 95% of dilated cardiomyopathy patients, and nonsustained VT may be seen in up to 30% to 40% of cases. Prophylactic administration of anti-arrhythmics is not effective and may actually increase mortality [96]. Therefore, their routine use to suppress asymptomatic ventricular arrhythmias is not warranted.

Observation unit disposition

OU patients may be discharged at any time, once there has been a good therapeutic response. Although there are very few studies that have determined predictors of successful ED discharge, a net volume output of greater than 1 L is associated with a higher rate of successful discharge from the ED OU [68].

Discharge criteria may aid in selecting candidates who may be sent home (Box 8). Most important in the disposition determination is the clinical assessment, but a post-treatment BNP level can help to guide this decision. If nesiritide

---

Box 8. Heart failure observation unit: discharge guidelines[a]

- Patient reports subjective improvement.
- If normally ambulatory, able to do so without significant orthostasis.
- Resting heart rate < 100 beats/min; Systolic BP > 80 mm Hg.
- Total urine output > 1 L, and urine output > 30 cc/h (or > 0.5 cc/kg/h).
- Room air oxygen saturation > 90% (unless on home oxygen).
- No angina.
- No electrocardiogram or cardiac marker evidence of myocardial ischemia/infarction.
- No new clinically significant arrhythmia.
- Normal electrolyte profile without increasing azotemia.

---

[a] Patients not meeting all of the guidelines should be considered for inpatient treatment (except as appropriate in the end-stage palliative care cohort).

---

has been used, it will be necessary to stop its infusion at least 4 half-lives (90 minutes) before its measurement.

Successful discharge of HF patients after an OU treatment course requires the coordination of a multimedication regimen that includes diuretics, digoxin, ACE inhibitors (or ARBs), and possibly spironolactone, and beta-blockers. Optimally, medications are adjusted to meet target-dosing recommendations [1,5,29]. Therefore, close consultation with the physician who will ultimately manage the outpatient course is necessary to provide the best outcomes. An aggressive management protocol may anticipate the discharge of approximately 75% of OU HF patients [4,58,59,65].

Discharge planning is critical in HF. A multidisciplinary team approach can produce significant improvements in HF outcomes by decreasing revisit rates, lowering inpatient length of stay, and reducing hospitalization costs [4,58,59,65,67, 97–100]. The team approach should provide the option of outpatient consultations with social work, dietetics, cardiology, and advance practice

nurses. Because noncompliance is estimated to cause 50% of HF re-hospitalizations [60,63, 64,66], patient education is a critical facet to be addressed during OU treatment.

Disposition from the OU is predicated on the relief of dyspnea, improvement of congestion without long-suffering orthostasis, and discharge to an adequate outpatient environment. If these goals cannot be met, inpatient hospitalization or placement in an assisted-living facility should be considered. Approximately 25% [4,58,59,65] of HF patients will require inpatient hospitalization after a 24-hour OU admission. Patients not meeting discharge criteria by the 24-hour OU LOS limit require inpatient admission. A lower threshold for admission is appropriate in the very elderly, those with poor social situations, and those with multiple co-morbidities. Even patients requiring admission after an OU stay derive a measurable benefit from its use. In patients admitted from the OU after failure of therapy, the mean hospitalization LOS, inclusive of their OU time, was 0.8 days less than patients admitted directly from the ED to the inpatient unit [4].

References

[1] Packer M, Cohn JN. Consensus recommendations for the management of chronic heart failure. Am J Cardiol 1999;83(2A):1A–38A.

[2] Massie BM, Shah NB. Evolving trends in epidemiologic factors of heart failure: rationale for preventative strategies and comprehensive disease management. Am Heart J 1997;133:703–12.

[3] CMS 2001 in-patient discharge data base: MEDPAR, DRG 427.

[4] Peacock WF 4th, Remer EE, Aponte J, et al. Effective observation unit treatment of decompensated heart failure. Congest Heart Fail 2002;8:68–73.

[5] USDHHS: Heart failure: evaluation and care of patients with left-ventricular systolic dysfunction (Clinical Practice Guideline, Number 11, AHCPR publication No. 94–0612). US Department of Health and Human Services, Washington, DC, June, 1994.

[6] Marantz PR, Tobin JN, Wassertheil-Smoller S, et al. The relationship between left ventricular systolic function and congestive heart failure diagnosed by clinical criteria. Circulation 1988;77: 607–12.

[7] Hobbs RE, Czerska MD. Congestive heart failure. Current and future strategies to decrease mortality. Postgrad Med 1994;96:167–72.

[8] Clemens LE, Almirez RG, Baudouin KA, et al. Pharmacokinetics and biological actions of

subcutaneously administered human brain natri-uretic peptide. J Pharmacol Exp Ther 1998;87: 67–71.

[9] Nakao K, Mukoyama M, Hosoda K, et al. Biosyn-thesis, secretion, and receptor selectivity of human brain natriuretic peptide. Can J Physiol Pharmacol 1991;59:1500–6.

[10] Cowie MR, Struthers AD, Wood DA, et al. Value of natriuretic peptides in assessment of patients with possible new heart failure in primary care. Lancet 1997;350:1349–53.

[11] Mair J, Thomas S, Puschendorf B. Natriuretic pep-tides in assessment of left-ventricular dysfunction. Scan J Clin Invest 1999;9(Suppl 230):132–42.

[12] Struthers AD. Ten years of natriuretic peptide re-search: a new dawn for their diagnostic and thera-peutic use? BMJ 1994;308:1615–9.

[13] Peacock WF, Emerman CL, Doleh M, et al. The in-cidence of elevated cardiac enzymes in decompen-sated heart failure. Acad Emerg Med 2001;5:552.

[14] Peacock WF, DeMarco T, Emerman CL, Wynne J. Heart failure with an elevated troponin is associated with increased morbidity and mortality: an AD-HERE registry analysis. Ann Emerg Med 2004; 44(4):S72.

[15] Remes J, Miettinen H, Reunanen A, et al. Validity of clinical diagnosis of heart failure in primary health care. Eur Heart J 1991;12:315–21.

[16] Stevenson LW. The limited availability of physical signs for estimating hemodynamics in chronic heart failure. JAMA 1998;261:884–8.

[17] Davis AP, Francis CM, Love MP, et al. Value of the electrocardiogram in identifying heart failure due to left ventricular systolic dysfunction. Br Med J 1996;312:222.

[18] Marantz PR, Kaplan MC, Alderman MH. Clinical diagnosis of congestive heart failure in patients with acute dyspnea. Chest 1990;97:776–81.

[19] Chakko S, Woska D, Marinez H, et al. Clinical, radiographic, and hemodynamic correlations in chronic congestive heart failure: conflicting results may lead to inappropriate care. Am J Med 1991; 90:353–9.

[20] Kono T, Suwa M, Hanada H, et al. Clinical signif-icance of normal cardiac silhouette in dilated cardiomyopathy; evaluation based upon echocar-diography and magnetic resonance imaging. Jpn Circ J 1992;56:359–65.

[21] Ruskin JA, Gurney JW, Thorsen MK, et al. Detec-tion of pleural effusions on supine chest radio-graphs. AJR Am J Roentgenol 1987;148:681–3.

[22] Chait A, Cohen HE, Meltzer LE, et al. The bedside chest radiograph in the evaluation of incipient heart failure. Radiology 1972;105:563–6.

[23] Butman SM, Ewy GA, Standen JR, et al. Bedside cardiovascular examination in patients with severe chronic heart failure: importance of resting or in-ducible jugular venous distention. J Am Coll Car-diol 1993;22:968–74.

[24] Marantz PR, Kaplan MC, Alderman MH. Clinical diagnosis of congestive heart failure in patients with acute dyspnea. Circulation 1993;88:107–15.

[25] Peacock WF, Kies P, Albert NM, et al. Bioimpe-dance monitoring for detecting pulmonary fluid in heart failure: equal to chest radiography? Congest Heart Fail 2000;6:86–9.

[26] Dao Q, Krishnaswamy P, Kazanegra R, et al. Util-ity of B-type natriuretic peptide in the diagnosis of congestive heart failure in an urgent-care setting. J Am Coll Cardiol 2001;37:379–85.

[27] McKee PA, Castelli WP, McNamara PM, et al. The natural history of congestive heart failure: The Framingham Study. N Engl J Med 1971;285: 1441–6.

[28] Francis CM, Caruana L, Kearney P, et al. Open ac-cess echocardiography in management of heart fail-ure in the community. BMJ 1995;310:634–6.

[29] ACC/AHA. ACC/AHA guidelines for the evalua-tion and management of chronic heart failure in the adult. [Cited March 18, 2002]. Avail-able from: http://www.acc.org/clinical/guidelines/failure/I_introduction.

[30] Wheeldon NM, MacDonald TM, Flucker CJ, et al. Echocardiography in chronic heart failure in the community. Q J Med 1993;86:255–61.

[31] Maeda K, Tsutamoto T, Wada A, et al. Plasma brain natriuretic peptide as a biochemical marker of high left ventricular end-diastolic pressure in patients with symptomatic left ventricular dysfunc-tion. Am Heart J 1998;135:825–32.

[32] Yamamoto K, Burnett JC, Jougasaki M, et al. Su-periority of brain natriuretic peptide as a humoral marker of ventricular systolic and diastolic dys-function and ventricular hypertrophy. Hyperten-sion 1996;28:988–94.

[33] Omland T, Aakvaag A, Bonarjee V, et al. Plasma brain natriuretic peptide as an indicator of left ven-tricular systolic function and long-term survival after acute myocardial infarction. Comparison with plasma atrial natriuretic peptide and N-termi-nal proatrial natriuretic peptide. Circulation 1996; 93:1963–9.

[34] Kazanegra R, Cheng V, Garcia A, et al. A rapid test for B-type natriuretic peptide correlates with falling wedge pressures in patients treated for decompen-sated heart failure: a pilot study. J Card Fail 2001;7:21–9.

[35] Jensen KT, Carstens J, Ivarsen P, et al. A new, fast and reliable radioimmunoassay of brain na-triuretic peptide in human plasma. Reference val-ues in healthy subjects and in patients with different diseases. Scand J Clin Lab Invest 1997; 57:529–40.

[36] Buckley MG, Markandu ND, Miller MA, et al. Plasma concentrations and comparisons of brain and atrial natriuretic peptide in normal subjects and in patients with essential hypertension. J Hum Hypertens 1993;3:345–50.

[37] Wallen T, Landahl T, Herner T, et al. Brain natriuretic peptide in an elderly population. J Intern Med 1997;242:307–11.

[38] Sayama H, Nakamura Y, Saito N, et al. Relationship between left ventricular geometry and brain natriuretic peptide levels in elderly subjects. Gerontology 2000;46:71–7.

[39] Lernfelt B. Aging and left ventricular function in elderly healthy people. Am J Cardiol 1991;68:547–9.

[40] Kohse KP. Differential regulation of brain and atrial natriuretic peptides in hemodialysis patients. Clin Nephrol 1993;40:83–90.

[41] McCullough PA, Duc P, Omland T, et al. B-type natriuretic peptide and renal function in the diagnosis of heart failure: an analysis from the Breathing Not Properly Multinational Study. Am J Kidney Dis 2003;41(3):571–9.

[42] Cheng V, Kazanagra R, Garcia A, et al. A rapid bedside test for B-type peptide predicts treatment outcomes in patients admitted for decompensated heart failure: a pilot study. J Am Coll Cardiol 2001;37:386–91.

[43] Tang WH, Girod JP, Lee MJ, et al. Plasma B-type natriuretic peptide levels in ambulatory patients with established chronic symptomatic systolic heart failure. Circulation 2003;108(24):2964–6.

[44] Niinuma H, Nakamura M, Hirarnori K. Plasma B-type natriuretic peptide measurement in a multiphasic health screening program. Cardiology 1998;90:89–94.

[45] Davis M, Espiner E, Richards G, et al. Plasma brain natriuretic peptide in assessment of acute dyspnoea. Lancet 1994;343:440–4.

[46] McDonagh TA, Robb SD, Morton JJ, et al. Biochemical detection of left-ventricular systolic dysfunction. Lancet 1998;351:9–13.

[47] Maisel AS, Krishnaswamy P, Nowak RM, et al. Breathing Not Properly Multinational Study Investigators. Rapid measurement of B-type natriuretic peptide in the emergency diagnosis of heart failure. N Engl J Med 2002;347:161–7.

[48] Bettencourt P, Ferreira A, Dias P, et al. Evaluation of brain natriuretic peptide in the diagnosis of heart failure. Cardiology 2000;93:19–25.

[49] Fujimora M, Yasumura Y, Ishida Y, et al. Improvement in left ventricular function in response to carvedilol is accompanied by attenuation of neurohumoral activation in patients with dilated cardiomyopathy. J Card Fail 2000;6:3–10.

[50] Nishikimi T, Matsuoka H, Ishikawa K, et al. Antihypertensive therapy reduces increased plasma levels of adrenomedullin and brain natriuretic peptide concomitant with regression of left ventricular hypertrophy in a patient with malignant hypertension. Hypertens Res 1996;19:97–101.

[51] Selvais P, Donckier J, Laloux R, et al. Cardiac natriuretic peptides for diagnosis and risk stratification in heart failure: influences of left ventricular dysfunction and coronary artery disease on cardiac hormonal activation. Eur J Clin Invest 1998;28: 636–42.

[52] Tsutamoto T, Wada A, Maeda K, et al. Plasma brain natriuretic peptide level as a biochemical marker of morbidity and mortality in patients with asymptomatic or minimally symptomatic left ventricular dysfunction. Eur Heart J 1999;20: 1799–807.

[53] Yu CM, Sanderson JE. Plasma brain natriuretic peptide—an independent predictor of cardiovascular mortality in acute heart failure. Eur J Heart Fail 1999;1:59–65.

[54] Hammerer-Lercher A, Neubauer E, Muller S, et al. Head-to-head comparison of N-terminal pro-brain natriuretic peptide, brain natriuretic peptide and N terminal pro-atrial natriuretic peptide in diagnosing left ventricular dysfunction. Clin Chim Acta 2001;310:193–7.

[55] Harrison A, Morrison LK, Krishnaswamy P, et al. B-type natriuretic peptide predicts future cardiac events in patients presenting to the emergency department with dyspnea. Ann Emerg Med 2002;39: 131–8.

[56] Arroliga AC. Noninvasive positive pressure ventilation in acute respiratory failure: does it improve outcomes? Cleve Clin J Med 2001;68:677–80.

[57] Peacock WF, Emerman CL, Costanzo MR, et al. Early initiation of intravenous therapy improves heart failure outcomes: an analysis from the ADHERE registry database. Ann Emerg Med 2003; 42(4):S26.

[58] Peacock WF 4th, Albert NM. Observation unit management of heart failure. Emerg Med Clin North Am 2001;19:209–32.

[59] Peacock WF, Aponte JH, Craig MT, et al. Inpatient versus emergency department observation unit management of heart failure. Ann Emerg Med 1998;32:S46.

[60] Fonarow GC, Adams KF Jr, Abraham WT, et al. The ADHERE Scientific Advisory Committee, Study Group, and Investigators. Risk stratification for in-hospital mortality in acutely decompensated heart failure: classification and regression tree analysis. JAMA 2005;293:572–80.

[61] Diercks DB, Kirk JD, Peacock WF, Weber JE. Identification of emergency department patients with decompensated heart failure at low risk for adverse events and prolonged hospitalization. J Cardiac Failure 2004;10(4):S114.

[62] Burkhardt J, Peacock WF, Emerman CL. Elevation in blood urea nitrogen predicts a lower discharge rate from the observation unit. Ann Emerg Med 2004;44(4):S99.

[63] Rich MW, Beckham V, Wittenberg C, et al. A multidisciplinary intervention to prevent the readmission of elderly patients with congestive heart failure. N Engl J Med 1995;333:1190–5.

[64] Rich MW, Vinson JM, Sperry JC, et al. Prevention of readmission in elderly patients with

congestive heart failure. J Gen Intern Med 1993;8: 585–90.

[65] Albert NM, Peacock WF. Patient outcome and costs after implementation of an acute heart failure management program in an emergency department observation unit. J Int Soc Heart Lung Transplant 1999;18:92.

[66] Vinson JM, Rich MW, Sperry JC, et al. Early readmission of elderly patients with congestive heart failure. J Am Geriatr Soc 1990;38:1290–5.

[67] Quaglietti SE, Atwood JE, Ackerman L, et al. Management of the patient with congestive heart failure using outpatient, home, and palliative care. Prog Cardiovasc Dis 2000;43:259–74.

[68] Peacock W, Aponte J, Craig M, et al. Predictors of unsuccessful treatment for congestive heart failure in the emergency department observation unit. Acad Emerg Med 1997;4:494.

[69] Cohn JN, Johnson G, Ziesche S, et al. A comparison of enalapril with hydralazine-isosorbide dinitrate in the treatment of chronic congestive heart failure. N Engl J Med 1991;325:303–10.

[70] Cohn JN, Archibald DG, Ziesche S, et al. Effect of vasodilator therapy on mortality in chronic congestive heart failure: results of the Veterans Administration Cooperative Study. N Engl J Med 1986; 314:1547–52.

[71] The SOLVD Investigators. Effect of enalapril on survival in patients with reduced left ventricular ejection fractions and congestive heart failure. N Engl J Med 1991;325:293–302.

[72] The CONSENSUS Trial Study Group. Effects of enalapril on mortality in severe congestive heart failure: Results of the Cooperative North Scandinavian Enalapril Survival Study (CONSENSUS). N Engl J Med 1987;315:1429–35.

[73] Marcus LS, Hart D, Packer M, et al. Hemodynamic and renal excretory effects of human brain natriuretic peptide infusion in patients with congestive heart failure. A double-blind, placebo-controlled, randomized crossover trial. Circulation 1996;94:3184–9.

[74] Abraham WT, Lowes BD, Ferguson DA, et al. Systemic hemodynamic, neurohormonal, and renal effects of a steady-state infusion of human brain natriuretic peptide in patients with hemodynamically decompensated heart failure. J Card Fail 1998;4: 37–44.

[75] Burger AJ, Horton DP, Elkayam U, et al. Nesiritide is not associated with the proarrhythmic effects of dobutamine in the treatment of decompensated CHF: The PRECEDENT Study. J Card Fail 1999;5(Suppl 1):178.

[76] Elkayam U, Silver MA, Burger AJ, et al. The effect of short-term therapy with nesiritide (B-type natriuretic peptide) or dobutamine on long-term survival. J Card Fail 2000;6(Suppl 2):169.

[77] Young JB, Stevenson LW, Abraham WT, et al. Rationale and design of the VMAC Trial: Vasodilation in the Management of Acute Congestive Heart Failure. J Card Fail 2000;6(Suppl 2):182.

[78] Colucci WS, Elkayam U, Horton DP, et al. Nesiritide Study Group: intravenous nesiritide, a natriuretic peptide, in the treatment of decompensated congestive heart failure. Nesiritide Study Group. N Engl J Med 2000;343:246–53.

[79] Silver MA, Ghali JK, Horton DP, et al. Effect of nesiritide versus dobutamine on short-term outcomes in the treatment of acutely decompensated heart failure. J Card Fail 1998;4(Suppl 1):150A.

[80] Peacock WF, Emerman CE, Young J, on behalf of the PROACTION study group. Safety and efficacy of nesiritide for the treatment of decompensated heart failure in emergency department observation unit patients. JACC 2003;4(6)(Suppl A):336A.

[81] Colucci WS, Packer M, Bristow MR, et al. US Carvedilol Study Group: carvedilol inhibits clinical progression in patients with mild symptoms of heart failure. Circulation 1996;94:2800–6.

[82] Tsuyuki RT, Yusuf S, Rouleau JL, et al. Combination neurohormonal blockade with ACE inhibitors, angiotensin II, antagonists and beta-blockers in patients with congestive heart failure: design of the Randomized Evaluation of Strategies for Left Ventricular Dysfunction (RESOLVED) pilot study (phase II). Eur Heart J 1998;19S:308.

[83] The International Steering Committee. Rationale, design, and organization of the Metoprolol CR/XL randomized intervention trial in heart failure (MERIT-HF). Am J Cardiol 1997;80(Suppl 9B): 54J–8J.

[84] CIBIS Investigators and Committees. A randomized trial of beta-blockade in heart failure: The Cardiac Insufficiency Bisoprolol Study (CIBIS). Circulation 1994;90:1765–73.

[85] Bristow MR, Gilbert EM, Abraham WT, et al. MOCHA Investigators: carvedilol produces dose-related improvements in left ventricular function and survival in subjects with chronic heart failure. Circulation 1996;94:2807–16.

[86] The Rales Investigators. Effectiveness of spironolactone added to an angiotensin-converting enzyme inhibitor and a loop diuretic for severe chronic congestive heart failure (The Randomized Aldactone Evaluation Study [RALES]). Am J Cardiol 1996; 78:902–7.

[87] Cioffi G, Pozzoli M, Forni G, et al. Systemic thromboembolism in chronic heart failure. A prospective study in 406 patients. Eur Heart J 1996; 17:1381–9.

[88] Baker DW, Wright RF. Management of heart failure. IV. Anticoagulation for patients with heart failure due to left ventricular systolic dysfunction. JAMA 1994;272:1614–8.

[89] Turpie AG. Thrombosis prophylaxis in the acutely ill medical patient: insights from the prophylaxis in MEDical patients with ENOXaparin (MEDENOX) trail. AJC 2000;86(12B):48M–52M.

[90] ACC/AHA. Guidelines for the evaluation and management of heart failure: report of the American College of Cardiology/American Heart Association task force on practice guidelines (Committee of Evaluation and Management of Heart Failure). Circulation 1995;92:2764–84.

[91] Elkayam U, Weber L, McKay C, et al. Spectrum of acute hemodynamic effects of nifedipine in severe congestive heart failure. Am J Cardiol 1985;56: 560–6.

[92] Barjon JN, Rouleau JL, Bichet D, et al. Chronic renal and neurohumoral effects of the calcium entry blocker nisoldipine in patients with congestive heart failure. J Am Coll Cardiol 1987;9:622–30.

[93] Elkayam U, Amin J, Mehra A, et al. A prospective, randomized, double-blind, crossover study to compare the efficacy and safety of chronic nifedipine therapy with that of isosorbide dinitrate and their combination in the treatment of chronic congestive heart failure. Circulation 1990;82:1954–61.

[94] Goldstein RE, Boccuzzi SJ, Cruess D, et al. Diltiazem increases late-onset congestive heart failure in post-infarction patients with early reduction in ejection fraction. The Adverse Experience Committee and the Multicenter Diltiazem Post-infarction Research Group. Circulation 1991;83:52–60.

[95] Batsford WP, Mickleborough LL, Elefteriades JA. Ventricular arrhythmias in heart failure. Cardiol Clin 1995;13:87–91.

[96] The Cardiac Arrhythmia Suppression Trail (CAST) Investigators. Preliminary report: effect of encainide and flecainide on mortality in a randomized trial of arrhythmia suppression after myocardial infarction. N Engl J Med 1989;321: 406–12.

[97] Albert NM. Manipulating survival and life quality outcomes in heart failure through disease state management. Crit Care Nurse Clin North Am 1999;11:121–41.

[98] Cline CMJ, Israelsson BYA, Willenheimer RB, et al. Cost effective management program for heart failure reduces hospitalization. Heart 1998;80: 442–6.

[99] Fonarow GC, Stevenson LW, Walden JA, et al. Impact of a comprehensive heart failure management program on hospital readmission and functional status of patients with advanced heart failure. J Am Coll Cardiol 1997;30:725–32.

[100] Gattis W, Hasselblad V, Whellan D, et al. Reduction in heart failure events by the addition of a clinical pharmacist to the heart failure management team. Arch Intern Med 1999;159:1939–45.

ELSEVIER
SAUNDERS

CARDIOLOGY
CLINICS

Cardiol Clin 23 (2005) 589–599

Cost Effectiveness of Chest Pain Units

Sandra Sieck, RN, MBA

Sieck HealthCare Consulting, 9431 Jeff Hamilton Road, Mobile, AL 36695, USA

Health care is undergoing unprecedented change resulting from increasing pressures to deliver quality care to greater numbers of people in a resource-constrained environment. Although all providers of care are affected, the acute hospital facility bears an inordinate amount of this pressure, often caught between decreasing global reimbursements and the need to care for sicker and more complex patients. The Chest Pain Unit (CPU) represents a venue that effectively merges the clinical needs of a segment of acute cardiac patients with the economic needs of the acute care facility.

Origin of the chest pain unit

Historically, the outpatient CPU concept was developed to heighten community awareness on the early warning signs of a heart attack and create an ease of hospital entry for the chest pain patient. CPUs experienced exponential growth from 1980 to 1998 but offered little more than successful marketing strategies to increase hospital admissions, a factor that often contributed to overcrowding in many community hospitals [1].

After, the CPU served as a temporary holding area, sorting out patients who were at low risk for developing a myocardial infarction. This "triage role" allowed for reduced use of acute inpatient stays by those patients who did not require a high level of care. This triaging allowed appropriate care to be provided to the low-risk chest pain patient while maintaining open bed availability in the intensive care unit (ICU) for patients requiring a higher level of service.

CPUs have continued to evolve to better meet the needs of the health care system and the acute cardiac patient. More recently, as a result of changing reimbursement patterns, CPUs also have been able to address some of the financial pressures placed on the acute care facility by third-party payers.

Financial pressures on acute care facilities

The Balanced Budget Act (BBA) of 1997 made sweeping changes to Medicare, generating savings that were critical to extending the life of the Medicare Trust Fund [2]. In the health care arena, most of these changes impacted the acute care facility most directly. Lacking a complete understanding of the impact of the BBA; however, many facilities failed to make the necessary changes to offset the new plan, resulting in overall decreased reimbursements in 1997. The fixed reimbursements of the diagnosis-related group (DRG) program began to adversely affect hospitals' revenues and profit margins.

In an effort to maintain economic viability, hospitals targeted two key areas for cost reduction efforts: bed days and staffing. Intense efforts were made at reducing average length of stay (LOS) and reducing the number of hospital employees. Although this strategy resulted in initial cost benefits, savings plateaued, and margins eroded further. By 1999, DRG reimbursement increased only 0.6%, and hospitals' overall average-operating margins had decreased to 2.76% [3]. These eroding profit margins, and a reduction in the number of acute care facilities as a result of mergers and acquisitions, created an unstable environment in which hospitals were struggling to remain solvent [3].

As revenues were held in check, another factor added to the burdens on the acute care facility: health care use continued to increase. During the

_____
E-mail address: ssieck@sieckhealthcare.com

decade leading to 2003, inpatient admissions increased nearly 10% while outpatient visits increased approximately 61% [3]. The number of emergency department (ED) visits increased steadily from 1997 to 2002, from 99.6 million to 114.2 million [3]. This immense growth and demand on emergency services led to an overwhelming reduction in the availability of these services and is considered a major contributor to the process and economic changes that are now occurring.

The ED is acknowledged as the most common point of entry into the health care system. As facilities begin to factor in the expected 8 million annual ED visits for chest pain predicted in the upcoming years, the emergence of the CPU—often termed ED Observation Unit—and other specialized short stay units are now under reconsideration to help alleviate some of the hospital system burdens, such as ED overcrowding, reduction of unnecessary admissions, and the opportunity to optimize revenue.

Acute coronary syndrome

Current bottlenecks in the ED are caused by the large, challenging group of patients who present with chest pain of possible cardiac origin, or "low-probability" patients as categorized by the America Heart Association and the American College of Cardiology (ACC/AHA) guidelines.

The ED itself is not the cause of overcrowding; rather, it is simply the unit most vulnerable to gridlock (Fig. 1) [4]. The lack of inpatient beds is the most commonly cited reason for crowding in the ED [4,5]. Although most chest pain patients are unlikely to have sustained a myocardial infarction or need treatment in an ICU, the high rate of acute hospital admission adds to the bed-day burden of the acute care facility.

Acute coronary syndrome (ACS) is a potentially lethal condition that affects approximately 2 million people in the United States. Most ACS patients seek care through an ED, and this patient volume is saturating these departments. Treatment delays, medical errors, poor outcomes, against medical advice, higher re-admissions, diversions, increasing costs, and threatened quality all play a role in the health care crisis.

ACS patients use a tremendous amount of resources initially in the ED, only to be admitted into an inpatient bed later for a 2- to 3-day LOS in the acute facility. From a DRG reimbursement perspective, all testing done in the ED arena is now debited from the total DRG payment for which the patient was admitted. If the admitting diagnosis DRG is not changed from DRG 143 (chest pain) to a higher acuity DRG 140 (unstable angina), it will most likely contribute negatively to the hospital bottom line (opportunity revenue loss of $1500–$2000).

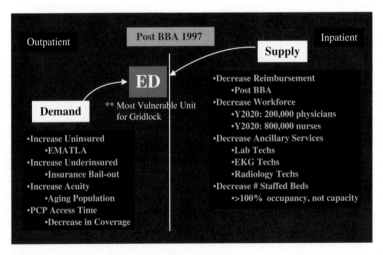

Fig. 1. Comparison between supply and demand affecting the health care systems access to care, hospital overcrowding and efficiency demands. Hospital overcrowding was considered a unit phenomenon tied to the emergency department. Issues surrounding the causes and solutions, overcrowding is increasingly perceived as a system problem. (*Adapted from* Joint Commission Resources. Managing patient flow: strategies and solutions for addressing hospital overcrowding. 2004. p. 11.)

Emergence of the "new" chest pain unit

The CPU is no longer merely a holding area for low-risk cardiac patients or a conduit to the inpatient service for the higher-risk group. A new CPU concept is emerging as a venue for addressing some of the previously mentioned clinical and economic pressures that face the acute care facility.

Use of a CPU can show resource advantages over the typical acute hospital admission. The typical chest pain patient spends an average of 2.1 days in the hospital; when seen and treated only in the CPU, this same patient can be discharged safely in 6 to 12 hours. Each outpatient bed frees 2.2 to 3.5 inpatient beds that can be allocated to high-acuity patients who require admission [6]. Additionally, quality measures can be improved also. For instance, the Impact on the Care of the Emergency Department Chest Pain Patient from the Chest Pain Evaluation Registry (CHEPER) study reported a significant reduction in missed myocardial infarctions from 4.5% to 0.4%, a change that enhances quality and directly impacts the high-cost medical/legal payouts and re-admissions from erroneous diagnoses [7].

Observation units for heart failure recently have shown a positive impact on reducing after-health-care use in patients who present with acute decompensated heart failure. Table 1 summarizes data from the Cleveland Clinic experience [8].

Future directions in acute coronary syndrome

Non–ST-segment elevation myocardial infarction (NSTEMI) and unstable angina (UA) patients represent the next challenging focus for optimizing cost-efficient acute cardiac care. These patients present to facilities earlier in the thrombosis progression model of the disease than STEMI patients, making them more difficult to

diagnose and treat, and essentially all are admitted to the acute care facility. They are often difficult to distinguish from non-ACS patients who present with chest pain.

The ACC/AHA guidelines highlight the role of CPUs and "short-stay ED coronary care units" to facilitate a more definitive evaluation while avoiding the unnecessary hospital admission of patients who have not developed ACS. Such evaluation also helps to avoid the inappropriate discharge of patients who develop active myocardial ischemia without ST-segment elevation. Personnel in these units use critical pathways or protocols designed to arrive at a decision about the presence or absence of myocardial ischemia and, if present, to characterize it further as UA or NSTEMI and to define the optimal next step in the care of the patient (eg, admission, acute intervention). The goal is to arrive at such a decision after a finite amount of time, which usually falls between 6 and 12 hours but may extend up to 24 hours, depending on the policies in individual hospitals. The time spent shifts from days of care to hours of care.

The difference between NSTEMI and UA also brings to light an important economic factor. If a physician diagnoses a patient who presents with elevated biomarkers with ST depression but fails to document the elevation of these cardiac markers, the facility is reimbursed as a UA payment. The difference in reimbursement for the NSTEMI and UA patients is approximately $4000 to $6000. Physician documentation can thus play a vital role in how the facilities and office practice coders submit for reimbursement.

CPUs are able to advance the STEMI and NSTEMI/UA patients through the system quickly and consistently while promptly facilitating safe discharge of the low-probability chest pain patients. The ultimate goal of the CPU is to transition many of the services now performed in the ICU setting to the CPU for earlier diagnosis and management—the true "short-stay coronary care unit."

Reimbursement issues

Centers for Medicare and Medicaid Services (CMS) is the third-party payer for most of the acute cardiac patients who are largely of Medicare age. CMS is now trying to shift unnecessary inpatient volume back to the point of entry for more efficient risk stratification, assessment, and more intense treatment. This approach

Table 1
Observation unit results for patients with heart failure

Utilization parameter	Change after OU	Percent change
Revisits	90%–51%	44% decrease
ED observation discharges	9%	
HF rehospitalizations	77%–50%	36% decrease
Observation hospitalizations	23% decreased LOS	

Abbreviations: HF, heart failure; OU, observation unit.

emphasizes the integration of observation unit services as a viable alternative to inpatient health care delivery and is being accomplished by shifting resources—or reimbursement—to the outpatient setting, most commonly the ED in a CPU or observation unit.

The facility payment for a CPU service is paid under a new observation code, the Ambulatory Patient Classification (APC) 0339. APC 0339 is a separate observation carve-out payment that CMS has agreed to pay as a third door opportunity for acute care facilities. One intention of APC 0339 is to offer an alternative pathway to diagnose, treat, and admit or discharge patients rapidly who are diagnosed with chest pain, congestive heart failure, and asthma. CMS selected these three medical conditions to focus on four mains areas of concern: (1) morbidity, (2) mortality, (3) appropriateness of admissions, and (4) reduction in inappropriate discharges. The current shift of this large class of patients from their traditional inpatient treatment protocol to a more efficient plan of care initiated in the CPU or ED observation unit has resulted in a significant economic impact on the acute care facility [9].

The CPU is shown to impact economics and clinical outcomes in several studies. One multicenter study demonstrated that observation in a CPU resulted in a lower incidence of missed myocardial infarction (0.4% versus 4.5%, $P <$ 0.001) and lower final rate of hospital admission (47% versus 57%, $P < 0.001$) [7]. These clinical benefits were accompanied by an average saving of more than $120 per patient (almost $2.9 million reduction in true costs for 23,407 patients seen in the ED for chest pain) [7]. In a prospective, randomized trial of patients seen at a CPU, no cases existed of missed primary cardiac events and no erroneous discharges, and use of resources was more efficient when ACS patients were seen at the CPU than when they were admitted by way of the ED to a cardiac care unit [10]. Practice standards specific to the institution represent another method of improving quality of care while controlling cost. Practice standards can promote adherence to regulatory directives, cost-containment measures, and evidence-based guidelines for diagnosis and treatment.

Hospitals have also reduced costs of treatment for inpatient stays for low-risk chest pain. Fig. 2 shows the effect of a quality-improvement initiative in fiscal year (FY) 2000 related to ACS patients. As part of the initiative, the acute care facility modified treatment protocols to adhere to the AHA/ACC guidelines for the management of ACS. From FY 2000 to 2002, inhospital mortality of ACS patients decreased from 4.8% to 1.9%, and LOS decreased from 5.9 days to 4.6 days. The average cost per case dropped from $11,777 to $10,623, saving $1,154 per ACS

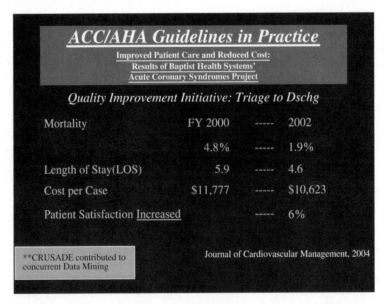

Fig. 2. Healthcare facilities increasing must provide high quality medicine at reasonable cost. (*Adapted from* Jackson S, Sistrunk H, Staman K, et al. Improved patient care and reduced costs: results of Baptist Heal Systems' acute coronary syndromes project. J Cardiovasc Manag 2003;14:4.)

patient. These results demonstrate that institutions can examine care patterns, change them, and maintain quality clinical outcomes [11].

Despite these cost savings, the DRG reimbursement system does not always result in full coverage of costs of care for an inpatient stay (Fig. 3). The following example demonstrates the full impact of reimbursement differences between DRG and APC coding for chest pain evaluation and treatment in a hospital.

The hospital analysis is based on 4000 chest pain patients, 289 of which qualified for APC 0339 outpatient observation versus an inpatient admission using DRG 143. In a 12-month retrospective analysis, the patients who were routed through the CPU generated a profit of $32,000 for the hospital, whereas the patients admitted under DRG 143 resulted in a loss, "costing" the system $188,000. By merely "transferring to observation" and at the time meeting minimal testing to meet the APC 0339 payment requirements, whereas in the outpatient CPU versus "admitting" to the inpatient system, a $220,000 variance was created. Fixed cost and variable cost was factored into these calculations to give a more accurate representation of the results.

Although this scenario does not reflect every hospital's situation, it underscores the potential adverse financial implications of providing higher-intensity care than is medically necessary. An evidence-based, protocol-driven CPU has the ability to route patients rapidly through rapid risk-stratification protocols to appropriate inpatient admissions while reducing missed myocardial infarctions and providing safe discharges with fewer returns. Careful up-front risk stratification not only results in increased efficiency of care, but also in cost advantages through a more favorable reimbursement situation.

Services, such as CPUs, can be structured to provide the resources necessary at the point-of-entry to diagnose and treat ACS patients efficiently, directing them into the proper service lines at maximum efficiency. High-acuity and moderate-risk patients are now admitted, and low-probability patients, who in the past would have been admitted, are diagnosed and released safely after only hours versus the past pattern of days. The study performed by Ross on the impact of an ED observation bed on inpatient bed availability [12] indicates that 1 patient treated in an observation unit bed equals 2.2 to 3.5 inpatient beds. This equation is one of the variables that contributes to the economic feasibility of CPUs. This 3:1 ratio increases the physician's productivity while driving down fixed and variable costs allocated to the outpatient services.

Federal regulations and the effect on chest pain units in 2005

The federal regulations continue to change to accommodate the shift in acuity to the outpatient setting. These regulations do not specify bricks

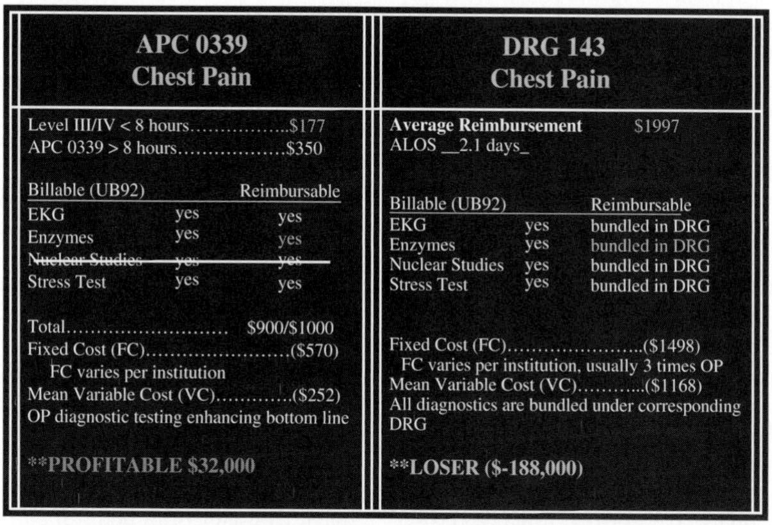

APC 0339 Chest Pain			DRG 143 Chest Pain		
Level III/IV < 8 hours................$177			**Average Reimbursement**		$1997
APC 0339 > 8 hours..................$350			ALOS __2.1 days_		
Billable (UB92)		Reimbursable	Billable (UB92)		Reimbursable
EKG	yes	yes	EKG	yes	bundled in DRG
Enzymes	yes	yes	Enzymes	yes	bundled in DRG
~~Nuclear Studies~~	~~yes~~	~~yes~~	Nuclear Studies	yes	bundled in DRG
Stress Test	yes	yes	Stress Test	yes	bundled in DRG
Total..........................		$900/$1000			
Fixed Cost (FC).......................($570)			Fixed Cost (FC)......................($1498)		
FC varies per institution			FC varies per institution, usually 3 times OP		
Mean Variable Cost (VC)...........($252)			Mean Variable Cost (VC)...........($1168)		
OP diagnostic testing enhancing bottom line			All diagnostics are bundled under corresponding DRG		
PROFITABLE $32,000			**LOSER ($-188,000)**		

Fig. 3. Comparison of inpatient DRG 143 (chest pain) coverage versus outpatient APC 0339 (chest pain). DRG, diagnosis-related group; APC, ambulatory patient classification; FC, fixed cost; VC, viable cost; OP, outpatient.

and mortar as part of the reimbursement criteria for APC 0339. A CPU or observation unit can be located within or near an ED or be a free-standing unit. It is not the location of a CPU that distinguishes its services from an ED but the type of care it provides.

These regulations are particularly influential from a reimbursement standpoint. Financial incentives have been put into play to ensure efficient care is provided in the CPU. These changes are more economically favorable to the hospitals that employ CPUs.

Specific excerpts from the Federal Register on the recent changes in the APC reimbursement as of January 2005 are summarized in Table 2 [13].

The main impacts of the regulatory changes are

- The duration of the CPU stay must be 8 to 48 hours.
- If an admission occurs after the CPU stay, the hospital is not financially disadvantaged.
- Previously required laboratory tests have been eliminated as part of the APC requirement (requires medical necessity).
- Any tests performed (medically necessary) as part of a CPU stay can be billed for in addition to the APC 0339 charge.

Quality implications of chest pain units

In an effort to support the dramatic restructuring of health care delivery, CMS has also revamped its image from an institution of strictly financial reimbursement to include a healthy plan of quality mixed into its evolving plan of health care delivery. CMS is crafting new aggressive approaches to facilitate implementation of a proactive strategy to provide resources for care aimed at earlier detection and treatment of acute cardiac conditions. In recent years, however, leaders and policy-makers have directed increased attention to strategies for achieving system-wide improvements in health care quality and patient safety that will lead to larger-scale, more rapid changes in professional and provider behavior than have been experienced to date.

Protocols designed around the ACC/AHA guidelines will allow facilities to meet or exceed certain quality indicators developed for these ACS patients, also creating greater patient satisfaction. CMS is developing pay-for-performance programs and a bonus reimbursement for meeting quality standards in certain clinical areas;

reducing reimbursement for those who do not meet the defined indicators; participating in the CMS/Premier Quality Demonstration Project initiative; and experimenting with a sliding scale concept that pays based on the number of quality indicators facilities meet (Fig. 4).

The pay-for-performance approach acknowledges the reality that financial rewards are among the most powerful tools for bringing about behavior change [1]. Also, the alignment of payment program incentives to support the provision of safe, high-quality care is a complex undertaking because it must simultaneously achieve fair reimbursement for necessary services, promote desired behavior change, and avoid unintended consequences. In the end, new payment policies and programs must work to the advantage of the patient and support the provision of patient-centered care.

In the near future, hospital reimbursement likely will be directly proportional to quality performances. CMS also has several efforts in progress to provide hospital quality information to consumers and others to improve the care provided by the nation's hospitals. These initiatives build on previous CMS and quality initiative strategies to identify illnesses or clinical conditions that affect Medicare beneficiaries to promote the best medical practice associated with the targeted clinical disorders; prevent or reduce further instances of these selected clinical disorders; and prevent related complications [2].

Trans-theoretic Y model application

The separation of quality and finance is no longer a viable plan of operation and must be redesigned to create an efficient plan focused on process to optimize clinical and financial outcomes. The business world has long recognized this tenet and has created models by which business units are aligned efficiently and strategically toward achieving a well-defined end product or service.

A new approach to understanding the entire concept of health care delivery from point-of-entry to discharge is the trans-theoretic Y-model (Fig. 5). This model emphasizes a multidisciplinary team approach to align the "care units" that affect a cardiac patient's progress through the current system (Fig. 6). By understanding how each care unit's operational strategies affect each subsequent care unit from point of entry to discharge, a seamless transfer of patient care in outpatient and inpatient settings can optimize quality

Table 2
Summary of federal regulation changes in 2005 [12]

Excerpts	Analysis/Comments
1. Beginning in early 2001, the APC Panel began discussing the topic of separate payment for observation services. In its deliberations, the APC Panel asserted that observation services following clinical and emergency room visits should be paid separately, and that observation following surgery should be packaged into the payment for the surgical procedure. For CY 2002, separate payment for observation services (APC 0339) was implemented under the OPPS for three medical conditions: chest pain, CHF, and asthma. A number of accompanying requirements were established: the billing of an evaluation and management visit in conjunction with the presence of certain specified diagnosis codes on the claim; hourly billing of observation care for a minimum of 8 hours up to a maximum of 48 hours; timing of observation beginning with the clock time on the nurse's admission note and ending at the clock time on the physician's discharge orders; a medical record documenting that the beneficiary was under the care of a physician who specifically assessed patient risk to determine that the beneficiary would benefit from observation care; and provision of specific diagnostic tests to beneficiaries based on their diagnoses.	APC 0339, outpatient observation, was developed in 2001 and implemented in April 2002 as a clinical and financial opportunity for facilities. This new outpatient observation differs from the traditional inpatient observation. Criteria, such as the inclusion of an E&M level code, must be billed with one of three conditions (chest pain, CHF, and asthma). Once the patient has been in observation for minimum of 8 hours up to a maximum of 48, beginning with the nurse's admission note and ending at the time on the physician's discharge orders. Physician must document progress notes during beneficiary's stay in observation. Diagnostic testing requirements have changed from 2002 to 2005 and are discussed later in Analysis # 2.
2. CMS received comments from the community and the APC Panel asserting that the requirements for diagnostic testing are overly prescriptive and administratively burdensome, and that hospitals may perform tests to comply with the CMS requirements, rather than based on clinical need.	Specifying which diagnostic tests must be performed as a prerequisite for payment of APC 0339 may be imposing an unreasonable reporting burden on hospitals and may, in some cases, result in unnecessary tests being performed. Therefore, beginning in CY 2005, the authors are proposing removal of the current requirements for specific diagnostic testing, and reliance on clinical judgment in combination with internal and external quality review processes to ensure that appropriate diagnostic testing (which the authors expect would include some of the currently required diagnostic tests) is provided for patients receiving high-quality, medically necessary observation care. *Accordingly, beginning in CY 2005, the following tests should no longer be required to receive payment for APC 0339 (observation):* For congestive heart failure, a chest radiograph (71010, 71020, 71030), and ECG (93005), and pulse oximetry (94760, 94761, 94762). For asthma, a breathing capacity test (94010) or pulse oximetry (94760, 94761, 94762). For chest pain, two sets of cardiac enzyme tests, two CPK (82550, 82552, 82553) or two troponins (84484, 84512), and two sequential ECGs (93005).

(continued on next page)

Table 2 (*continued*)

Excerpts	Analysis/Comments
3. Hospitals and the APC panel further suggested that the method for accounting for the beneficiary's time in observation care be modified.	In an effort to reduce hospitals' administrative burden related to accurate billing, counting time in observation care should end at the time the outpatient is actually discharged from the hospital or admitted as an inpatient. Twentyfour hours is adequate for the clinical staff to determine what further care the patient needs. In CY 2005, separate payment should continue to be made for observation care based on claims meeting the requirement for payment of HCPCS code G0244 (observation care provided by a facility to a patient with CHF, chest pain, or asthma, minimum 8 hours, maximum 48 hours). However, do not include claims reporting more than 48 hours of observation care in calculating the final payment rate for APC 0339. In CY 2005, OPPS payments for observation care should increase over CY 2004 levels for two reasons. First, the proposal to eliminate the requirement that specific diagnostic tests be performed to receive separate payment for observation care will result in more observation stays being paid for under APC 0339. Several CY 2003 claims with packaged observation services reported for CHF, asthma, and chest pains would qualify for separate payment. Adopting the proposed changes, the volume of claims for payment under APC 0339 should increase in CY 2005. This volume increase, combined with the slightly higher median cost calculated for APC 0339 based on CY 2003 claims, would likely result in higher aggregate Medicare payments to hospitals for observation care in CY 2005 than in previous years. The payment is approximately $403.93, which translates into a 12% increase over 2004.
4. The beneficiary must be in the care of a physician during the period of observation, as documented in the medical record by admission, discharge, and other appropriate progress notes that are timed, written, and signed by the physician.	The medical record must include documentation that the physician explicitly assessed patient risk to determine that the beneficiary would benefit from observation care.

Abbreviations: CHF, congestive heart failure; CY, calendar year; OPPS, outpatient prospective payment system; E&M, evolution and management; CPK, creatine phosphokinase; HCPCS, healthcare common procedure coding system.

improvement and positive economic value. Without each care unit providing vital information to others in this holistic approach, moving patients efficiently through the system is challenged.

The trans-theoretic Y-model places an emphasis on process improvement while targeting two end points: quality and contribution margin (Fig. 7). This concept begins at the point of entry and ends at discharge and marries a clinical and financial strategy that meets quality indicators while producing desirable profit margins. This plan can be implemented on any disease state, particularly chest pain or ACS patients. Beginning in the ED, this concept emphasizes an efficient, rapid assessment and action centered on a seamless integration of ancillary services, such as the laboratory, diagnostic imaging, and skilled nursing while understanding the economic impacts on decisions made as the patient is directed through the system. The failure of any one of these services could bring the ED to a halt, thus supporting the notion that the ED is not

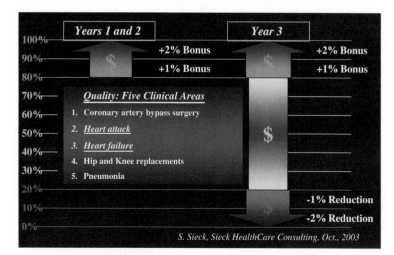

Fig. 4. Principles for the construct of pay-for-performance.

necessarily the cause of the gridlock; rather, it is the unit that becomes most vulnerable to it [4].

Compare the hospital setting to an industrial setting. Without uncertainty industrial facilities can detail the route from raw material to finished product with pinpoint accuracy. Checks and balances and alternative plans for the unexpected exist throughout the process. At every opportunity, dollars and time are being shaved—cost-avoidance. The end product is priced to the market based on the operating costs within the process. If the process varies and these costs or resource use climb, actions are taken to control the variances. If not, the contribution margin is eroded and eventually could become negative. The objective is to keep the contribution margin at its maximum without compromising quality. If the quality team does not communicate its concerns to the profitability team, then major issues of conflict arise and the system does not operate at optimal efficiency (see Fig. 6). Without question, the top industry leaders can pick a point randomly within their process and report on the variables within.

Until health care delivery systems take an internal look at their plan of operation and the economic plan that coincides, reimbursement will continue its current path. The Joint Commission on Accreditation of Health care Organizations

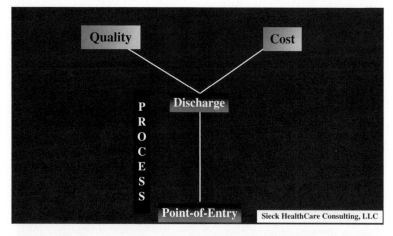

Fig. 5. Trans-theoretical Y Model: a new approach to understanding the entire concept of health care delivery from point-of-entry to discharge.

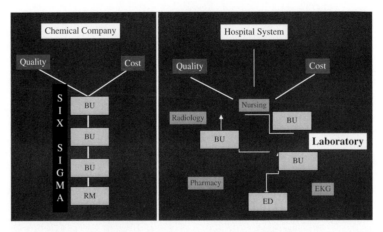

Fig. 6. Comparison of hospital system, Zig-Zag model to industry leaders, Vertical model.

(JCAHO) is looking for efficiency from point-of-entry to discharge, and CPUs can assist in this process because the ED is the most common point of entry into the system. JCAHO has developed a new standard, LD.3.15, to monitor the management of patient flow, attempting to alleviate overcrowding, effective January 1, 2005. Its main focus is identifying and mitigating impediments to efficient patient flow throughout the hospital [4].

Health care is a service industry and is learning to operate like an efficient and quality-driven business. The CPU represents an early step in this learning that can be applied throughout the point-of-care continuum. The Institute of Medicine in its recent report *Crossing the Quality Chasm* [14], concluded that in order for the health system to meet the future demands of the population of the United States and provide quality care, drastic reinvention is required; trying to "fix" the current system is insufficient. The principles used in the redesign of the CPU and the overall shift of care to the outpatient setting represent initial stages in that direction.

Summary

Acute care facilities are struggling to maintain economic viability in an environment of cost-constraints, declining reimbursements, and increasingly expensive technology. Two-thirds of facilities are operating at 1% or less, and one third of all hospitals have reported operating margins in the negative [15]. To survive, hospitals are being challenged to reinvent the way acute care is delivered. The experience and evolution of CPUs for the treatment of certain segments of the acute cardiac patient offer insight into the

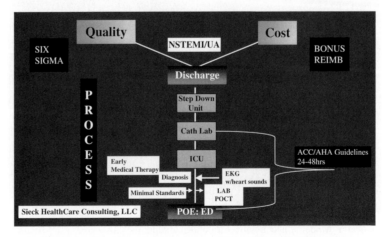

Fig. 7. Applying disease management to Trans-Theoretical Y model.

development of new models of acute care that can blend cost-efficiency with quality.

CPUs have taken on a new role with clinical outcomes and quality improvement at their core. The new federal regulations and APC coding provide re-allocation of resources and dollars to outpatient services to identify and treat patients rapidly, thus enhancing the role of the CPU as a cost-efficient entry for acute cardiac patients.

The CPU offers an alternative clinical and financial strategy to hospitals and physicians in the emerging health care reform model. Third-party payers will continue to assess the impact on morbidity and mortality as the transition to outpatient services progresses. In order for hospitals to take advantage of outcomes-based financial incentives offered by the government, realignment of the business units must occur to maximize efficiency by including all departments, such as ancillary services.

Strategies that emphasize focused care-process improvement initiatives while targeting quality and economic margins are the wave of the future. The CPU represents the first wave of the new model for patients who experience chest pain and heart failure. As this model is refined and shown to impact cost and quality favorably, this experience is likely to extend to other cardiac conditions.

References

[1] Bayley MD, Schwartz JS, Shofer FS, et al. The financial burden of ED congestion and hospital overcrowding for chest pain patients awaiting admission. Acad Emerg Med 2002;9:367–8.

[2] Centers for Medicare and Medicaid Services. Available at: http://www.cms.hhs.gov/media/press/release.asp?Counter=351. Accessed February 22, 1999.

[3] Modern Healthcare, By the Numbers: Health of our nation's hospitals, 2004. p. 12.

[4] Joint Commission Resources. Managing patient flow: strategies and solutions for addressing hospital overcrowding. 2004, p. 11.

[5] National Center for Health Statistics/Center for Disease Control and Prevention. National Hospital Discharge Survey. 1998, Series 12, No. 14. September, 2000.

[6] Ross M, Wilson AG, McPherson M, et al. The impact of an ED observation unit on inpatient bed capacity. Ann Emerg Med 2001;8:576.

[7] Graff LG, Dallara J, Ross MA, et al. Impact on the care of the emergency department chest pain patient from the Chest Pain Evaluation Registry (CHEPER) Study. Am J Cardiol 1997;80(5):563–8.

[8] Peacock WF, Emerman CL. Management of acute decompensated heart failure in the emergency department. J Am Coll Cardiol 2003;4(Suppl A): 336A.

[9] Sieck S. Best practice ACS. Journal of Critical Pathways in Cardiology 2002;1(4):223–30.

[10] Farouh ME, Smars PA, Reeder GS, et al. A clinical trial of a chest-pain observation unit for patients with unstable angina. Chest Pain Evaluation in the Emergency Room (CHEER) Investigators. N Engl J Med 1998;339(26):1882–8.

[11] Jackson S, Sistrunk H, Staman K. Improved patient care and reduced costs: results of Baptist Health Systems' acute coronary syndromes project. J Cardiovasc Manag 2003;14:4.

[12] Ross M. Maximizing use of the emergency department observation unit: a novel hybrid design. Ann Emerg Med 2001;37:267–74.

[13] Centers for Medicare and Medicaid Services. Medicare: Hospital outpatient prospective payment system and 2005 CY payment rates, 50447–50973 [04–18427]. Available at: http://www.access.gpo.gov/su_docs/fedreg/a040816c.html. Accessed August 16, 2004.

[14] Berwick SM. A user's manual for the IOM's 'Quality Chasm' Report. Health Aff 2002;21:80–90.

[15] Advancing Health in America. Promises Under Pressure: Pressures Threaten Prescriptions or Change; The Care for Hospital Payment Improvement. Available at: www.mhanet.org/i4a/pages/index/fcm?pageid=459. Accessed May 21, 2003.

Medical Error Prevention in ED Triage for ACS: Use of Cardiac Care Decision Support and Quality Improvement Feedback

Denise H. Daudelin, RN, MPH[a,b], Harry P. Selker, MD, MSPH[a,b,*]

[a]Tufts University School of Medicine, Boston, MA, USA
[b]Institute for Clinical Research and Health Policy Studies, Tufts-New England Medical Center,
750 Washington Street, Box 63, Boston, MA 02111, USA

Acute coronary syndromes (ACS) is the most common serious condition requiring emergency and acute care. Among the 8 million patients who present to emergency departments (EDs) in the United States each year with symptoms consistent with a cardiac problem, about 25% prove to have actual ACS. About one third (8%) of the presenting group prove to have acute myocardial infarction (AMI), of whom approximately 40%, or 3% of the overall group, have early-stage AMI deserving reperfusion treatment. The problem for the ED physician, therefore, is to identify, triage, and treat promptly and accurately the small proportion of patients who require immediate emergency care while efficiently dealing with the great majority who do not have ACS. This issue has been a focus of the time-insensitive predictive instrument (TIPI) approach to improving ED triage and treatment decision-making [1–5] and the TIPI Information System (TIPI-IS) feedback reporting system.

In the care of such patients, errors are made; thus, important opportunities exist for improvement in these ED triage and treatment decisions.

In ED *triage* in the United States each year, about 12,000 patients who present with AMI and 14,000 who present with unstable angina (UA) are mistakenly sent home from the ED [6], which nearly doubles their expected mortality rates [6]. Reflecting this problem is that ED cases of missed ACS perennially represent one of the largest cost categories of adult malpractice claims in the United States. In ED *treatment* of patients who present with AMI, the lifesaving impact of coronary reperfusion therapy is directly related to the timeliness of implementation [7,8], yet many are not treated promptly and about 90,000 per year are not treated at all. These errors in triage and treatment for ACS are critical to the patient and occur on a scale that makes them a public health issue. Thus, they present important opportunities to reduce medical errors.

Reducing these medical errors requires innovative changes to patient care processes, existing equipment, and performance improvement activities that can be achieved through the use of information technology (IT).

Computerized physician order entry systems and electronic medical error reporting software are patient safety systems that require changes to, or additional layers in, the patient care workflow. These systems prove challenging to introduce effectively and without disruption to patient care. More easily introduced is IT that is seamlessly built into workflow and that enhances existing patient care and performance improvement activities. Representing this approach, the conventional computerized electrocardiograph is

This article was supported by Grant Numbers RO1 HS/HL07360, RO1 HS 08212, and U18 HS11200 from the Agency for Healthcare Research and Quality.

* Corresponding author. Institute for Clinical Research and Health Policy Studies Tufts-New England Medical Center 750 Washington Street, Box 63 Boston, MA 02111.

E-mail address: hselker@tufts-nemc.org (H.P. Selker).

an IT tool that can be adapted to improve patient safety by providing clinical decision support in real-time, without changing the patient care process. The device also provides workflow tools to prevent medical error and identifies patients for inclusion in performance and outcome measurement systems.

Development of real-time decision support, concurrent event alerts, and retrospective feedback reporting

A series of decision support and risk reduction tools for real-time use in the ED have been developed in addition to an information system to provide concurrent missed AMI event alerting and retrospective feedback reports for improvement of the management of ACS patients. The core of this approach is the ability of a "time-insensitive predictive instrument" (TIPI) to compute, for every ED patient on presentation, a 0% to 100% probability that a patient truly has acute cardiac ischemia (ACI), and if having an AMI, the likely outcome benefits of thrombolytic therapy. A key feature of this prediction is the "*time-insensitive*" aspect of TIPIs, which refers to the fact that they compute, for a given ED patient, the *same* probability of value when used in the *real-time* ED setting or when used *retrospectively* for review of medical care. As now available in conventional electrocardiographs, besides printed on the ECG header as a decision aid for the physician the computed TIPI probabilities are stored in the electrocardiograph's computer, can be saved in a database, and then used to trigger concurrent flags about ongoing care and to generate retrospective reports and feedback for clinicians.

Real-time decision support for emergency department triage: the original acute coronary ischemia predictive instrument

The original ACI predictive instrument [1] was developed to be an easy-to-use method to improve ED physician triage decisions so that fewer patients *without* ACI would be admitted to cardiac care units (CCUs), but without decreasing proper admission of those with ACI. Reasoning that a 0% to 100% probability value might be incorporated easily into physicians' clinical decision-making, based on prospectively collected data on 2801 patients seen in six divergent hospitals' EDs for 1 year, a logistic regression equation was developed that used seven variables and was

applicable to all six hospitals. Using a programmed calculator, a patient's 0% to 100% probability of having ACI could be computed in 20 seconds. In a 2320-patient 11-month prospective controlled trial of the predictive instrument's impact on ED care, its use markedly improved physicians' diagnostic specificity ($P = .002$), with no significant change in sensitivity. The false positive diagnosis rate improved significantly ($P = .004$), whereas the false negative diagnosis rate did not change. Accordingly, ED triage dispositions for patients who proved to have ACI were not changed from the appropriately high CCU admission rates, but for patients *without* ACI, CCU admission rates dropped from 24% during the control periods to 17%, and their ED discharge rates to home increased from 44% during the control periods to 51% ($P = .003$), *a 30% reduction in CCU admissions for patients without ACI*. The predictive instrument's need for a calculator, however, was cumbersome. Thus, for better ease of use and attractiveness to clinicians, the authors designed the ACI-TIPI, its revised version, to be programmed into conventional computerized electrocardiographs.

Development of the acute coronary ischemia time-insensitive predictive instrument for real-time and retrospective decision support

Although improvement of CCU use might be done by real-time and retrospective interventions, the latter has had little formal evaluation. Use of real-time test results and decision aids are more familiar to clinicians than feedback systems. Attractive and clinically relevant reports on triage and treatment decisions, however, should facilitate continuous quality improvement by emergency medical services (EMS), physicians and institutions self-assessment. (Also, payors and organizations responsible for hospital and CCU use for coronary disease need a fair and accurate retrospective tool by which the appropriateness of CCU use can be measured.) Thus, there is a need for a clinically valid attractive measure for feedback on ACI/AMI care.

Ideally, a *single* tool should be able to serve prospective and retrospective purposes. Generally, however, tools designed for real-time use, such as our original ACI predictive instrument, have not been validated for retrospective medical record review, and tools for retrospective review of care have not been applicable to real-time use, limiting clinicians' interest and confidence in their use. Thus, the authors developed a "*time-insensitive* predictive instrument" for ACI (ACI-TIPI), valid for prospective real-time clinical use *and* retrospective medical record review, that accurately computes a patient's likelihood of having ACI at the time of presentation [2]. Not only theoretically desirable as a tool usable by clinicians, administrators, and payors, the ACI-TIPI might have the added benefit of promoting cooperation between these groups. This ACI-TIPI was tested on the 2320 patients seen at the six study hospitals' EDs during the second year, along with the original instrument, and both were compared with ED physician diagnostic performance [2]. Calculation of the receiver-operating characteristic (ROC) curve areas, which simultaneously evaluate sensitivity and specificity of a continuous scale test, yielded values of 0.88–0.89 for the ACI-TIPI and the original instrument, demonstrating excellent and similar diagnostic performance by both. Besides the ACI-TIPI, all subsequent predictive instruments, for mortality from ACI/AMI [3], for mortality from congestive failure [4], and the TPI [5] (see later discussion) meet TIPI criteria.

Incorporating acute coronary ischemia time-insensitive predictive instrument into electrocardiographs to support real-time emergency department/emergency medical services care

Convinced that the predictive instrument's probability would be used more were it automatically printed in the text header on ECGs (Fig. 1), the ACI-TIPI was programmed into a computerized electrocardiograph [9]. To do this, an ACI-TIPI was written using Hewlett-Packard (now Philips) ElectroCardiographic Language [9,10]. This activity was done in repeating iterative cycles of programming ECG waveform-based measurement criteria and then comparing the program's performance on sample ECGs to readings by the ECG reader who designed the original ACI-TIPI ECG variables (HPS).

Because it was felt that the ACI-TIPI and the approach of incorporating a predictive instrument into a computerized electrocardiograph would not benefit a maximal number of patients if restricted, we published all details of the ACI-TIPI's formula and the incorporation of a TIPI into an electrocardiograph was put into the public domain. Marketed or prototype ACI-TIPI/TPI electrocardiographs

exist by all United Stated EMS electrocardiograph manufacturers.

Besides enabling presentation of the ACI-TIPI on the ECG, its incorporation into a computerized electrocardiograph allows transfer of patients' ACI probabilities into a database, which is central to the development of a performance measurement and feedback system, the TIPI information system (TIPI-IS). Thus, the probability, ECG, and data entered into the electrocardiograph in clinical use (age, sex, presenting symptoms, physician, location) can be combined with other data and used for reports and analyses. This information allows clinicians and operations personnel of EMS and hospital organizations to use the same clinically valid risk-adjusted outcome predictions/measures (without medical record review).

The multicenter acute coronary ischemia time-insensitive predictive instrument clinical trial

In our 10-hospital, 10,689-patient clinical trial of the ACI-TIPI electrocardiograph's impact on ED triage of patients with symptoms suggestive of ACI conducted in public, private, community, and tertiary hospitals in urban, suburban, and semi-rural areas, the ACI-TIPI improved ED triage [11]. In doing so, it demonstrated differential impact depending on whether patients had ACI or not, whether the hospital had high or low cardiac telemetry unit capacity, and whether the triaging ED physician was an unsupervised resident or not. Even as the ACI-TIPI reduced unnecessary admissions, it did not reduce appropriate hospital and cardiac unit admission for patients with true ACI, either UA or AMI. This result further confirmed the ACI-TIPI's safety and effectiveness in ED use. Given that about 6% of ED patients presenting with symptoms suggesting ACI prove to have stable angina, such reductions would correspond yearly in the United States to approximately 30,000 fewer hospitalizations and 20,000 fewer CCU admissions, and about $728 million saved [11].

Studies of failure to hospitalize emergency department patients with acute coronary ischemia

Among our studies of factors contributing to ED triage and treatment errors [12–24], the authors have sought the causes for failing to hospitalize ED patients who have ACI [6,25,26]. In the authors' first such study, based on the care at the hospitals that participated in the original

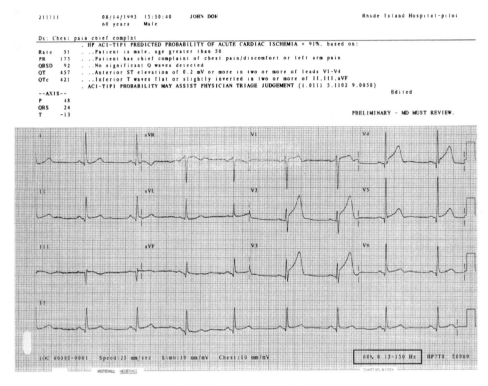

Fig. 1. ACI-TIPI ECG header.

ACI predictive instrument trial, approximately 2% of ED patients with AMI were sent home mistakenly [25], most commonly related to problems in physician use of the ECG [6,25]. Among ED patients sent home with AMI, 35% had ECG abnormalities consistent with ACI *noted* by the physician but not given sufficient weight in the triage decision [25]. Additionally, 25% had ECG abnormalities suggesting AMI (ST elevation) that were *missed* by the ED physician [25]. Analyses showing errors in physician ECG reading of ST segments and T waves contributing to suboptimal ED triage supported these findings [26].

In the authors' study of failure to hospitalize ED patients with ACI (AMI or UAP) in the ACI-TIPI Trial hospitals, the results were consistent with earlier findings [6]. Among the 10,689 ED patients studied, of those with AMI (n = 889), 2.1% were sent home, and of those with UAP (n = 966), 2.3% were not hospitalized. Yearly in the United States, this corresponds to 26,000 ED patients with ACI mistakenly not hospitalized: 12,000 with AMI and 14,000 with UAP. Of note, failure to hospitalize for ACI was more likely if the patient was nonwhite (2.2 times more likely, and 4.5 times more likely if having an AMI), a woman

under age 55 (6.7 times more likely) had a primary symptom of shortness of breath rather than chest pain (2.7 times more likely), or a normal or nondiagnostic ECG (3.3 times more likely, and 7.7 times more likely if having an AMI). These failures to hospitalize showed a statistical trend for greater mortality: nonhospitalized patients with AMI were 1.9 times more likely to die than similar patients who were hospitalized, and nonhospitalized patients with UAP were 1.7 times more likely to die than similar patients who were hospitalized.

These findings possibly reflected physicians' overdependence on generalities. Among ED patients, it is true that ACI is less likely in younger women, African-Americans, those without chest pain, and those with normal ECGs; but some such patients do have ACI. Physicians must be careful not to over-generalize about certain groups, and for these patients, the ACI-TIPI and TPI may help (see later discussion of TPI Trial on use of coronary reperfusion therapy for women). The wide range in hospitals' rates of failure to hospitalize (0%–11%) suggests that hospitals should monitor, and continually improve, their ED performance. Of note, "chest pain centers" did not have better performance; it seems that what is important is not the ED label, but that its physicians fully evaluate the entire patient, and understand the proper use of diagnostic technologies and receive feedback about diagnostic performance [27,28].

Acute coronary ischemia time-insensitive predictive instrument risk management tool: an ECG-based form for avoiding medical errors

Based on these studies, cases of patients who presented with AMI and mistakenly sent home were reviewed to devise a way to reduce such errors. A "risk management form" was developed and integrated into ACI-TIPI software so the form is generated and partially filled-out automatically by the electrocardiograph at the time of the patient's initial ECG (Fig. 2) [29]. The intent was that the form prompt consideration and documentation of the key clinical factors for such cases, be immediately and conveniently available for real-time use, and include the electrocardiograph's computerized interpretation in its text, along with the ACI-TIPI probability of ACI, to lessen the likelihood that ECG abnormalities and high-risk patients would be missed.

To assess the potential impact of the risk management form, the form was retrospectively applied to 20 cases that came to malpractice litigation. This information was also compared with what the impact would be were the form not automatically generated by the electrocardiograph, to see whether this approach was warranted. With the electrocardiograph-generated version, 61% of cases were seen as much less likely or certain to not come to malpractice litigation, versus 37% for the nonautomatic version ($P = .001$). Moreover, for those that would have come to litigation, had the automatic electrocardiograph-generated version been used, 80% would have had a significantly better outcome, including 59% who were judged to be likely to have a better outcome ($P = .001$). The provision of the ACI-TIPI probability should help the clinician appreciate the importance of such ECG abnormalities as contributors to the patient's likelihood of having ACI. The clinical information needed to fill out the rest of the form should provide the kind of documentation that better reveals appropriate care, and the process of filling-in the items was created in the hopes that it deter suboptimal care in the process of such documentation. Based

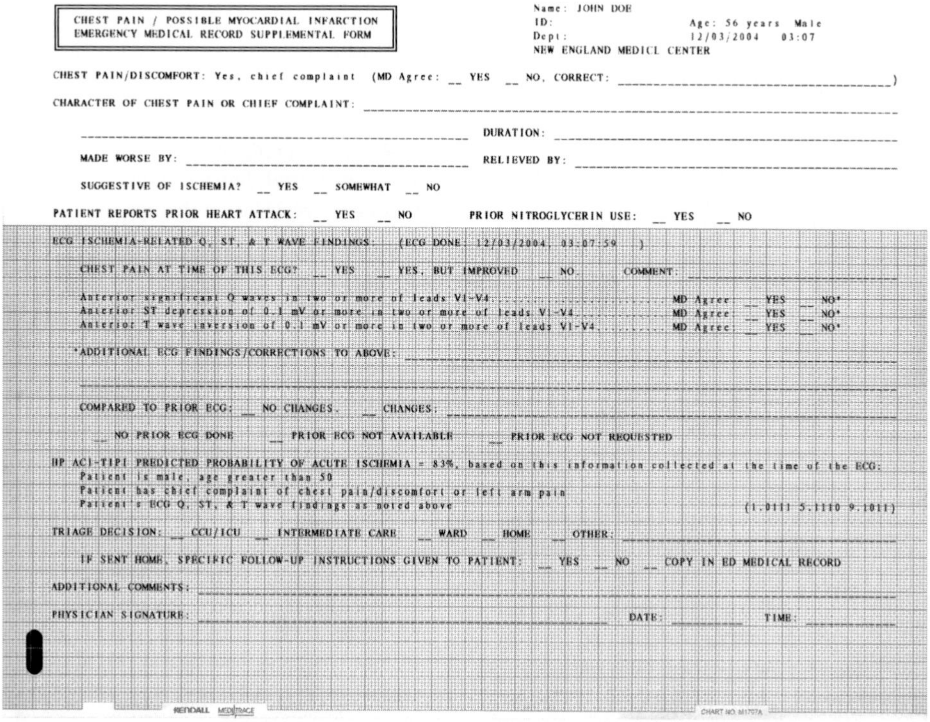

CHEST PAIN / POSSIBLE MYOCARDIAL INFARCTION
EMERGENCY MEDICAL RECORD SUPPLEMENTAL FORM

Name: JOHN DOE
ID: Age: 56 years Male
Dept: 12/03/2004 03:07
NEW ENGLAND MEDICL CENTER

CHEST PAIN/DISCOMFORT: Yes, chief complaint (MD Agree: __ YES __ NO, CORRECT: ______)

CHARACTER OF CHEST PAIN OR CHIEF COMPLAINT: ______

______ DURATION: ______

MADE WORSE BY: ______ RELIEVED BY: ______

SUGGESTIVE OF ISCHEMIA? __ YES __ SOMEWHAT __ NO

PATIENT REPORTS PRIOR HEART ATTACK: __ YES __ NO PRIOR NITROGLYCERIN USE: __ YES __ NO

ECG ISCHEMIA-RELATED Q, ST, & T WAVE FINDINGS: (ECG DONE: 12/03/2004, 03:07:59)

CHEST PAIN AT TIME OF THIS ECG? __ YES __ YES, BUT IMPROVED __ NO. COMMENT: ______

Anterior significant Q waves in two or more of leads V1-V4. .... MD Agree: __ YES __ NO*
Anterior ST depression of 0.1 mV or more in two or more of leads V1-V4. .... MD Agree: __ YES __ NO*
Anterior T wave inversion of 0.1 mV or more in two or more of leads V1-V4. .... MD Agree: __ YES __ NO*

*ADDITIONAL ECG FINDINGS/CORRECTIONS TO ABOVE: ______

COMPARED TO PRIOR ECG: __ NO CHANGES. __ CHANGES: ______

__ NO PRIOR ECG DONE __ PRIOR ECG NOT AVAILABLE __ PRIOR ECG NOT REQUESTED

HP ACI-TIPI PREDICTED PROBABILITY OF ACUTE ISCHEMIA = 83%, based on this information collected at the time of the ECG:
Patient is male, age greater than 50
Patient has chief complaint of chest pain/discomfort or left arm pain
Patient's ECG Q, ST, & T wave findings as noted above (1.0111 5.1110 9.1011)

TRIAGE DECISION: __ CCU/ICU __ INTERMEDIATE CARE __ WARD __ HOME __ OTHER: ______

IF SENT HOME, SPECIFIC FOLLOW-UP INSTRUCTIONS GIVEN TO PATIENT: __ YES __ NO __ COPY IN ED MEDICAL RECORD

ADDITIONAL COMMENTS: ______

PHYSICIAN SIGNATURE: ______ DATE: ______ TIME: ______

KENDALL MEDITRACE CHART NO. M1707A

Fig. 2. ECG risk management form.

on this, the authors worked with Hewlett-Packard (now Philips) to incorporate the automatic form into their electrocardiograph.

Financial implications of the impact of the form exist. For the 12 case records for which complete financial data were available, the legal and processing expenses averaged $45,000 and settlements averaged $337,000 [29]. With the form automatically generated by the electrocardiograph, the mean projected savings per case was $382,000, corresponding to $1.2 billion yearly savings in the United States. These savings should serve to make the ACI-TIPI approach attractive to hospitals, especially those with their own "captive" malpractice companies.

Development of the thrombolytic predictive instrument to assist recognition and treatment of ST-elevation myocardial infarction

Emergent coronary reperfusion therapy, used promptly, can be lifesaving for patients with ST-elevation myocardial infarction (STEMI) [7,30–32]. In emergency settings, however, this can be difficult, especially for less obvious candidates, and when key physician decision-makers are not on-site. Intensive efforts by physician leaders, the National Heart Attack Alert Program, organizations interested in quality of care, and others [32–41], have helped increase use and promptness of coronary reperfusion therapy [42]. Further improvement is needed [42,43], especially for other than anterior STEMI, the category of AMI for which thrombolytic therapy was first recognized as effective [7,30] and for women, who have received less coronary reperfusion therapy than men [43,44]. Also, a need remains for ways to support prompt and accurate coronary reperfusion therapy decisions in hospitals and prehospital EMS settings where consultation with off-site physicians is required.

To assist treatment decisions, the TPI was developed, a collection of five component predictive instruments designed to accurately assess the likely patient-specific benefits and risks from the use of thrombolytic therapy for STEMI. This tool helps clinicians identify patients for coronary reperfusion therapy based on their probabilities of benefits and complications and facilitates earliest possible use of coronary reperfusion therapy [5,45]. With manufacturers, programs were developed for conventional computerized electrocardiographs, so that when significant ST-segment elevation of STEMI is detected, TPI predictions

are automatically computed and printed on the ECG header. These predictions include probabilities for acute (30-day) mortality if and if not treated with thrombolytic therapy; 1-year mortality rates if and if not treated with thrombolytic therapy; cardiac arrest if and if not treated with thrombolytic therapy; thrombolytic therapy-related stroke and major bleeding requiring transfusion.

The TPI database, on which the TPI's five component models were developed and tested, include the original data on patients who presented with AMI from 13 clinical trials and registries, including 107 hospitals of all types throughout the United States, totaling 4911 patients [1,45–57]. Separate logistic regression predictive instruments were developed for each outcome. For each, clinically important and statistically significant variables were selected for preliminary models, alternative forms and combinations of these variables were investigated, and models reformulated to optimize performance while preserving parsimony. This included creating two special ECG variables to reflect two determinants of the impact of thrombolytic therapy: a measure of AMI size and an indicator of "earliness" in the AMI's course [56]. In addition, to satisfy the need for a regression method that could accommodate the rapidly changing influence of ECG-based infarct size, QT interval, and coronary reperfusion therapy use in the first hours of ACI/AMI, a new method of regression was devised [58].

Thrombolytic predictive instrument clinical effectiveness trial: impact on use and promptness of coronary reperfusion therapy

To test whether the electrocardiograph-based TPI improves ED selection of patients for coronary reperfusion therapy and promptness of treatment, a 22-month randomized controlled clinical effectiveness trial was run on the use and impact of thrombolytic therapy and overall coronary reperfusion therapy. Given our interest and the demonstrated need for improvement in the use of coronary reperfusion therapy [42,43], especially for other than anterior AMI [7,30] and for women [43,44], our study hypotheses focused on these groups, and also on hospitals where consultation with off-site physicians was required. Study endpoints were percentages of patients receiving (a) thrombolytic therapy; (b) thrombolytic therapy within 1 hour of ED presentation; and (c) all coronary reperfusion therapy, either by thrombolytic therapy or percutaneous transluminal coronary angioplasty (PTCA). The trial ran in EDs at 28 urban, suburban, and rural hospitals across the United States, from major cardiac centers to small community hospitals.

Included in the trial were all consenting patients at least 35 years old presenting to any study hospital with STEMI. At participating hospitals, software-generating TPI predictions was installed on conventional computerized electrocardiographs. When a significant ST-elevation characteristic of STEMI was automatically detected, the electrocardiograph randomly assigned the patient to the control or intervention group. If assigned to the intervention group, the electrocardiograph automatically prompted the user to enter information needed to compute the TPI predictions: age, sex, history of hypertension or of diabetes, blood pressure, and time since ischemic symptom onset. The remaining variables, based on ECG waveform measurements, were automatically acquired by the electrocardiograph. Then the ECG was printed with TPI predictions on its header (Fig. 3). If variables were missing, TPI predictions were not calculated, but an alert listing missing variables was printed, allowing entry of missing data, if available. For patients in the control

group, the ECG had only the header text customarily used in that ED.

Collected data included: sociodemographic data; initial and follow-up clinical features; ECGs and cardiac biomarker test results; triaging physician training level, specialty, and whether ED-based; whether on-site or off-site (telephone) consultation was used for the coronary reperfusion therapy decision; whether the patient received thrombolytic therapy or PTCA; and how long after chest pain onset was the therapy received. TPI software automatically acquired clinical variables required for TPI calculations and ECG Q-wave, ST-segment, and T-wave measurements. Site physicians, blinded to study group, assigned confirmed diagnoses based on presentation, clinical course, initial and follow-up ECGs, and biomarker tests, using the World Health Organization criteria [59]. Patients' ED care was classified by whether consultation with an off-site physician was used in making the treatment decision. Hospital size, type, whether having on-site ED staff, and physician type were used as potential explanatory variables.

Of 2875 patients who presented with AMI at the participating hospitals, 1243 (43%) had

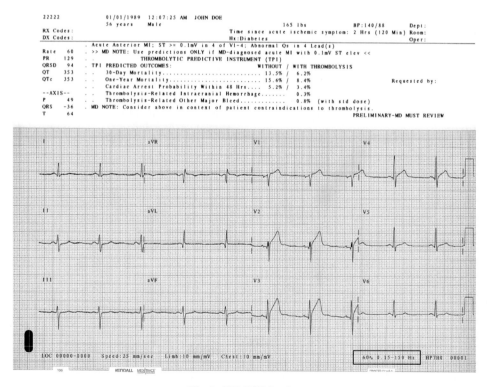

Fig. 3. TPI ECG header.

ST-segment elevation. Of these, 1197 were randomly assigned to study groups; 732 (61%) had
inferior STEMI, and 465 (39%) had anterior
STEMI. Of patients with inferior STEMI in the
control group, compared with the TPI group,
61% compared with 68% ($P = .03$) received
thrombolytic therapy; 53% compared with 59%
($P = .08$) received thrombolytic therapy within 1
hour; and 68% compared with 75% ($P = .03$) received coronary reperfusion therapy overall, either as thrombolytic therapy or primary PTCA.
Of patients with anterior STEMI in the control
group compared with the TPI group, 60% compared with 54% ($P > .2$) received thrombolytic
therapy; 51% compared with 45% ($P > .2$) received thrombolytic therapy within 1 hour; and
68% compared with 64% of TPI patients ($P >
.2$) received overall coronary reperfusion therapy.
Among women (n = 398) in the control group
compared with the TPI group, 48% compared
with 58% ($P = .03$) received thrombolytic therapy; 41% compared with 48% ($P = .10$) received
thrombolytic therapy within 1 hour; and 56%
compared with 66% ($P = .04$) received overall
coronary reperfusion therapy. Of patients who
required physician consultation by telephone
(n = 271) in the control group compared with
the TPI group, 47% compared with 63%
($P = .01$) received thrombolytic therapy; 41%
compared with 54% ($P = .04$) received thrombolytic therapy within 1 hour; and 51% compared
with 66% ($P = .01$) received overall coronary reperfusion therapy. Thus, the trial showed that
the TPI increased use of thrombolytic therapy,
use of thrombolytic therapy within 1 hour, and
use of overall coronary reperfusion therapy by
11% to 12% for patients with inferior STEMI,
18% to 22% for women, and 30% to 34% for patients with an off-site physician. The TPI's effect
was minimal on patients who exhibited high baseline coronary reperfusion therapyrates, such as for
men who presented with anterior STEMIs. For
the targeted groups (those more often missed,
women and those with less obvious STEMIs,
and situations in which physicians were off-site),
however, the TPI increased recognition of STEMI
and use and timeliness of coronary reperfusion
therapy.

In the TPI Trial, it is of interest that the TPI's
impact was not seen among patients with anterior
STEMI, and when combining STEMI locations, it
was not seen among men. This is thought to be
because anterior STEMIs have received longer-
standing emphasis for coronary reperfusion

therapy and are more easily recognized in the precordial leads of the conventional ECG, and thus
physicians already do a good job of detecting
them as appropriate candidates for coronary
reperfusion therapy, and treat them. Similarly,
AMI presents more "classically" in men and is
already better recognized (and treated) in men
than women [6,60,61]. The high rates of coronary
reperfusion therapy for anterior STEMI and men
when seen in experienced centers may require little
improvement. Less than 5% of the TPI Trial's patients, however, were seen in hospitals without on-
site ED physicians, and no patients were included
while in transit by way of EMS (when all physician input would be remote). Thus, it is important
that the TPI did improve the speed and use of
coronary reperfusion therapy among all patients
who presented with AMI (including anterior and
men) when the ED physician or needed physician
consultants are off-site. Because many hospitals'
EDs still are not staffed 24 hours daily, and, especially in rural settings, long transport times may
mandate EMS use of thrombolytic therapy or
a decision for direct transport to one of the
20% of United States hospitals that are primary
PTCA-capable [62], it seems likely that the
TPI may improve coronary reperfusion therapy
use for patients with anterior STEMI in these
settings.

The TPI is particularly attractive for EMS use.
Prehospital thrombolytic therapy is indicated for
situations in which transport times are long [63–
66], and the recent availability of single bolus
thrombolytic therapy [67–69] and the increasing
use of 12-lead ECGs in ambulances [70–74]
provide a foundation for this approach [75–77].
The provision of TPI predictions for patients
with STEMI in the field can support EMS use
of thrombolytic therapy. Also, for patients who
present with contraindications to thrombolytic
therapy, *pre*hospital identification as a reperfusion
candidate by the TPI can help avoid transport to
a facility lacking primary PTCA capability, avoiding the need for re-transport to a PTCA-capable
center. Clarifying reperfusion needs and options
in the field, especially in rural areas, can save
time, and improve patient outcomes [78]. That
the TPI increased overall coronary reperfusion
therapy use suggests it should facilitate decision-
making for both types of reperfusion in prehospital EMS use. Also, even with hospital-based
coronary reperfusion therapy, advance notice by
EMS, as in the MITI Trial [63], prompted by
the TPI, should reduce delays after arrival.

Time-insensitive predictive instrument information system cardiac error reduction system based on acute coronary ischemia time-insensitive predictive instrument demonstration project

Having shown that ACI-TIPI's predictions on ECGs provide effective real-time decision support, the TIPI-IS demonstration project was undertaken. An ACI-TIPI-IS was created to measure the impact of real-time, concurrent, and retrospective ACI-TIPI interventions on medical errors in ED triage. Also, through a series of user tests, the system's attractiveness and use for various users was evaluated, and its reports were modified to improve their usefulness in identifying and addressing medical error.

In the ACI-TIPI-IS demonstration project [79], the TIPI-IS provided concurrent and retrospective reporting and feedback for ED physicians and their hospitals. Implemented and used at five hospitals, the project provided a range of concurrent alerts and feedback reports to over 70 physicians at these facilities. This project has been successful in demonstrating the use of the ACI-TIPI probabilities within an information system providing concurrent alerting and retrospective feedback reports.

A prototype TIPI-IS database and web server-based user interface was created to (1) aggregate the ECG Management System data, ADT, Lab and ICD9 diagnostic coding data into a data warehouse database; and (2) create a TIPI-IS web server to distribute TIPI-IS reports and allow physicians (using a standard web browser) to explore the underlying patient data (Fig. 4). The web-based user interface was fully redesigned after repeated usability testing and enhanced with additional outcome information, including confirmed diagnoses of ACI after inpatient evaluation and whether patients had cardiac catheterization, PTCA or coronary bypass surgery. The system evaluation process included an iterative review with ED physicians leading to the redesign of screens and reports. Reports for comparison and benchmarking across groups of hospitals and for drill-down within a hospital were created and were additionally reviewed and revised by health plans and malpractice insurers to ensure that the reports met the requirements for risk reduction and medical error prevention programs (Fig. 5).

Implementation of the TIPI-IS had five major components: (1) preparation of the ECG equipment and ECG computerized management system; (2) installation of the TIPI-IS server within each hospital's intranet; (3) linking and integrating each

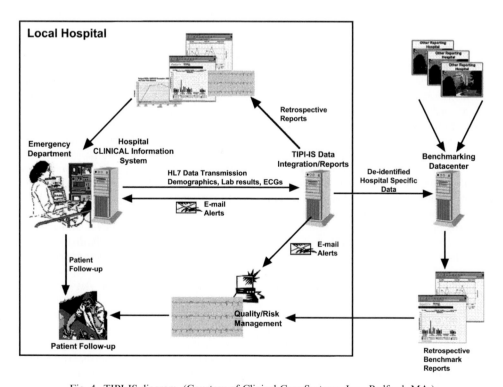

Fig. 4. TIPI-IS diagram. (Courtesy of Clinical Care Systems, Inc., Bedford, MA.)

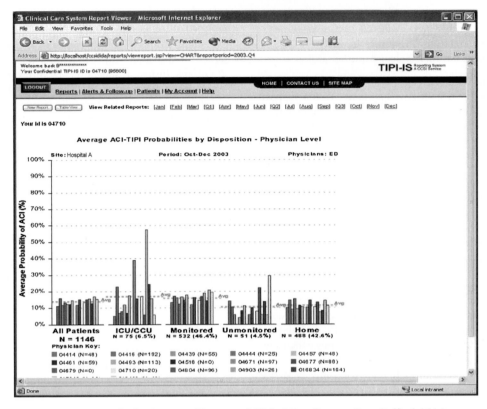

Fig. 5. TIPI-IS feedback report. (Courtesy of Clinical Care Systems, Inc., Bedford, MA.)

hospital's key computerized databases through electronic data interfaces to the TIPI-IS server; (4) testing of interface data; and (5) user training. Testing interfaces from feeder systems to the TIPI-IS at each site was conducted to ensure TIPI-IS captured data completely and mapped key data elements accurately for subsequent reporting. Electronic data collection eased the resources required to compile a large database, but also posed challenges in collecting accurate data because it depended on the diligence of staff entering the data for operational purposes rather than research purposes.

Access to data and reports through the web-based interface improved availability of data, and despite user testing and redesign of the original system, the web-based system continued to be available for use. Frequent users of the system were project staff and ED department Quality Improvement (QI) staff who had operational needs to access the data. When new reports or information were posted on the website, each physician received an e-mail with the link to the web page. A key advantage of the TIPI-IS approach,

which was successfully demonstrated, is the ability to compile large amounts of information for feedback reporting and error reduction through an automatic electronically compiled database. This process leveraged the clinical information systems already in place and minimized the resources required to collect and analyze data.

During the intervention period, ED QI nurses and physicians were given a general overview of the project and training in the use of the TIPI-IS, the content and significance of the concurrent alerts and feedback reports. These meetings were conducted with the ED physician leader who distributed physician-specific feedback reports with information from baseline data collection and a secure password to access their reports online.

Concurrent alerts were designed within the database system to signal patient cases that met criteria for immediate follow-up to prevent possible missed diagnosis of ACI. These thresholds included patients sent home from the ED with an ACI-TIPI value in the high-risk category or with a positive cardiac biomarker. The alert triggered an e-mail or pager message to the ED and ED physician indicating a patient required follow-up/review (Fig. 6). The results of follow-up on these alerts were entered into the alert follow-up screen. Patients were contacted to return to the EDs if needed and hospitalized for further evaluation when appropriate.

Retrospective review of a sample of patients sent home from the ED with moderate- to high-risk ACI-TIPI probabilities was conducted to identify cases of missed diagnosis of ACI. This review, conducted at each site by the ED director, identified a series of issues ranging from incomplete documentation to variations in practice, sometimes within, though sometimes not within, standard expectations of that ED. Results were addressed with staff during monthly morbidity and mortality review, in individual feedback discussions, and in some cases, by changes in the ED's practices.

Summary

Medical errors in the care of patients who present with ACS include errors in ED triage, such as the decision to send home a patient from the ED

who presents with ACS or to hospitalize a patient who does not prove to be experiencing ACS to the CCU, and errors in treatment, such as the failure to promptly use reperfusion therapy for patients with ST-elevation AMI. ECG-based ACI-TIPI and TPI predictive instruments, with a linked TIPI-IS, provide real-time, concurrent, and retrospective decision support tools and feedback for the prevention of medical errors in the care of patients who present with ACS. In real-time, ACI-TIPI probabilities printed on the ECG header for the ED physician, provide an additional piece of information for triage decision making, and the ACI-TIPI risk management form reduces liability risk by prompting consideration and documentation of key clinical factors in the diagnosis of ACI. Also in real-time, the TPI increases overall coronary reperfusion therapy use. Concurrent flagging by TIPI-IS uses electronically acquired ECG and hospital data to provide concurrent alerts about potential misdiagnosis or mis-triage of patients with ACS. Retrospectively TIPI-IS–based feedback reports allow performance improvement. These examples of information technology tools, integrated into ECG equipment already used in hospitals to deliver patient care, demonstrate the potential to adapt other existing equipment or other patient care activities to enhance patient safety and error reduction.

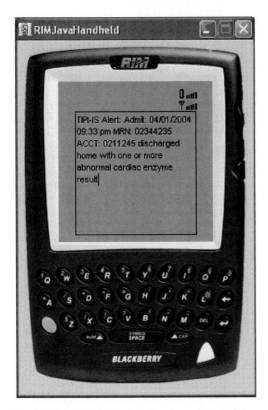

Fig. 6. TIPI-IS alert message. (Courtesy of Clinical Care Systems, Inc., Bedford, MA.)

References

[1] Pozen MW, D'Agostino RB, Selker HP, et al. A predictive instrument to improve coronary unit admission practices in acute ischemic heart disease. N Engl J Med 1984;310:1273–8.

[2] Selker HP, Griffith JL, D'Agostino RB. A tool for judging coronary care unit admission that is appropriate for both real-time and retrospective use: a time-insensitive predictive instrument (TIPI) for acute cardiac ischemia: a multicenter study. Med Care 1991;29:610–27.

[3] Selker HP, Griffith JL, D'Agostino RB. A time-insensitive predictive instrument for acute myocardial infarction mortality: a multicenter study. Med Care 1991;29:1196–211.

[4] Selker HP, Griffith JL, D'Agostino RB. A time-insensitive predictive instrument for acute mortality due to congestive heart failure: development, testing, and use for comparing hospitals: a multicenter study. Med Care 1994;32:1040–52.

[5] Selker HP, Griffith JG, Beshansky JR, et al. Patient-specific predictions of outcomes in myocardial infarction for real-time emergency use: a thrombolytic predictive instrument. Ann Intern Med 1997;127:538–48.

[6] Pope JH, Aufderheide TA, Ruthazer R, et al. A multicenter prospective study of missed diagnoses of acute myocardial infarction and unstable angina pectoris in the emergency department. N Engl J Med 2000;342:1163–70.

[7] Gruppo Italiano per lo Studio Della Streptochinasi Nell'Infarcto Miocardico (GISSI). Effectiveness of intravenous thrombolytic therapy in acute myocardial infarction. Lancet 1986;1:397–401.

[8] Weaver WB, Eisenberg MS, Martin JS, et al. Myocardial infarction triage and intervention project phase I: patient characteristics and feasibility of prehospital initiation of thrombolytic therapy. J Am Coll Cardiol 1990;15:925–31.

[9] Cairns CB, Niemann JT, Selker HP, et al. A computerized version of the time-insensitive predictive instrument: use of the Q wave, ST segment, T wave and patient history in the diagnosis of acute myocardial infarction by the computerized ECG. J Electrocardiol 1991;24:S46–9.

[10] Lobodzinski SM, Laks MM. Present and future concepts in computerized electrocardiography. Intern Med Specialist 1987;8:152–92.

[11] Selker HP, Beshansky JR, Griffith JL, et al. Use of the acute cardiac ischemia time-insensitive predictive instrument (ACI-TIPI) to assist emergency department triage of patients with chest pain or other symptoms suggestive of acute cardiac ischemia: a multicenter controlled clinical trial. Ann Intern Med 1998;129:845–55.

[12] Selker HP, Griffith JL, Dorey FJ, et al. How do physicians adapt when the coronary care unit is full? A prospective multicenter clinical study. JAMA 1987;257:1181–5.

[13] McCarthy BD, Wong JB, Selker HP. Detecting acute cardiac ischemia in the emergency department: a review of the literature. J Gen Intern Med 1990;5:365–73.

[14] Fleming C, D'Agostino RB, Selker HP. Is coronary care unit admission restricted for elderly patients? A multicenter study. Am J Public Health 1991;81:1121–6.

[15] Jayes RL, Beshansky JR, D'Agostino RB, et al. Do patients' coronary risk factors predict acute cardiac ischemia in the emergency room? J Clin Epidemiol 1992;45:621–6.

[16] Georgeson S, Linzer M, Griffith JL, et al. Acute cardiac ischemia in patients with syncope: importance of the initial electrocardiogram. J Gen Intern Med 1992;7:379–86.

[17] Larsen GC, Griffith JL, Beshansky JR, et al. Electrocardiographic left ventricular hypertrophy in patients with suspected acute cardiac ischemia—its influence on diagnosis, triage and short-term prognosis: a multicenter study. J Gen Intern Med 1994;9:666–73.

[18] Maynard C, Beshansky JR, Griffith JL, et al. The influence of sex on the use of cardiac procedures in patients presenting to the emergency department:

a prospective multicenter study. Circulation 1996;94:93–8.

[19] Maynard C, Beshansky JR, Griffith JL, et al. Causes of chest pain and symptoms suggestive of acute cardiac ischemia in African American patients presenting to the emergency department: a multicenter study. J Natl Med Assoc 1997;89:665–71.

[20] Picken HA, Zucker DR, Griffith JL, et al. Insurance type and the transportation to emergency departments of patients with acute cardiac ischemia: the ACI-TIPI insurance study. Am J Man Care 1998;4:821–7.

[21] Feldman JA, Fish SS, Beshansky JR, et al. Acute cardiac ischemia in patients with cocaine-associated complaints: results of a multicenter trial. Ann Emerg Med 2000;36:469–76.

[22] Udelson JE, Beshansky JR, Ballin DS, et al. Emergency department assessment of Tc-99m sestamibi imaging for evaluation and triage of patients with suspected acute cardiac ischemia: a randomized, multicenter, controlled clinical trial. JAMA 2002;288:2693–700.

[23] Pope JH, Ruthazer R, Kontos MC, et al. The impact of electrocardiographic left ventricular hypertrophy and bundle branch block on the triage and outcome of emergency department patients with a suspected acute coronary syndrome: a multicenter study. Am J Emerg Med 2004;22(3):156–63.

[24] Coronado BE, Pope JH, Griffith JL, et al. Clinical features, triage and outcome of patients presenting to the emergency department with a suspected acute coronary syndrome but without pain: a multicenter study. Am J Emerg Med 2004;22(7):568–74.

[25] McCarthy BD, Beshansky JR, D'Agostino RB, et al. Missed diagnoses of acute myocardial infarction in the emergency department: results from a multicenter study. Ann Emerg Med 1992;22:579–82.

[26] Jayes RL, Larsen GC, Beshansky JR, et al. Physician electrocardiogram reading in the emergency department—accuracy and effect on triage decisions: findings from a multicenter study. J Gen Intern Med 1992;7:387–92.

[27] Zalenski RJ, Rydman RJ, Ting S, et al. A national survey of emergency department chest pain centers in the United States. Am J Cardiol 1998;81:1305–9.

[28] Zalenski RJ, Selker HP, Cannon CP, et al. National Heart Attack Alert Program position paper: chest pain centers and programs for the evaluation of acute cardiac ischemia. Ann Emerg Med 2000;35:462–71.

[29] Selker HP, Beshansky JR, Pozen JD, et al. Electrocardiograph-based emergency department risk management tool based on the ACI-TIPI; potential impact on care and malpractice claims. J Healthc Risk Manag 2002;11–8.

[30] Fibrinolytic Therapy Trialists' (FTT) Collaborative Group. Indications for fibrinolytic therapy in suspected acute myocardial infarction: collaborative overview of early mortality and major morbidity

results from all randomized trials of more than 1000 patients. Lancet 1994;343:311–22.

[31] ISIS-2 (Second International Study of Infarct Survival) Collaborative Group. Randomized trial of intravenous streptokinase, oral aspirin, both, or neither among 17,187 cases of suspected acute myocardial infarction: ISIS-2. Lancet 1988;2:349–60.

[32] Cannon CP, Antman EM, Walls R, et al. Time as an adjunctive agent to thrombolytic therapy. J Thromb Thrombolysis 1994;1:27–34.

[33] National Heart Attack Alert Program Coordinating Committee 60 Minutes to Treatment Working Group. Emergency department: rapid identification and treatment of patients with acute myocardial infarction. Ann Emerg Med 1994;23:311–29.

[34] National Heart Attack Alert Program Coordinating Committee Access to Care Subcommittee. Emergency medical dispatching: rapid identification and treatment of acute myocardial infarction. Am J Emerg Med 1995;13:67–73.

[35] National Heart Attack Alert Program Coordinating Committee Access to Care Subcommittee. 9-1-1: rapid identification and treatment of acute myocardial infarction. Am J Emerg Med 1995;13:188–95.

[36] Rogers WJ, Bowlby LJ, Chandra NC, et al. Treatment of myocardial infarction in the United States (1990 to 1993) observations from the national registry of myocardial infarction. Circulation 1994;90:2103–14.

[37] National Heart Attack Alert Program Coordinating Committee Access to Care Subcommittee. Access to timely and optimal care of patients with acute coronary syndromes–community planning considerations: a report by the National Heart Attack Alert Program. J Thromb Thrombolysis 1998;6:19–36.

[38] National Heart Attack Alert Program Coordinating Committee Working Group on Educational Strategies to Prevent Prehospital Delay in Patients at High Risk for Acute Myocardial Infarction. Educational strategies to prevent prehospital delay in patients at high risk for acute myocardial infarction: a report by the National Heart Attack Alert Program. J Thromb Thrombolysis 1998;6:47–61.

[39] Sims RJ, Topol EJ, Holmes DR, et al. Link between the angiographic substudy and mortality outcomes in a large randomized trial of myocardial reperfusion: importance of early and complete infarct artery reperfusion. Circulation 1995;91:1923–8.

[40] Ryan TJ, Anderson JL, Antman EM, et al. ACC/AHA guidelines for the management of patients with acute myocardial infarction: a report for the American College of Cardiology/American Heart Association Task Force on Practice Guidelines (Committee on Management of Acute Myocardial Infarction). J Am Coll Cardiol 1996;28:1328–428.

[41] Ryan TJ, Antman EM, Brooks NH, et al. 1999 update: ACC/AHA guidelines for the management of patients with acute myocardial infarction: executive summary and recommendations: a report of the American College of Cardiology/American Heart Association Task Force on Practice Guidelines (Committee on Management of Acute Myocardial Infarction). Circulation 1999;100:1016–30.

[42] Rogers WJ, Canto JG, Lambrew CT, et al, for the Investigators in the National Registry of Myocardial Infarction 1, 2, and 3. Temporal trends in the treatment of over 1.5 million patients with myocardial infarction in the US from 1990 through 1999. J Am Coll Cardiol 2000;36:2056–63.

[43] Berger AK, Radford MJ, Krumholtz HM. Factors associated with delay in reperfusion therapy in elderly patients with acute myocardial infarction: analysis of the cooperative cardiovascular project. Am Heart J 2000;139:985–92.

[44] Barron HV, Bowlby LJ, Breen T, et al, for the National Registry of Myocardial Infarction 2 Investigators. Use of reperfusion therapy for acute myocardial infarction in the United States. Data from the National Registry of Myocardial Infarction 2. Circulation 1998;97:1150–6.

[45] Selker HP, Griffith JL, Beshansky JR, et al. The thrombolytic predictive instrument project: combining clinical study databases to take medical effectiveness research to the streets. Washington DC: AHCPR, DHHS; 1992.

[46] Kennedy JW, Martin GV, Davis KB, et al. The Western Washington intravenous streptokinase in acute myocardial infarction randomized trial. Circulation 1988;77:345–52.

[47] Proceedings of symposium on rapid identification and treatment of acute myocardial infarction. National Heart, Lung and Blood Institute, DHHS, USA, 1992.

[48] Weaver WB, Eisenberg MS, Martin JS, et al. Myocardial infarction triage and intervention project phase I: Patient characteristics and feasibility of prehospital initiation of thrombolytic therapy. J Am Coll Cardiol 1990;15:925–31.

[49] Pozen MW, D'Agostino RB, Mitchell JB, et al. The usefulness of a predictive instrument to reduce inappropriate admissions to the coronary care unit. Ann Intern Med 1980;92:238–42.

[50] Rosati RA, McNeer JF, Starmer CF, et al. A new information system for medical practice. Arch Intern Med 1975;135:1017–24.

[51] Pryor DP, Califf RM, Harrell FE, et al. Clinical databases: Accomplishments and unrealized potential. Med Care 1985;23:623–47.

[52] Topol EJ, Califf RM, George BS, et al. A randomized trial of immediate versus delayed elective angioplasty after intravenous tissue plasminogen activator in acute myocardial infarction. N Engl J Med 1987;317:581–8.

[53] Topol EJ, Califf RM, George BS, et al. Coronary arterial thrombolysis with combined infusion of recombinant tissue-type plasminogen activator and urokinase in patients with acute myocardial infarction. Circulation 1988;77:1100–7.

[54] Topol EJ, George BS, Kereiakes DJ, et al. A randomized controlled trial of intravenous tissue plasminogen activator and early intravenous heparin in acute myocardial infarction. Circulation 1989;79: 281–6.

[55] Wall TC, Strickland J, Masoud J, et al. Thrombolytic therapy on the homefront: intravenous urokinase in community hospitals. N C Med J 1989;50:363–6.

[56] Califf RM, Topol EJ, Stack RS, et al. Evaluation of combination thrombolytic therapy and timing of cardiac catheterization in acute myocardial infarction: results of the thrombolysis and angioplasty in myocardial infarction-phase 5 randomized trial. Circulation 1991;83:1543–56.

[57] Althouse R, Maynard C, Cerqueira MD, et al. The Western Washington myocardial infarction registry and emergency department tissue plasminogen activator treatment trial. Am J Cardiol 1990;66: 1298–303.

[58] Schmid CH, D'Agostino RB, Griffith JL, et al. A logistic regression model when some events precede treatment: the effect of thrombolytic therapy for acute myocardial infarction on the risk of cardiac arrest. J Clin Epidemiol 1997;50:1219–29.

[59] Gillum RF, Fortmann SP, Prineas RJ, et al. International diagnostic criteria for acute myocardial infarction and acute stroke. Am Heart J 1984;108:150–8.

[60] Zucker DR, Griffith JL, Beshansky JR, et al. Presentations of acute myocardial infarctions in men and women: results from a prospective, multicenter study. J Gen Intern Med 1997;12:79–87.

[61] Coronado BE, Griffith JL, Beshansky JR, et al. Hospital mortality in women and men with acute cardiac ischemia: a prospective multicenter study. J Am Coll Cardiol 1997;29:1490–6.

[62] Lange RA, Hillis LD. Should thrombolysis or primary angioplasty be the treatment of choice for acute myocardial infarction? N Engl J Med 1996; 335:1311–7.

[63] Weaver WD, Cerqueira M, Hailstrom AP, et al. Prehospital-initiated vs. hospital initiated thrombolytic therapy the myocardial infarction triage and intervention trial. JAMA 1993;270:1211–6.

[64] Selker HP, Zalenski RJ, Antman EM, et al. An evaluation of technologies for identifying acute cardiac ischemia in the emergency department: a report from a national heart attack alert working group. Ann Emerg Med 1997;29:1–87.

[65] Rawles J. Halving of mortality at 1 year by domiciliary thrombolysis in the Grampian Region Early Anistreplase Trial (GREAT). J Am Coll Cardiol 1994;23:1–5.

[66] The European Myocardial Infarction Project Group. Prehospital thrombolytic therapy in patients with suspected acute myocardial infarction. N Engl J Med 1993;329:383–9.

[67] Cannon CP, Gibson CM, McCabe CH, et al, for the Thrombolysis in Myocardial Information (TIMI) 10B Investigators. TNK-tissue plasminogen activator compared with front-loaded alteplase in acute myocardial infarction. Results of the TIMI 10B trial. Circulation 1998;98:2805–14.

[68] Van de Werf F, Cannon CP, Luyten A, et al. Safety assessment of single bolus administration of TNK-tPA in acute myocardial infarction. The ASSENT-1 trial. Am Heart J 1999;137:786–91.

[69] Fong WC, Fox NL, Cannon CP, et al. Determination of a weight-adjusted dose of TNK-tissue plasminogen activator. Am Heart J 2001;141:33–40.

[70] Aufderheide TP, Hendley GE, Thakur RK, et al. The diagnostic impact of prehospital 12-lead electrocardiography. Ann Emerg Med 1990;19:1280–7.

[71] Karagounis L, Ipsen SK, Jessop MR, et al. Impact of field-transmitted electrocardiography on time to in-hospital thrombolytic therapy in acute myocardial infarction. Am J Cardiol 1990;66:786–91.

[72] Canto JG, Rogers WJ, Bowlby LJ, et al. The prehospital electrocardiogram in acute myocardial infarction: is its full potential being realized? J Am Coll Cardiol 1997;29:498–505.

[73] Kereiakes DJ, Gibler WB, Martin LH, the Cincinnati Heart Project Study Group, et al. Relative importance of emergency medical system transport and the prehospital electrocardiogram on reducing hospital time delay to therapy for acute myocardial infarction. A preliminary report from the Cincinnati Heart Project. Am Heart J 1992;123:835–40.

[74] Kudenchuk PJ, Maynard C, Cobb LA, et al. Utility of the prehospital electrocardiogram in diagnosing acute coronary syndromes: the Myocardial Infarction Triage and Intervention (MITI) project. J Am Coll Cardiol 1998;32:17–27.

[75] Cannon CP, Sayah AJ, Walls RM. Prehospital thrombolysis: an idea whose time has come. Clin Cardiol 1999;22:10–9.

[76] Amit G, Weiss T, Zahger D. Coronary angioplasty or intravenous thrombolysis: the dilemma of optimal reperfusion in acute myocardial infarction: a critical review of the literature. J Thromb Thrombolysis 1999;8:113–23.

[77] Stern R, Arntz HR. Prehospital thrombolysis in acute myocardial infarction. Eur J Emerg Med 1998;5:471–9.

[78] Widimsky P, Groch L, Zelizko M, et al, on behalf of the PRAGUE Study Group Investigators. Multicentre randomized trial comparing transport to primary angioplasty vs. immediate thrombolysis vs. combined strategy for patients with acute myocardial infarction presenting to a community hospital without a catheterization laboratory. The PRAGUE study. Eur Heart J 2000;21:823–31.

[79] Daudelin D, Selker H, Kwong M, et al. Information technology to reduce errors in emergency cardiac care. In: Henriksen K, Battles JB, Marks E, et al, editors. Advances in patient safety: from research to implementation. Vol. 3. Implementation issues. Rockville, MD: Agency for Healthcare Research and Quality; 2005 in press.

Cumulative Index 2005

Note: Page numbers of article titles are in **boldface** type.

A

Accelerated diagnostic protocols (ADPs), in CPUs, 504

Accident(s), diving, patent foramen ovale and, history of, 98

ACCORD trial, in prevention of cardiovascular outcomes in type 2 diabetes, 215

ACE inhibitors. See *Angiotensin-converting enzyme (ACE) inhibitors.*

ACI. See *Acute coronary ischemia (ACI).*

ACI predictive instrument. See *Acute coronary ischemia (ACI) predictive instrument.*

Acid(s), fatty, free, unbound, as biomarker of cardiac ischemia, 496

ACI-TIPI, for real-time and retrospective decision support, 602–603

ACI-TIPI clinical trial, multicenter, 603

ACI-TIPI demonstration project, TIPI information system cardiac error reduction system based on, 608–611

ACI-TIPI management tool, in medical error prevention, 605–606

ACSs. See *Acute coronary syndromes (ACSs).*

Acute care facilities, financial pressures on, 589–590

Acute coronary ischemia (ACI), ED patients with, failure to hospitalize, studies of, 603–605

Acute coronary ischemia (ACI) predictive instrument, original, 602

Acute coronary syndromes (ACSs), **401–409**
  clinical presentation of, chest discomfort in, 425–426
  ED demands of, 590
  ED triage for, medical error prevention in, **601–614**

ACI-TIPI for real-time and retrospective decision support in, 602–603
decision support and risk reduction tolls for real-time use in, 602
ECG in, 603
multicenter clinical trial, 603
original ACI predictive instrument in, 602
future directions in, 589
in ED and CPUs, troponin for, 455–456
missed diagnoses of, in ED, **423–451**
  angina pain equivalents and, 426–427
  atypical presentation–related, 427–428
  biochemical markers and, 435–437
  biomarkers of neurohumoral activation and inflammation and, 437
  cardiac imaging–related, 437–438
  central aortic pressure–related, 438
  chest discomfort–related, 425–426
  clinical presentation–related factors, 425
  computer-based decision aids and, 438–440
  creatine kinase and, 435–436
  described, 423–424
  ECG-related. See also under *Electrocardiography (ECG).*
  ECG–related, 430–435
  Goldman Chest Pain Protocol–related, 438–439
  in women, causes of, 439–440
  methodologic issues related to, 424–425
  myocardial performance index–related, 438
  myoglobin and, 436–437
  outcomes of, 441–443
  past medical history–related, 428–429
  physical examination–related, 429–430
  Q wave–related, 432
  race-related, 440–441
  technetium-99m sestamibi myocardial perfusion imaging–related, 438
  troponin and, 436
prevalence of, 401, 601
risk scores, 403–404
risk stratification for, 402

0733-8651/05/$ - see front matter © 2005 Elsevier Inc. All rights reserved.
doi:10.1016/S0733-8651(05)00091-3

cardiology.theclinics.com

Acute coronary (*continued*)
  suspected, evaluation of, imaging in,
    517–530
    acute myocardial perfusion imaging,
      517–518
    cost-effectiveness of, 525
    diagnostic value in, 518–522
    in special populations, 524–525
    incorporation into chest pain evaluation,
      525–527
    negative predictive value and prognosis,
      519–521
    radiopharmaceutical issues in, 522–523
    sensitivity in, 518–519
    tracer injection timing in, 523–524
    troponin and, 523
  treatment of, 404–407
    antithrombotic agents in, 404–405
    reperfusion therapy in, 407
    STEMI–related, 406
    thrombolysis in, 406–407
  without myocardial infarction, evaluation of,
    imaging in, 519

Acute myocardial infarction, diabetes mellitus
  and, management of, intensive glycemic
  control in, **111–128**

Acute myocardial perfusion imaging, in suspected
  ACS evaluation, 517–518

ADHF. See *Heart failure, acute decompensated.*

ADPs. See *Accelerated diagnostic protocols
  (ADPs).*

α-Adrenergic agonists, for diabetes and
  hypertension, 144

ADVANCE trial, in prevention of cardiovascular
  outcomes in type 2 diabetes, 214–215

Albumin, ischemia modified, as biomarker of
  cardiac ischemia, 496

Albuminuria, cardiovascular disease in diabetics
  and, 132

Aldosterone antagonists, in ADHF management
  in EDOU, 583

Amplatzer atrial septal defect occluder, in patent
  foramen ovale closure, 78–79

Amputation, for peripheral arterial disease in
  CKD, 231

Amyloidosis, cardiac, NOCAD due to, 562

Anemia
  CKD and, 354

management of, in cardiovascular disease in
  renal transplant recipients, 338

Aneurysmal patent foramen ovale, 40–41

Angel Wings device, in patent foramen ovale
  closure, 79–80

Angina, described, 559

Angina pain, equivalents of, in ACS presentation,
  428–429

Angioplasty, for cardiovascular disease in CKD,
  305–307

Angiotensin, in diabetes mellitus prevention, 174

Angiotensin II–receptor blockers, for diabetes and
  hypertension, 144–145

Angiotensin-converting enzyme (ACE) inhibitors,
  for diabetes and hypertension, 142–143

Ankle brachial index less than 0.90, peripheral
  arterial disease in CKD and, prevalence of, 226

Anticoagulant(s), in ADHF management in
  EDOU, 583

Antihypertensive and Lipid-Lowering Treatment
  to Prevent Heart Attack Trial, 347

Anti-inflammatory drugs, nonsteroidal
  in ADHF management in EDOU, 583
  in hypertension, 240–241

Antioxidant(s)
  in dialysis, studies of, 325–326
  in uremia, 324–325

Antiplatelet agents
  for cardiovascular disease in renal transplant
    recipients, 337
  for peripheral arterial disease in CKD, 230

Antithrombotic agents, for ACSs, 404–405

Arterial disease, CKD and, 277

Arteriosclerotic cardiovascular disease, uremia-
  related factors for, 354

Arteriovenous fistulae
  for vascular access in hemodialysis, 249–250
    failure of, pathology of, 257–258
    prevalence of, 254–255
    rationale for, 256
    surveillance of, 256–257
    venous stenosis in, pathogenesis of, 260–262

Artery(ies), central, renal failure effects on, 313

Atherogenesis, accelerated, renal failure and, 313

Atherosclerosis, oxidative stress and, 320–321

Atherothrombosis, inflammation and, biomarkers of, 491–492

Atrial septal defect closure, in pediatric patients, 42–43

Atrial septal defect occlusion system, in patent foramen ovale closure, 81–82

Atrial septum, anatomy of, 36–37

B

Balanced Budget Act (BBA), 589

Balloon occlusion, temporary, trial of, 37–39

BARI 2D study, in prevention of cardiovascular outcomes in type 2 diabetes, 216

BBA. See *Balanced Budget Act (BBA).*

Beta-blockers
for ADHF in EDOU, 583
for cardiovascular disease in renal transplant recipients, 337
for CHF in CKD, 279
for diabetes and hypertension, 144

Biguanide(s), in prevention of cardiovascular disease in diabetics, 127–128

Binding proteins, fatty acid, in ED and CPUs, 455

Biochemical markers, missed diagnosis of ACS in ED due to, 437–439

Biomarkers
in ED and CPUs, **453–465**
background of, 453–455
creatine kinase myocardial band, 455
fatty acid binding protein, 455
for patients with ST elevation and myocardial infarction, 456–457
ischemia-related, 455–456
myoglobin, 455
troponin, 453–455
for high-risk patients with ACSs, 457–458
for intermediate and low risk patients, 458–460
for patients with ST elevation and myocardial infarction, 456–457
for renal failure patients, 460–461
of atherothrombosis and inflammation, 491–492
of CAD, **491–501**
of cardiac ischemia, 495–497

B-type (brain) natriuretic peptide, 496–497
ischemia modified albumin, 496
unbound free fatty acid, 496
of inflammation
CD40 ligand, 494–495
C-reactive protein, 492–494
IL-6, 494
IL-10, 495
lipoprotein-associated phospholipase A2, 494
selectins, 495
serum amyloid A, 495
of neurohumoral activation and inflammation, missed diagnoses of ACS in ED due to, 439
of plaque instability or rupture, 497–498

Blood pressure
management of
for peripheral arterial disease in CKD, 229
in cardiovascular disease in renal transplant recipients, 336
in prevention of cardiovascular outcomes in type 2 diabetes, 218–219
renal replacement therapy effects on, 386–387
target, in diabetics with hypertension, 148
thiazolidinediones effects on, in prevention of cardiovascular disease in diabetics, 129–130

Body weight, cardiovascular disease in diabetics and, 132

B-type (brain) natriuretic peptide
as biomarker of cardiac ischemia, 496–497
vs. filling pressures, in ADHF management in EDOU, 575

B-type (brain) natriuretic peptide assays, in ADHF management in EDOU, 574–575

B-type (brain) natriuretic peptide confounders, in ADHF management in EDOU, 575

Buttoned device, in patent foramen ovale closure, 79

Bypass Angioplasty Revascularization Investigation 2 Diabetes Trial, 190–191

C

CAD. See *Coronary artery disease (CAD).*

Calcification, vascular
CKD and, 357
in renal failure, **373–384.** See also *Renal failure, vascular calcification in.*

Calcium channel blockers
  for diabetes and hypertension, 144
  in ADHF management in EDOU, 583

Calcium–phosphate metabolism, renal
  replacement therapy effects on, 387–388

Cardiac amyloidosis, NOCAD due to, 562

Cardiac biomarker POCT
  applications of, 474–476
  in CPUs, **467–490**
    algorithmic strategies, 479–481
    cost-effectiveness of, 479–481
    customer satisfaction, 481–482
    multimarkers, 479–481
    planning and implementation of, 482–484
    risk management, 481–482
    timeliness in, 478–479
    TTAT in, 477–478
  technologies for, 469–477
  types of, 470–472

Cardiac ischemia, biomarkers of, 495–497. See
  also *Biomarkers, of cardiac ischemia.*

Cardiac valvular abnormalities, in CKD, 350

Cardiologist(s), pediatric, in patent foramen ovale
  closure, **35–45**. See also *Patent foramen ovale,
  closure of, pediatric cardiologist in.*

Cardiomyopathy
  CKD and, 276
  microvascular dysfunction and, NOCAD due
    to, 561

CardioSEAL septal occluder, in patent foramen
  ovale closure, 74–77

Cardiovascular diseases
  arteriosclerotic, uremia-related factors for, 354
  CKD and, **343–362, 363–372.** See also *Chronic
    kidney disease (CKD), cardiovascular
    disease due to.*
  diabetes mellitus and
    prevention of, **121–139.** See also *Diabetes
      mellitus, cardiovascular disease
      associated with, prevention of.*
    type 2, prevention of. See also *Diabetes
      mellitus, type 2, cardiovascular outcomes
      in, prevention of.*
  diabetes melltius and, type 2, prevention of,
    213–222
  ESRD and, 311, 349–350
    mortality due to, 385
  in renal replacement therapy patients,
    349–350

in renal transplant recipients, management of,
  331–342. See also *Renal transplant
  recipients, cardiovascular disease in,
  management of.*
renal failure and, pathophysiology of, **311–317.**
  See also *Renal failure, cardiovascular disease
  and, pathophysiology of.*

Cardiovascular events, renal replacement therapy
  and, 388–389

Cardiovascular Health Study, 345–346, 353

Cardiovascular risk factors, in diabetics,
  comprehensive risk reduction of, **195–212.** See
  also *Diabetes mellitus, cardiovascular risk
  factors in patients with, comprehensive risk
  reduction of.*

Catheter(s)
  cuffed double-lumen silicone, for vascular
    access in hemodialysis, 251–252
  in patent foramen ovale closure, 41–42

CD40 ligand, as biomarker of inflammation,
  494–495

Centers for Medicare and Medicaid Services
  (CMS), 591–593

Central aortic pressure, missed diagnoses of ACS
  in ED due to, 440

Central arteries, renal failure effects on, 313

Chest discomfort, in ACS presentation, 427–428

Chest pain
  evaluation of, imaging of suspected ACS in,
    525–527
  in ED
    EBCT for triaging patients with, **541–548**
    MSCT for triaging patients with, 545
  stimulant use–related, in CPUs, 554–555
  with normal coronary angiogram,
    management of, **559–568.** See *Chest pain
    with normal coronary angiogram
    (NOCAD).*

Chest pain centers (CPCs). See *Chest pain units
  (CPUs).*

Chest pain units (CPUs)
  ADPs in, 504
  biomarkers in, **453–465.** See also *Biomarkers,
    in ED and CPUs.*
  concept of, **411–421**
  cost effectiveness of, 418–419, **589–599**
  described, 504
  echocardiography in, **531–539**

efficacy of, 415–418
emergence of, 591
examples of, 414–415
exercise testing in, **503–516**
  as indicator of low clinical risk, 503–504
  described, 507–510
  early
    current guidelines for, 505–506
    initial recommendations for, 504–505
    initial studies of, 506–507
  immediate, 510–513
  in special groups, 512
  issues related to, 512–513
  vs. myocardial scintigraphy, 511–512
federal regulations for, 593–594, 595–596
for acute coronary syndrome patients, 591
for special patients, **549–557**
  CAD–related, 551–553
  chest pain related to stimulant use, 554–555
  diabetics, 553–554
  women, 549–551
implementation of, 411–414
origin of, 589
quality implications of, 594
reimbursement issues related to, 591–593
synonyms for, 504
trans-theoretic Y model application in, 594, 596–598
women in, management of, 549–551

Chest pain with normal coronary angiogram (NOCAD)
cardiomyopathy and, 561
coronary spasm and, 561, 563–564
differential diagnosis of, 560
endothelial dysfunction and, 559–561, 563
epicardial disease and, 560–561
hypertension and, 561
management of, **559–568**
microvascular disease and, 561–562, 565
microvascular dysfunction and, 560, 565
  idiopathic, 562
microvascular endothelial dysfunction and, 561, 565
myocardial bridging due to, 561, 564–565
noncoronary causes of, 560, 562
  diagnosis of, systemic approach to, 562–563
pathophysiology of, 559–560
prognosis of, 563–565
valvular disease and, 562

CHF. See *Congestive heart failure (CHF)*.

Children, atrial septal defect closure in, 42–43

Choline, whole blood, as biomarker of plaque instability or rupture, 497

Chronic kidney disease (CKD)
anemia and, 354
arterial disease due to, 277
CAD in, **285–298**
  assessment of, 285–286
  outcomes of, 293–294
  risk factors for
    in dialysis patients, 286–287
    in nondialysis patients, 287–289
cardiac valvular abnormalities in, 350
cardiovascular disease due to, **343–362, 363–372**
  accelerated, pathophysiology of, 350–357
  Antihypertensive and Lipid-Lowering Treatment to Prevent Heart Attack Trial, 347
  British population-based study, 346
  Cardiovascular Health Study, 345–346
  described, 345–347
  Framingham Offspring community study, 346
  Hoorn study, 345
  HOPE study, 346
  managed care group database analysis, 346–347
  management of
    medical therapy in, 307–308
    primary angioplasty in, 305–307
    rationale for, 304–305
  pathophysiology of, 276–277
  percutaneous coronary interventions for, **299–310**
    creatinine levels after, outcome-related, 300–301
  renal protection for, rationale for, 301
  risk factors for, 299–300
  Second National Health and Nutrition Examination Survey mortality study, 346
  studies of, 345–347
    conclusions from, 347–349
CHF in, **275–284**
  epidemiology of, 277
  management of, 278–280
    beta-blockers in, 279
    diabetes management in, 279
    dialysis in, 279
    digoxin in, 279
    diuretics in, 279
    erythropoietin in, 279
    hypertension management in, 278–279

Chronic kidney disease (CKD) (*continued*)
      nephrology referral in, 279
      renin-angiotensin system interruption in,
         279
      smoking cessation in, 279
      statins in, 279
    pathophysiology of, 276–277
    risk factors for, 277–278
  chronic microinflammation and, 355–357
  coronary pathobiology in, 304
  diabetes mellitus and, 351, 365
  dyslipidemia in, 351–353, 364–365
    interactions between, mechanisms for, 366
    treatment of, 366–367
  erythropoietin for, 354–355
  health care perspective on, 275
  hypertension in, **237–248**, 350. See also
    Hypertension, in CKD.
  inflammation in, markers of, 353
  ischemic heart disease due to, 276–277
  left ventricular hypertrophy and, 355
  lipids and, 365
  microalbuminuria and, 350–351
  myocardial stress in, biomarkers of, 357–358
  nontraditional modifiable factors in, 353
  oxidative pathways in, **319–330**. See also
    Oxidative stress.
  oxidative stress and, 355–357
  patient perspective on, 275–276
  peripheral arterial disease in
    ankle brachial index less than 0.90 due to,
      prevalence of, 226
    diagnostic testing for, 226–227
    epidemiology of, 225–228
    impact of, 228
    incidence of, 227–228
    intermittent claudication due to, prevalence
      of, 225–226
    management of, **225–236**
      amputation in, 231
      antiplatelet agents in, 230
      blood pressure–lowering agents in, 229
      cilostazol in, 230
      exercise in, 230
      revascularization in, 230–231
      smoking cessation in, 229–230
      statin therapy in, 228–229
      surgical, 230–231
    prevalence of, 225
  peripheral vascular disease in
    outcomes of, 290–293
    risk factors for, 289–290
  proteinuria and, 350–351

  stages of, 343–344, 364
    impact on cardiovascular biology, 344–345
  valve replacement in, 350
  vascular calcification and, 357

Cilostazol, for peripheral arterial disease in CKD,
  230

CKD. See *Chronic kidney disease (CKD).*

Claudication, intermittent, peripheral arterial
  disease in CKD and, prevalence of, 225–226

CMS. See *Centers for Medicare and Medicaid
  Services (CMS).*

Coagulation, cardiovascular disease in diabetics
  and, 131

Cocaine, in hypertension, 240

Computer-based decision aids, missed diagnoses
  of ACS in ED due to, 440–442

Congenital heart disease, patent foramen ovale
  and, 37–39

Congestive heart failure (CHF)
  cardiovascular disease in renal transplant
    recipients due to, 333–334
  in CKD, **275–284**. See also *Chronic kidney
    disease (CKD), CHF in.*

Consent, informed, for patent foramen ovale
  closure, 18–19

Contrast-induced nephropathy
  pathophysiology of, 301–302
  prevention of, 302–304

Coronary angiogram, normal, chest pain and,
  management of, **559–568**. See also *Chest pain
  with normal coronary angiogram (NOCAD).*

Coronary artery bypass grafting, percutaneous
  coronary intervention *vs.*, in diabetics,
  187–193. See also *Diabetes mellitus,
  percutaneous coronary intervention vs. coronary
  artery bypass grafting in.*

Coronary artery disease (CAD)
  biomarkers of, **491–501**
  in CKD, **285–298**. See also *Chronic kidney
    disease (CKD), CAD in.*
  likelihood of, 402–403
  management of, in CPUs, 551–553
  prevalence of, 402–403

Coronary revascularization, in diabetics, 187

Coronary spasm, NOCAD due to, 561, 563–564

CPUs. See *Chest pain units (CPUs).*

C-reactive protein, as biomarker of inflammation, 492–494

Creatine kinase, missed diagnoses of ACS in ED due to, 437–438

Creatine kinase myocardial band, in ED and CPCs, 455

Cuffed double-lumen silicone catheters, for vascular access in hemodialysis, 251–252

Cyclosporine, in hypertension, 240

D

Diabetes mellitus
  acute myocardial infarction with, management of, intensive glycemic control in, **111–128**
  as coronary hear disease risk-equivalent, 155
  burden of, 167
  cardiovascular disease associated with
    albuminuria and, 132
    body weight and, 132
    coagulation and, 131
    fibrinolysis and, 131
    glycemic control effects on, 122–123
    inflammation and, 131
    insulin resistance effects on, 122–123
    insulin sensitizing agents effects on, 123
    prevalence of, 121
    prevention of, **121–139**
      insulin secretagogues in, 123–126
      insulin sensitizing agents in, 127–132
      metformin in, 128
      nonsulfonylurea secretagogues in, 127
      thiazolidinediones in, 128–131
    treatment of, 132–133
  cardiovascular risk factors in patients with
    comprehensive reduction of, **195–212**
    current state of affairs, 209–210
    dyslipidemia, 197–199
    future directions related to, 209–210
    hyperglycemia, 202–203
    hypertension, 199–202
    increased thrombotic tendency, 203–204
    multiple risk factor intervention for, 204–208
    practical considerations related to, 208–209
  CKD and, 351, 365
  coronary revascularization in, 187
  ESRD due to, 363
  hypertension and, **141–153**
    described, 141–142
    renal failure with, treatment of, 147
    target blood pressure in patients with, 148

    treatment of
      ACE inhibitors in, 142–143
      α-adrenergic agonists in, 144
      angiotensin II–receptor blockers in, 144–145
      antihypertensive agents in, 145–147
      ß-blockers in, 144
      calcium channel blockers in, 144
      combination therapy in, 148–150
      drugs in, 142–150
      surrogate markers in, 147
      thiazide diuretics in, 143–144
  lipid management in, **155–164**
    combination therapy in, 161–162
    evidence from, 156–157
    goals in, 159
    principles of, 159–161
  lipoprotein abnormalities associated with, 155–156
  management of
    in CHF in CKD, 279
    in CPUs, 553–554
    renin-angiotensin system in, 168–170
  new onset, renin angiotensin system in, 176–177
  percutaneous coronary intervention *vs.*
    coronary artery bypass grafting in, **187–193**
    Bypass Angioplasty Revascularization Investigation 2 Diabetes Trial, 190–191
    described, 187–189
    emerging therapies, 191–192
    repeat vascularization, 189
  prevention of
    lifestyle modifications in, 168, 174–176
    renin angiotensin system in, **167–185**
  renin-angiotensin system in, **167–185**
    activation of, 170–172
    as preventive agent, **167–185**
    as therapeutic agent, **167–185**
    in endothelial function, 174
    in new onset diabetes, 176–177
    in vascular endothelial function, 172–173
    interaction between angiotensin, endothelium, and insulin resistance, 174, 177–180
  risk factors for, 167–168
  triglyceride and high-density lipoprotein intervention in, 157–159
  type 2
    cardiovascular outcomes in, prevention of, **213–222**
      blood pressure interventions in, 218–219

Diabetes mellitus (*continued*)
  clinical trials examining glycemic
    management techniques in,
    215–218
  clinical trials examining glycemic targets
    in, 214–215
  lifestyle interventions in, 219–220
  lipids in, 218–219
  nonglycemic therapies in, 218–220
  revascularization interventions in, 218
  described, 213

Diagnostic value
  in suspected ACS evaluation, 518–522
  incremental, in suspected ACS evaluation,
    521–522

Dialysis
  antioxidants in, studies of, 325–326
  hypertension in patients on, 241–242
  in CHF in CKD management, 279

Digoxin
  in ADHF management in EDOU, 583
  in CHF in CKD management, 279

Diuretic(s)
  in ADHF management in EDOU, 581–582
  in CHF in CKD management, 279
  thiazide, for diabetes and hypertension,
    143–144

Diving, patent foramen ovale and, **97–104.** See
  also *Patent foramen ovale, diving and.*

Diving accidents, patent foramen ovale and,
  history of, 98

DREAM study, in prevention of cardiovascular
  outcomes in type 2 diabetes, 217–218

Drug(s), in hypertension, 240–241

Dyslipidemia
  in CKD, 351–353, 364–365
    mechanisms for, 366
    treatment of, 366–367
  in diabetes mellitus, 197–199

E

EBCT. See *Electron beam CT (EBCT).*

ECG. See *Electrocardiography (ECG).*

Echocardiographer(s), in placement of patent
  foramen ovale closure devices, **53–64**

Echocardiography
  in CHCs, **531–539**

intracardiac, in placement of patent foramen
    ovale closure devices, pertinent views to
    obtain with, 57–60
  missed diagnoses of ACS in ED due to,
    439–440
  three-dimensional
    in patent foramen ovale diagnosis, 51
    in placement of patent foramen ovale
      closure devices, 60–64
  transesophageal
    in patent foramen ovale diagnosis, 49–50
    in placement of patent foramen ovale
      closure devices, 54–57
  transthoracic, in patent foramen ovale
    diagnosis, 47–49

ED. See *Emergency department (ED).*

EDOU. See *Emergency department (ED)
  observation unit (OU).*

Education
  family, patent foramen ovale closure
    device–related, 18–19
  patient, patent foramen ovale closure
    device–related, 18–19

Electrocardiography (ECG)
  continuous/serial ECG, in ACS diagnosis, 437
  diagnostic accuracy of, in ACS diagnosis,
    432–437
  exercise stress, in ACS diagnosis, 437
  "nondiagnostic" patterns of, in ACS diagnosis,
    434
  non–standard lead, in ACS diagnosis, 437
  normal, in ACS diagnosis, 434
  prehospital 12-lead, in ACS diagnosis,
    434–437
  with ACI-TIPI for real-time and retrospective
    decision support in medical error
    prevention in ED triage for ACS, 603

Electrolyzed-reduced water treatment, for
  hemodialysis, 326

Electron beam CT (EBCT), for triaging patients
  presenting to ED with chest pain, **541–548**

Emergency department (ED)
  acute coronary syndrome demands on, 588
  biomarkers in, **453–465.** See also *Biomarkers,
    in ED and CPUs.*
  chest pain in patients presenting to, EBCT for
    triaging, **541–548**
  missed diagnoses of ACSs in, **423–451.** See also
    *Acute coronary syndromes (ACSs), missed
    diagnoses of, in ED.*

Emergency department (ED) observation unit (OU), in ADHF management, **569–588.** See also *Heart failure, acute decompensated.*
aldosterone antagonists in, 583
anticoagulants in, 583
beta-blockers in, 583
B-type natriuretic peptide assays in, 574–575
B-type natriuretic peptide confounders in, 575
B-type natriuretic peptide *vs.* filling pressures in, 575
calcium channel blockers in, 583
candidates for, 578–581
diagnostic evaluation in, 572
digoxin in, 583
diuretics in, 581–582
early management, benefits of, 578
economics of, 569–570
general support in, 577–578
neurohormones in, 572–573
NSAIDs in, 583
N-terminal pro–B-type natriuretic peptide in, 576–577
OU disposition in, 583–584
vasodilators in, 582

Emergency department (ED) triage, for ACS, medical error prevention in, **601–614.** See also *Acute coronary syndrome (ACS), ED triage for, medical error prevention in.*

Endothelial function, renin angiotensin system in, 174

Endothelial sodding/seeding, for venous neointimal hyperplasia in dialysis access, 265–266

Endothelium
dysfunction of, NOCAD due to, 559–561, 563
function of, 559–560
in diabetes mellitus prevention, 174

End-stage renal disease (ESRD)
cardiovascular disease in, 349–350
cardiovascular risk in, 311
death due to, causes of, 385
diabetes and, 363

Epicardial disease, NOCAD due to, 560–561

Erythropoietin
for CKD, 354–355
in CHF in CKD management, 279
in hypertension, 240

ESRD. See *End-stage renal disease (ESRD).*

Exercise, for peripheral arterial disease in CKD, 230

Exercise testing, in CPUs, **503–516.** See also *Chest pain units (CPUs), exercise testing in.*

F

Family education, patent foramen ovale closure device–related, 18–19

Fatty acid(s), free, unbound, as biomarker of cardiac ischemia, 496

Fatty acid binding protein, in ED and CPCs, 455

Fibrinolysis, cardiovascular disease in diabetics and, 131

Fistula(ae), arteriovenous. See *Arteriovenous fistulae.*

Free fatty acid(s), unbound, as biomarker of cardiac ischemia, 496

G

Gene therapy, for venous neointimal hyperplasia in dialysis access, 265

Glycemic control, intensive, for acute myocardial infarction in diabetics, **111–118**

Glycemic management techniques, in prevention of cardiovascular outcomes in type 2 diabetes, clinical trials of, 215–218

Glycemic targets, in prevention of cardiovascular outcomes in type 2 diabetes, clinical trials of, 214–215

Goldman Chest Pain Protocol, missed diagnoses of ACS in ED due to, 440–441

H

Headache(s), migraine, patent foramen ovale in, **91–96.** See also *Patent foramen ovale, in migraine headache.*

Heart, renal failure effects on, 313–314

Heart disease
congenital, patent foramen ovale and, 37–39
ischemic
cardiovascular disease in renal transplant recipients due to, 334–335
CKD and, 276–277

Heart failure
acute decompensated
clinical features of, 573

Heart failure (*continued*)
  diagnostic evaluation of, 7–8, 574
  differential diagnosis of, 573–574
  management of, in EDOU, **569–588.** See
    also *Emergency department (ED)
    observation unit (OU), in ADHF
    management.*
  pathophysiology of, 571–572
  prognosis of, 576
  epidemiology of, 569–571
  vascular access in hemodialysis and,
    253–254

Heart Outcome and Prevention Evaluation
  (HOPE) study, subgroup analyses of, 346

Helex device, in patent foramen ovale closure, 81

Hemodialysis
  electrolyzed-reduced water treatment for, 326
  home, nocturnal, cardiovascular
    improvements and, physiologic link
    between, 389
  hypertension in, reverse epidemiology of,
    243–244
  vascular access in, **249–273**
    arteriovenous fistulae, 249–250
      pathology of, 257–258
      prevalence of, 254–255
      rationale for, 256
      surveillance of, 256–257
      venous stenosis in, pathogenesis of,
        260–262
    clinical standard of care for, 254–257
    complications of, 252–254
    cuffed double-lumen silicone catheters,
      251–252
    dysfunction of, management of, lack of
      effective therapies in, 262–264
    future directions in, 266–267
    heart failure due to, 253–254
    infections due to, 252–253
    polytetrafluoroethylene grafts, 250–251
      venous stenosis in, pathogenesis of,
        260–262
    types of, 249–254
    venous neointimal hyperplasia in, novel
      therapies for, 264–266

Hemodialyzer(s), vitamin E–bonded, 326

Home hemodialysis, nocturnal, cardiovascular
  improvements and, physiologic link between,
  389

Homocysteine, levels of, renal replacement
  therapy effects on, 388

Hoorn study, 345

HOPE study, subgroup analyses of, 346

Hypercoagulable states, in patent foramen ovale,
  65–71

Hyperglycemia, in diabetes mellitus, 202–203

Hyperparathyroidism, renal replacement therapy
  effects on, 387–388

Hypertension
  diabetes mellitus and, **141–153,** 199–202. See
    also *Diabetes mellitus, hypertension and.*
  in CKD, **237–248,** 350
    management of, 241, 278–279
      agents in, 242–243
  in dialysis patients, 241–242
  in hemodialysis, reverse epidemiology of,
    243–244
  microvascular dysfunction and, NOCAD due
    to, 559
  pathophysiology of, 237–241
    circulating inhibitors of nitric oxide in,
      239
    cocaine in, 240
    cyclosporine in, 240
    drugs in, 240–241
    erythropoietin in, 240
    lead in, 240
    nitric oxide in, 239
    NSAIDs in, 240–241
    oxidative stress in, 238–239
    renin-angiotensin system in, 238
    sodium and water in, 237–238
    sympathetic nervous system in, 239–240
    toxins in, 240

Hypoxemia, nocturnal, renal replacement therapy
  and, 388

I

IL. See *Interleukin(s) (IL).*

Imaging, in suspected ACS evaluation,
  517–530. See also specific modalities and
  *Acute coronary syndromes (ACSs),
  suspected, evaluation of, imaging in.*

Incremental diagnostic value, in suspected ACS
  evaluation, 521–522

Infection(s), vascular access in hemodialysis and,
  252–253

Infiltrative disease, microvascular dysfunction
  and, NOCAD due to, 562

Inflammation
  atherothrombosis and, biomarkers of, 491–492
  biomarkers of, 491–495. See also *Biomarkers, of inflammation.*
  missed diagnoses of ACS in ED due to, 439
  cardiovascular disease in diabetics and, 131
  oxidative stress and, in CKD, 323–324

Informed consent, for patent foramen ovale closure, 18–19

Insulin resistance
  cardiovascular disease in diabetics and, 122–123
  in diabetes mellitus prevention, 174, 177–180

Insulin secretagogues, 123–126
  in prevention of cardiovascular disease in diabetics, **121–139**
  sulfonylureas, 123–126

Insulin sensitizing agents, 127–132
  in prevention of cardiovascular disease in diabetics, **121–139**
  biguanides, 127–128

Interleukin(s) (IL)
  IL-6, as biomarker of inflammation, 494
  IL-10, as biomarker of inflammation, 495

Intracardiac echocardiography, in placement of patent foramen ovale closure devices, pertinent views to obtain with, 57–60

Intracardiac shunt, closure of, effect on migraines, 94

Ischemia
  cardiac, biomarkers of, 455–456, **491–501.** See also *Biomarkers, of cardiac ischemia.*
  myocardial, in ED and CPU patients, troponin for, 456–457

Ischemia modified albumin, as biomarker of cardiac ischemia, 496

Ischemic heart disease
  cardiovascular disease in renal transplant recipients due to, 334–335
  CKD and, 276–277

K

Kidney disease. See *Renal disease.*

L

Lead, in hypertension, 240

Left ventricular hypertrophy

cardiovascular disease in renal transplant recipients due to, 332–333
  CKD and, 355

Lifestyle modifications
  in diabetes prevention, 168, 174–176
  in prevention of cardiovascular outcomes in type 2 diabetes, 219–220

Ligand(s), CD40, as biomarker of inflammation, 494–495

Lipid(s)
  CKD due to, 365
  in diabetes, management of, **155–164.** See also *Diabetes mellitus, lipid management in.*
  in prevention of cardiovascular outcomes in type 2 diabetes, 218–219
  renal failure due to, 365–366
  renal replacement therapy effects on, 387

Lipoprotein(s)
  abnormalities associated with, diabetes-related, 155–156
  low-density, malondialdehyde-modified, as biomarker of plaque instability or rupture, 497–498

Lipoprotein-associated phospholipase A2, as biomarker of inflammation, 494

Low-density lipoprotein, malondialdehyde-modified, as biomarker of plaque instability or rupture, 497–498

M

Malondialdehyde-modified low-density lipoprotein, as biomarker of plaque instability or rupture, 497–498

Medical errors, in ED triage for ACS, prevention of, **601–614.** See also *Acute coronary syndrome (ACS), ED triage for, medical error prevention in.*

Metformin, in prevention of cardiovascular disease in diabetics, 128

Microalbuminuria, CKD and, 350–351

Microinflammation, chronic, CKD and, 355–357

Microvascular disease, NOCAD due to, 561–562

Microvascular dysfunction
  cardiomyopathy and, NOCAD due to, 561
  hypertension and, NOCAD due to, 561
  idiopathic, NOCAD due to, 562
  infiltrative disease and, NOCAD due to, 562

Microvascular dysfunction (*continued*)
  NOCAD due to, 560–562, 565
  valvular disease and, NOCAD due to, 562

Microvascular endothelial dysfunction, NOCAD
  due to, 561, 565

Microvascular system, function of, 560

Migraine(s)
  closure of intracardiac shunt effects on, 94
  patent foramen ovale in, **91–96.**
    See also *Patent foramen ovale,
    in migraine headache.*

MSCT, for triaging patients presenting to ED
  with chest pain, 545

Myeloperoxidase, oxidative stress and
  inflammation in uremic patients through,
  323–324

Myocardial bridging, NOCAD due to, 561,
  564–565

Myocardial infarction, ACS without, evaluation
  of, imaging in, 519

Myocardial ischemia, in ED and CPU patients,
  troponin for, 456–457

Myocardial performance index, missed diagnoses
  of ACS in ED due to, 440

Myocardial perfusion imaging, acute, in suspected
  ACS evaluation, 517–518

Myocardial scintigraphy, *vs.* exercise testing, in
  CPUs, 511–512

Myocardial stress, in CKD, biomarkers of,
  357–358

Myoglobin
  in ED and CPUs, 455
  missed diagnoses of ACS in ED due to,
  438–439

N

NAVIGATOR trial, in prevention of
  cardiovascular outcomes in type 2 diabetes,
  217

Negative predictive value, in suspected ACS
  evaluation, 519–521

Nephropathy, contrast-induced
  pathophysiology of, 301–302
  prevention of, 302–304

Nesiritide, in ADHF management in EDOU,
  582

Neurohormone(s), in ADHF management in
  EDOU, 572–573

Neurohumoral activation, biomarkers of, missed
  diagnoses of ACS in ED due to, 439

Nitric oxide
  circulating inhibitors of, in hypertension, 239
  in hypertension, 239

NOCAD. See *Chest pain with normal coronary
  angiogram (NOCAD).*

Nocturnal home hemodialysis, cardiovascular
  improvements and, physiologic link between,
  389

Nocturnal hypoxemia, renal replacement therapy
  and, 388

Nonglycemic therapies, in prevention of
  cardiovascular outcomes in type 2 diabetes,
  218–220

Non–ST elevation ACS, treatment of
  acute, 405
  invasive *vs.* conservative, 405

Nonsulfonylurea secretagogues, 127

NSAIDs. See *Anti-inflammatory drugs,
  nonsteroidal.*

N-terminal pro–B-type natriuretic peptide, in
  ADHF management in EDOU, 576–577

O

ORIGIN trial, in prevention of cardiovascular
  outcomes in type 2 diabetes, 217

Oxidative pathways, in CKD, **319–330**

Oxidative stress
  described, 319–320
  in atherosclerosis, 320–321
  in CKD, 355–357
    prevalence of, 321–323
  in hypertension, 238–239
  inflammation and, in CKD, 323–324

P

Pain, chest, in ED
  EBCT for triaging patients with, **541–548**
  MSCT for triaging patients with, 545

Patent foramen ovale, **1–6**
  aneurysmal, 40–41
  closure devices for
    assessment of, randomized trials of, 16–17
    described, 13–14

indications for, 17–18
operator skills with, 19–20
overview of, 14–15
patient and family education related to,
    18–19
placement of
    echocardiographer's role in, **53–64**
    echocardiography in, general approach
        to, 53–54
    intracardiac echocardiography in,
        pertinent views to obtain with, 57–60
    three-dimensional echocardiography in,
        60–64
    transesophageal echocardiography in,
        54–57
published reports of, 15–16
closure of, **73–83**
    atrial septal anatomy effects on, 39–40
    atrial septal defect–related, in pediatric
        patients, 42–43
    cardiac catheterization laboratory set-up
        for, 21–22
    catheter approach to, 41–42
    closure devices for, **13–35**
    complications of
        management of, 30–32
        prevention of, 30–32
        recognition of, 30–32
congenital heart disease and, 37–39
decompression pathology related to, 99–100
defined, 1–2
diagnosis of, **47–52**
    three-dimensional echocardiography in, 51
    traditional methods in, 47
    transesophageal echocardiography in,
        49–51
    transthoracic echocardiography in, 47–49
diving and, **97–104**
    accidents related to, history of, 98
    changing patency over time, 100–102
    increased risk with, 98–99
        prospective evaluation of, 100
effectiveness of, 43
hand-off back to referring physician after,
    29–30
hematologic ramifications of, **65–71**. See also
    *Patent foramen ovale, hypercoagulable
    state in.*
    medical therapy for, 69–70
historical perspective of, 35–36, **73–83**
    Amplatzer atrial septal defect occluder,
        78–79
    Angel Wings device, 79–80

atrial septal defect occlusion system, 81–82
    buttoned device, 79
    CardioSEAL septal occluder, 77
    Helex device, 81
    percutaneous devices, 74–77
    STARFlex septal occluder, 78
    transcatheter patch occlusion, 80–81
hypercoagulable state in, **65–71**
    arterial, 66–67
    implications of, 67–68
    testing for, 68–69
    venous, 65–66
in migraine headache, **91–96**
    positive effect of, 93–94
    prevalence of, 91–93
in special patient populations, 32–33
informed consent for, 18–19
mechanisms for, 5
out-patient follow-up issues, 29–30
pathophysiology of, 2–5
patient preparation for, 21
pediatric cardiologist in, **35–45**
    future role of, 44
percutaneous devices in, historical perspective
    of, 74–77
platypnea-orthodeoxia syndrome and,
    85–89. See also *Platypnea-orthodeoxia
    syndrome.*
postprocedure care, 28–29
procedure of, 22–28
risks associated with, 43–44
shunt detection in, traditional, 47
size of, 5
stroke and, **7–11**
    prevalence of, 7–8
temporary balloon occlusion trial in, 37–39

Patient education, patent foramen ovale closure
    device–related, 18–19

Peptide(s), B-type (brain) natriuretic, as
    biomarker of cardiac ischemia,
    494–495

Percutaneous coronary intervention, coronary
    artery bypass grafting *vs.*, in diabetics,
    187–193. See also *Diabetes mellitus,
    percutaneous coronary intervention vs. coronary
    artery bypass grafting in.*

Percutaneous devices, in patent foramen ovale
    closure, historical perspective of, 74–77

Percutaneous patent foramen ovale, closure of,
    13–35. See also *Patent foramen ovale,
    closure of.*

Peripheral arterial disease, in CKD, management of, **225–236.** See also *Chronic kidney disease (CKD), peripheral arterial disease in, management of.*

Peripheral vascular disease, in CKD, risk factors for, 289–290

Perivascular drug delivery, local, for venous neointimal hyperplasia in dialysis access, 265

Phospholipase A2, lipoprotein-associated, as biomarker of inflammation, 494

Plaque instability or rupture, biomarkers of, 497–498

Plasma protein-A, pregnancy-associated, as biomarker of plaque instability or rupture, 497

Platypnea-orthodeoxia syndrome
  clinical entities associated with, 85–86
  diagnosis of, 87–88
  noncardiac mechanisms of, 86–87
  patent foramen ovale and, **85–89**
  pulmonary perfusion abnormalities with, 87
  underlying mechanisms of, 85–86

POCT. See *Point-of-care testing (POCT).*

Point-of-care testing (POCT)
  cardiac biomarker. See *Cardiac biomarker POCT.*
    in CPUs, **467–490.** See also *Cardiac biomarker POCT, in CPUs.*
  defined, 467–468
  goals of, 467–468
  trends in, 467–468

Polytetrafluoroethylene grafts
  failure of, pathology of, 258–260
  for vascular access in hemodialysis, 250–251
    venous stenosis in, pathogenesis of, 260–262

Predictive value, negative, in suspected ACS evaluation, 519–521

Pregnancy-associated plasma protein-A, as biomarker of plaque instability or rupture, 497

PROactive trial, in prevention of cardiovascular outcomes in type 2 diabetes, 216

Protein(s)
  binding, fatty acid, in ED and CPUs, 455
  C-reactive, as biomarker of inflammation, 492–494
  fatty acid binding, in ED and CPUs, 455

Protein-A, plasma, pregnancy-associated, as biomarker of plaque instability or rupture, 497

Proteinuria, CKD and, 350–351

Pulmonary perfusion abnormalities, platypnea-orthodeoxia syndrome and, 87

Q

Q waves, in ACS diagnosis, 434

R

Race, as factor in missed diagnoses of ACS in ED, 442–443

Radiation therapy, for venous neointimal hyperplasia in dialysis access, 264–265

Radiopharmaceutical issues, in suspected ACS evaluation, 522–523

RECORD study, in prevention of cardiovascular outcomes in type 2 diabetes, 216

Reimbursement issues, CPU-related, 591–593

Renal disease
  chronic, hypertension in, **237–248.** See also *Hypertension, in CKD.*
  high-risk, percutaneous coronary interventions for, **299–310**
  incipient, cardiovascular risk in, 311–312
    risk factor profile, 312–313

Renal failure
  cardiovascular disease and, pathophysiology of, **311–317**
    accelerated atherogenesis in, 313
    central arteries in, 313
    heart in, 313–314
    risk factor profile in, 312–313
  in diabetics with hypertension, treatment of, 147
  in ED and CPUs, troponin for, 460–461
  lipids and, 365–366
  vascular calcification in, **373–384**
    described, 373
    detection of, 376–380
    mechanisms of, 374–376
    prognosis of, 380

Renal replacement therapy
  blood pressure effects of, 386–387
  calcium–phosphate metabolism effects of, 387–388
  cardiovascular disease in patients on, 349–350
  cardiovascular events due to, 388–389
  effects on cardiac geometry, 387
  effects on systolic function, 387
  future directions in, 389

homocysteine levels and, 388
hyperparathyroidism effects of, 387–388
lipid profile effects of, 387
newer paradigms in, **385–391**
nocturnal hypoxemia and, 388

Renal transplant recipients, cardiovascular
disease in
causes of, 331–335
CHF and, 333–334
incidence of, 332
ischemic heart disease and, 334–335
left ventricular hypertrophy and, 332–333
management of, **331–342**
anemia management in, 338
antiplatelet agents in, 337
beta-blockers in, 337
blood pressure targets in, 336
cholesterol reduction in, 335–336
lifestyle modification in, 335
renin-angiotensin antagonists in, 336–337
revascularization in, 338–339
risk-factor modification in, 335–338
prevalence of, 332
risk factors for, 332–335
nontraditional, 338

Renin-angiotensin antagonists, in cardiovascular
disease in renal transplant recipients
management, 336–337

Renin-angiotensin system
in diabetes mellitus, **167–185.** See also *Diabetes
mellitus, renin-angiotensin system in.*
in hypertension, 238
interruption of, in CHF in CKD management,
279

Reperfusion therapy, for ACSs, 407

Revascularization interventions, in prevention of
cardiovascular outcomes in type 2 diabetes,
218

S

Scintigraphy, myocardial, *vs.* exercise testing, in
CPUs, 511–512

Second National Health and Nutrition
Examination Survey mortality study, 346

Secretagogue(s)
insulin, 123–126. See also *Insulin
secretagogues.*
nonsulfonylurea, 127
limitations of, 127
mechanism of action of, 127

Selectin(s), as biomarker of inflammation, 495

Sensitivity, in suspected ACS evaluation, 518–519

Septum, atrial, anatomy of, 36–37

Serum amyloid A, as biomarker of inflammation,
495

Shunt(s), intracardiac, closure of, effect on
migraines, 94

Smoking cessation
for CHF in CKD, 279
for peripheral arterial disease in CKD,
229–230

Sodium, in hypertension, 237–238

Spasm, coronary, NOCAD due to, 561, 563–564

ST elevation, in ED and CPU patients, troponin
for, 456–457

STARFlex septal occluder, in patent foramen
ovale closure, 78

Statin(s)
for CHF in CKD, 279
for cholesterol reduction, in cardiovascular
disease in renal transplant recipients
management, 335–336
for peripheral arterial disease in CKD,
228–229

ST-elevation myocardial infarction (STEMI),
recognition and treatment of, thrombolytic
predictive instrument in, 606

STEMI. See *ST-elevation myocardial infarction
(STEMI).*

Stent(s), coated, for venous neointimal
hyperplasia in dialysis access, 265

Stress, oxidative. See *Oxidative stress.*

Stroke
described, 7
patent foramen ovale and, **7–11**

Sulfonylurea(s), 123–126
described, 123–124
mechanism of action of, 124–126

Sympathetic nervous system, in hypertension,
239–240

T

Technetium-99m sestamibi myocardial perfusion
imaging, missed diagnoses of ACS in ED due
to, 440

Therapeutic turnaround time (TTAT), in cardiac biomarker POCT, 477–478

Thiazide diuretics, for diabetes and hypertension, 143–144

Thiazolidinedione(s), in prevention of cardiovascular disease in diabetics, 128–131
  blood pressure effects of, 129–130
  described, 128
  endothelial function effects of, 130–131
  lipid metabolism and oxidation in, 129
  mechanism of action of, 128–129
  vascular reactivity effects of, 130–131
  vascular wall abnormalities due to, 130–131

Three-dimensional echocardiography
  in patent foramen ovale closure device placement, 60–64
  in patent foramen ovale diagnosis, 51

Thrombolysis, for ACSs, 406–407

Thrombolytic predictive instrument
  clinical effectiveness trial, 606–608
  in recognition and treatment of STEMI, 604

Thrombosis, in diabetes mellitus, 203–204

Time-insensitive predictive instrument (TIPI) information system cardiac error reduction system, based on ACI-TIPI demonstration project, 608–611

Timeliness, in cardiac biomarker POCT, 478–479

TIPI. See Time-insensitive predictive instrument (TIPI).

Toxin(s), in hypertension, 240

Tracer injection, in suspected ACS evaluation, timing of, 523–524

Transcatheter patch occlusion, in patent foramen ovale closure, 80–81

Transesophageal echocardiography
  in patent foramen ovale closure device placement, 54–57
  in patent foramen ovale diagnosis, 49–50

Trans-theoretic Y model application, of CPUs, 594, 596–598

Transthoracic echocardiography, in patent foramen ovale diagnosis, 47–49

Troponin
  in ED and CPUs, 453–455
    for high-risk patients with ACSs, 457–458

  for intermediate and low risk patients, 458–460
  for patients with ST elevation and myocardial infarction, 456–457
  for renal failure patients, 460–461
  in suspected ACS evaluation, 523
  missed diagnoses of ACS in ED due to, 438

Troponin I, myocardial stress and, 357–358

Troponin T, myocardial stress and, 357–358

TTAT. See Therapeutic turnaround time (TTAT).

U

Unbound free fatty acid, as biomarker of cardiac ischemia, 496

Uremia
  antioxidants in, 324–325
  arteriosclerotic cardiovascular disease and, 354
  oxidative stress and inflammation in, myeloperoxidase and, 323–324

V

VADT trial, in prevention of cardiovascular outcomes in type 2 diabetes, 215

Valve replacement, in CKD, 350

Valvular disease, microvascular dysfunction and, NOCAD due to, 562

Vascular calcification
  CKD and, 357
  in renal failure, **373–384.** See also Renal failure, vascular calcification in.

Vascular endothelial function, renin angiotensin system in, in diabetes mellitus, 172–173

Vasodilator(s), in ADHF management in EDOU, 582

Venous neointimal hyperplasia, in dialysis access, novel therapies for, 264–266

Vitamin E–bonded hemodialyzers, 326

W

Water, in hypertension, 237–238

Weight, body, cardiovascular disease in diabetics and, 132

Whole blood choline, as biomarker of plaque instability or rupture, 497

Women, in CPUs, management of, 549–551

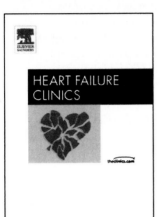

Changing Your Address?

Make sure your subscription changes too! When you notify us of your new
address, you can help make our job easier by including an exact copy of your
Clinics label number with your old address (see illustration below.) This
number identifies you to our computer system and will speed the processing of
your address change. Please be sure this label number accompanies your old
address and your corrected address—you can send an old Clinics label with
your number on it or just copy it exactly and send it to the address listed below.

We appreciate your help in our attempt to give you continuous coverage.
Thank you.

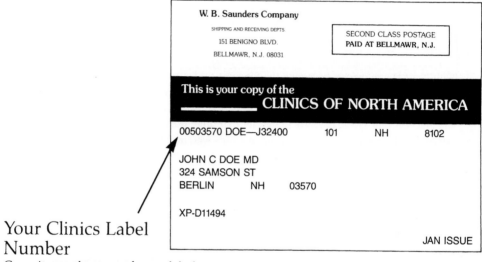

W. B. Saunders Company

SHIPPING AND RECEIVING DEPTS.

151 BENIGNO BLVD.

BELLMAWR, N.J. 08031

SECOND CLASS POSTAGE
PAID AT BELLMAWR, N.J.

This is your copy of the

_____ **CLINICS OF NORTH AMERICA**

00503570 DOE—J32400   101   NH   8102

JOHN C DOE MD
324 SAMSON ST
BERLIN   NH   03570

XP-D11494

JAN ISSUE

Your Clinics Label Number

Copy it exactly or send your label
along with your address to:
W.B. Saunders Company, Customer Service
Orlando, FL 32887-4800
Call Toll Free 1-800-654-2452

Please allow four to six weeks for delivery of new subscriptions and for
processing address changes.